NO MORE MEASLES!

The Truth About Vaccines and Your Health

NO MORE MEASLES!

The Truth About Vaccines and Your Health

Laurie Endicott Thomas

KERMIT PRESS
Veritas Vos Liberabit

Kermit Press
PO Box 425
Chatham, NJ 07928

Cover and Interior designer, David Moratto

ISBN: 978-0-9968818-1-4

NO MORE MEASLES!

The Truth About Vaccines
and Your Health

Contents

Introduction

When I was a child, I loved the television show *Gilligan's Island*. It was about seven people stranded on a desert island somewhere near Hawaii. My favorite character was the Professor. His name was supposedly Roy Hinkley. However, his fellow castaways never called him anything but Professor.

Despite having advanced degrees from several universities, the Professor was a humble high school science teacher. The other characters trusted him. They respected his intelligence, his education, his honesty, and his decency. The other castaways knew that the Professor sought knowledge for its own sake. They understood that he used his knowledge and wisdom unselfishly to help them.

Russell Johnson, the actor who played the Professor, had movie-star good looks. Since then, however, the entertainment industry in the United States has trained Americans to think that smart, educated people are unsexy "nerds." As a result, many Americans feel contempt for real professors. Many Americans would rather listen to the glamorous and seductive but uneducated Ginger Grant. They would rather be seduced by a sexy celebrity than learn from a professor. Thus, when they want information about childhood vaccinations, they ignore scientists. Instead, they turn to uneducated but glamorous celebrities like Jenny McCarthy, who was Playboy Playmate of the Year in 1994.

Jenny McCarthy has no scientific or medical training, although she quips that she got "a degree in autism" from "the University of Google." McCarthy claimed that her son had autism and that his autism resulted from his measles-mumps-rubella (MMR) vaccination. McCarthy argued, "Think of autism like a fart, and vaccines are the finger you pull to make it happen." Yet as I will explain in chapter 16, the scientific evidence clearly shows that vaccinations have nothing to do with autism. To use McCarthy's crude metaphor, people will pass the same amount of gas whether their finger is pulled or not. Likewise, vaccination has no effect on a child's risk of getting autism.

Ironically, McCarthy's son might not have had autism to begin with. One neurologist, Daniel B. Rubin, MD, PhD, suggested that the diagnosis of autism was probably wrong in McCarthy's son's case. Dr. Rubin noted that the boy's condition started with seizures. After the seizures were treated, the boy's condition improved. In the August 7, 2008 issue of *Neurology Today*, Dr. Rubin explained, "This would be more consistent with Landau-Kleffner syndrome, which is often misdiagnosed as autism." Landau-Kleffner syndrome looks like autism because it affects the speech centers of the brain. If Dr. Rubin is right, then McCarthy's claim that she knows something about how to prevent or cure autism is bogus.

Today, we live in the Information Age. The Internet gives scientists like the Professor and even science writers like me quick and easy access to the world's scientific literature. Thus, the Internet makes it far easier for educated people to base their opinions on scientific evidence. Yet the Internet also enables fools, liars, and snake-oil merchants to broadcast nonsense to a worldwide audience. The Internet provides the 21st century version of the old-fashioned traveling medicine show, in which salesmen used showmanship to sell worthless and possibly dangerous potions.

Today, much of the antivaccination rhetoric comes from people who are trying to sell you something that is probably worthless. The people who invest the money to build Web sites and produce documentaries to scare you away from vaccinating your children are nearly always selling something. Some of them sell high-priced dietary supplements that nobody really needs. Some sell homeopathic medicines that are really nothing but water. Some sell herbal products that are probably useless and are sometimes harmful. Some sell services such as spinal adjustment or "energy healing" that would have no effect on bacterial or viral infections.

Of course, conventional medicine is also an industry. For that reason, many people suspect that it serves the needs of its investors, rather than the needs of patients. These suspicions are sometimes well-founded. As I explained in my book *Thin Diabetes, Fat Diabetes*, doctors often use expensive drugs and surgical procedures instead of simple dietary advice to deal with problems that result from an unhealthy diet.

To see through the hype coming from both the conventional healthcare industry and the alternative medicine industry, you need to know some basic facts about history and biology. You also need to know how to think logically. Unfortunately, our public schools have generally been doing a poor job of teaching history and biology. Few even attempt to teach logic. This kind of educational neglect is no accident. As I explained in my book *Not Trivial: How Studying the Traditional Liberal Arts Can Set You Free*, our public schools in the United States have been deliberately dumbed down. Many schools use a method of reading instruction that does not work. Even for the children who somehow learn to read, most schools deliberately neglect the classical trivium of grammar, logic, and rhetoric.

In this book, I want to give people the biology and history lessons that they need in order to make rational decisions about vaccinations:

- What bacteria and viruses are, and how they attack our bodies.
- How the human body tries to defend itself against infection.
- How scientists prove that a particular disease is the result of infection by a particular germ.

- How government protects the public against the most dangerous infectious diseases.
- How the Food and Drug Administration decides which vaccines should be available in the United States.
- How the Centers for Disease Control and Preventions make recommendations about vaccination.
- How state governments decide what vaccines a child must receive before he or she can enter school.

Along the way, I get to tell some fascinating stories about the men and women who solved the mystery of infectious disease. I devote a chapter to each of the major vaccine-preventable diseases, including a discussion of the risks and benefits of the vaccines used to prevent them.

My goal in writing *Not Trivial* was to explain how to wipe out dyslexia and to put an end to racism and war. My goal in writing *Thin Diabetes, Fat Diabetes* was to reduce the death toll from diabetes. My goal in writing *No More Measles* is to inspire people to work together to drive measles, mumps, rubella, and a few other infectious diseases into extinction.

Many of the vaccine-preventable diseases reproduce only in human beings. If we can drive such a disease out of the human population through vaccination, the disease will be extinct forever. At that point, we can safely stop vaccinating people against it. Thus, we can save money and avoid even the small risk associated with using that vaccine. So far, vaccination campaigns have already driven smallpox and an animal disease called rinderpest into extinction. Another vaccination campaign has driven polio to the brink of extinction.

For more than a thousand years, smallpox was a major cause of death in Africa, Asia, and Europe. After 1492, smallpox devastated the populations of the Americas. Even in the 20th century, smallpox killed hundreds of millions of people. Yet thanks to the smallpox eradication campaign, there have been no cases of smallpox anywhere in the world since the 1970s. That's why we no longer vaccinate children against smallpox.

After we drive measles, mumps, and rubella into extinction, there will no longer be any need to give anyone the MMR vaccine. The eradication of these and several other horrible diseases is a tremendous gift that we can give to future generations.

Today, the biggest obstacle that stands in the way of disease eradication is fear. People are more afraid of the vaccines and of the vaccinators than they are of the diseases that the vaccines prevent. Yet as President Franklin Delano Roosevelt told us back in the depths of the Great Depression, the only thing we have to fear is fear itself.

Roosevelt had a particular interest in polio. In 1921, at the age of 39, he became permanently paralyzed by an illness that may have been polio. Because of his compassion for paralyzed children, FDR launched a fundraising campaign that was eventually called the March of Dimes. The March of Dimes not only helped children and adults who had been paralyzed by polio, it provided funding for the scientists who ultimately isolated the poliovirus and developed the vaccine that has come close to eradicating polio.

After polio was eliminated from the United States, the March of Dimes turned its attention to a new mission: preventing birth defects. It was a logical transition because a viral disease called rubella was known to be a major cause of miscarriage, stillbirth, and severe birth defects. (I will talk more about the history of polio and the March of Dimes in chapter 21. I will talk about rubella in chapter 24.)

An article published in 2003 in the *Journal of Medical Biography* suggested that Roosevelt's paralysis might have been due to Guillain-Barré syndrome, rather than polio. (Back then, there were no laboratory tests to confirm the diagnosis of polio.) We will never know for sure what caused Roosevelt's paralysis. But if Roosevelt had not received the diagnosis of polio, history might have been much different. If there had been no March of Dimes, the development of the polio vaccine might have been delayed for decades. As a result, hundreds of thousands more would have died or become paralyzed.

As I write this, a Global Polio Eradication Initiative is on the brink of driving poliovirus into extinction. This campaign is being funded and carried out by a public-private partnership involving international organizations such as the World Health Organization, UNICEF, the

CDC, national governments, and private organizations such as Rotary International.

The Global Polio Eradication Initiative has solved many hard technical problems, such as keeping the vaccine refrigerated in remote rural areas. However, the biggest hurdle it faces is fear and distrust in many communities where poliovirus is still circulating. Much of this fear and distrust is an understandable response to recent political events. War has always led to famine, pestilence, and death. If you want to fight infectious disease, you must work for peace.

So far, the Global Polio Eradication Initiative seems to have eradicated the type 2 strain of poliovirus. Type 2 poliovirus has not been found in any human being since 1999. As a result, the type 2 strain is being phased out of the oral polio vaccine. As I write this, type 1 and type 3 poliovirus continue to circulate in three countries: Afghanistan, Nigeria, and Pakistan. Unfortunately, poliovirus can easily be exported from those countries, especially because so many people from those countries make a religious pilgrimage to Mecca, in Saudi Arabia.

Fear and distrust are also leading to outbreaks of other vaccine-preventable diseases in the United States and other industrialized countries. There have always been religions that forbid any kind of medical care. Yet today, much of the resistance to vaccination is secular.

Many parents have been led to believe that the vaccines are worthless and possibly dangerous. Parents are being told that the government's vaccination recommendations are made to increase the profits of the vaccine makers, not to protect children's health. Many people oppose vaccination because they view vaccination as a tool of capitalism. They seem to be unaware that Communist countries, particularly the Soviet Union and Cuba, warmly embraced vaccination, clearly without a profit motive.

The disease eradication programs that are currently being supported by the Rotary International and the Bill and Melinda Gates Foundation will actually be bad for vaccine sales in the long run. Once an infectious disease has been driven into extinction, the sales of the vaccine to prevent that disease drop to zero overnight. The vaccine makers would make more money if the number of unvaccinated people stays just high enough to keep the diseases circulating. So the campaigns to eradicate diseases like smallpox and polio are driven by compassion, not greed.

To control the spread of a vaccine-preventable disease, we need to vaccinate nearly everyone. Unfortunately, a growing number of parents are refusing to allow their children to be vaccinated. In many places, the number of unvaccinated people is large enough to allow serious diseases such as whooping cough to circulate. For humanity to win the battle against measles and other eradicable infectious diseases, wisdom must triumph over fear.

Part I

Scientific and Political Debates

Vaccination has become a hotly debated topic. Like many debates, this one is ugly—for a simple, understandable reason. The people on both sides of the debate feel that their opponents are exposing children to danger. Doctors, scientists, and public health officials insist that the vaccines are necessary and that the benefits of vaccination far outweigh the risks. They feel that people who refuse to vaccinate are neglecting their own children and exposing other people to danger. In contrast, many antivaccination activists insist that the vaccines are unnecessary and pose unacceptable risks. Many of them believe that the vaccine makers are engaged in a criminal conspiracy to poison children, either simply for profit or as part of some attempt at genocide (even though vaccination has clearly saved lives).

The only way to put an end to this nasty bickering is to eradicate as many of the vaccine-preventable diseases as possible. Once a disease becomes extinct, there is no need to vaccinate any more people against it. As a result, children will need fewer shots and adults will be able to avoid many pointless arguments. Nowadays, no children are being vaccinated against smallpox. An international vaccination campaign drove smallpox into extinction in the 1970s. But to drive an infectious disease into extinction, you need to vaccinate a huge percentage of the population. Such high vaccination rates can be achieved only if the vaccines are mandatory.

Many people are against mandatory vaccination. They feel that the individual has a right to reject unwanted medical treatments. Yet the vaccines for the most serious diseases are given only during childhood. Thus, when adults reject vaccination, they are making that decision mainly for their children, not for themselves. Thus, the real issue is not self-determination. It's about who should make the decisions that affect a child's health.

When should the state step in to protect a child and the larger community? That is an ethical and legal question. But to answer it, we must first answer the scientific questions of how effective and how safe the vaccines are. I'll discuss the relationship between science and democracy in chapter 1.

To make good decisions about vaccination, you need to know something about biology. It also helps to know something about history and politics. The medical profession has existed for thousands of years. Yet for most of its history, the medical profession had remarkably little of any value to offer to patients with an infectious disease. In chapter 2, I'll explain how scientists discovered germs. In chapter 3, I'll explain how modern governments have made great progress in preventing and treating the diseases that are caused by germs.

As I explain in chapter 4, some of the forms of alternative medicine that are still popular today arose because many of the medical treatments that were being taught in even the top universities in the 18th and 19th centuries were ineffective and dangerous. Since then, of course, medical science has had astounding success in developing safe and effective ways to prevent and treat many serious diseases.

Modern medicine has gotten particularly good at preventing and treating infections. In 1900, most of the top ten causes of death in the United States were infectious diseases. But in 2010, only one of the top ten causes of death was infectious: influenza and pneumonia, which together ranked ninth as a cause of death. In chapter 29, I'll explain why influenza is so hard to conquer. In contrast, the medical profession and our public health agencies have done a poor job of managing the chronic diseases that result from lifestyle choices, such as our rich diet, cigarette smoking, and alcohol abuse.

It is puzzling that so many people campaign so hard against vaccination. The benefits of vaccination clearly outweigh the risks for nearly anyone. The people who campaign against vaccination seldom have a science education, and they never offer persuasive scientific evidence in support of their views.

We really do need citizen activists to keep an eye on how medicine is being practiced. But first, the general public must have a clear understanding of the relationship between science and democracy.

1

Science and Democracy

Like many Americans, I was brought up to believe that democracy is a good thing and that free and open debates are essential to democracy. Unfortunately, something seems to be going wrong with the way we in the United States engage in debates. Our debates seem to be generating more heat than light. Our debates about vaccination have been particularly ugly. Vaccine researchers have received verbal abuse and even death threats. Can you imagine the other castaways on *Gilligan's Island* treating the Professor that way?

The word *science* comes from the Latin word for knowledge, but it refers to knowledge of a particular kind. *Science* refers to knowledge that is gained through a logical analysis of careful observations, including the results of experiments. *Science* can also refer to that process for gaining knowledge. A scientist is someone who dedicates his or her life's work to gaining knowledge in that way.

The word *democracy* means rule by the people. In a democracy, ordinary people get to take part in making the decisions that affect them. These decisions are made in public through some process that involves public discussions. Sometimes, democracies make rules that put limits on an individual's freedoms. For example, traffic rules limit your freedom to drive however and wherever you wish. Yet those rules are generally accepted because they improve public health and safety.

As I discuss in chapter 5 of *Not Trivial*, there are several different kinds of discussion, each of which serves a different purpose. The political discussions within a democracy deal with two kinds of questions: scientific questions (i.e., questions about what is true) and policy questions (i.e., questions about what should be done, and who should do it).

To make good policy decisions, the people must first find reliable answers to some scientific questions, so that they can predict what the effects of various policies would be. Then, they must use a process of negotiation to come to a consensus on what should be done, and by whom. In discussions about vaccination policy, we seem to get stuck on the scientific questions. Unfortunately, many people are ignoring the scientists. Too many of us are listening instead to attention-seeking celebrities and profit-seeking entrepreneurs instead of to professors.

To get reasonable answers to scientific questions, one must use facts and logic. As John Adams, who later became the second President of the United States, once wrote, "Facts are stubborn things; and whatever may be our wishes, our inclinations, or the dictates of our passion, they cannot alter the state of facts and evidence." The rules of logic are also stubborn. When you have a given set of facts, the rules of logic sometimes lead to conclusions that you do not like. You may choose to deny the facts, but denial does not change reality.

Nonscientists often do not understand or appreciate what goes on in scientific debates. They may not understand that there are rules for deciding who wins, just as there are rules for deciding who wins a card game. Yet the rules in a card game were designed to make the game fun. Science is not a game, and the rules that scientists follow were not made up for fun. They were developed through a long and sometimes painful process of recognizing and correcting mistakes.

When people with no scientific training try to take part in scientific discussions, they often make errors of fact and errors in reasoning. They are simply unaware of many important facts. Nor do they know how to draw reasonable conclusions from the facts. In other words, they make mistakes because they lack knowledge and thinking skills. Yet because of their lack of knowledge and thinking skills, they cannot spot their own mistakes.

Of course, scientists face the same problem. Scientists don't always know all the facts that they need to know. They can also make errors in reasoning. Yet the scientific community has ways to solve those problems. Scientists take part in scientific discussions so that they can share their knowledge with each other and correct each other's mistakes. These discussions help scientists develop theories that provide a better description of reality, as well as finding better ways to solve practical problems.

Because of their knowledge and thinking skills, scientists can make important contributions to other kinds of discussions. For example, journalists often interview scientists when covering stories about scientific issues. Likewise, lawyers often hire scientists to serve as expert witnesses in court cases. Of course, judges don't allow just anyone to serve as an expert witness. To serve as an expert witness in a court case, you generally have to have some sort of expertise. You need qualifications, such as special training and experience.

When journalists choose sources for an article about some scientific question, they should be just as picky as a judge. Unfortunately, journalists often use an approach called false balance, in which they interview some crank who has kooky, provocative views about some important topic and then provide a comment or two from a genuine expert, supposedly for balance. Although this approach may seem to be fair, it is misleading. It can give fools and liars far more publicity than they deserve. The fact that their comments are given at the top of the story even lets them outshine the real experts.

As I'll explain in chapter 1, scientists are valuable members of a democratic society. Yet science itself is not democratic. Facts, being stubborn things, do not obey the will of the people. You cannot make something true by persuading the majority of the population to believe it. Nor is everyone created equal when it comes to a scientific debate. People who have dedicated their careers to studying a particular scientific discipline are likely to know far more than the average person about that subject. A wise person listens carefully to scientists.

To have a reasonable discussion about who should get what vaccines, you need to know something about history and biology. You also need to know something about the basic rules for how to have a reasonable discussion. In the following chapters, I'll give you an overview of how scientific medicine arose. I'll also explain how and why some popular alternative approaches to modern medicine were developed. I'll also explain why you are usually better off listening to scientists than to uneducated people, at least when any sort of scientific question is involved.

2

The Rise of Scientific Medicine

There have always been people who refuse for religious reasons to have any medical treatment, including vaccination. But today, many people speak out against vaccination for what they claim are scientific reasons. At first, some of these people sound as if they might have valid concerns about a particular vaccine. Yet when you cross-examine them, or simply listen to them carefully, you often find that they are against all vaccinations, as a matter of principle. Often, they recommend some other kind of treatment, such as homeopathy or chiropractic, as an alternative to vaccination. Yet those "alternative" treatments have no effect on infections.

To understand why some people support vaccination while others oppose it, you need to understand the role that medical theories play in medical practice. To understand medical theories, you must think of medicine as a way to solve problems. When you have a problem, the approach that you take to solving it will depend on what you think the cause of the problem is.

Throughout most of human history, people looked to the supernatural to explain the cause of disease. People assumed that if you were sick, you were being attacked by evil spirits. Maybe a witch had cast a spell on you. Or maybe you were being punished by God. If you think that you are being attacked by evil spirits or witchcraft, you are likely to use some sort of magic to ward off evil. For help, you would turn to some sort of magician. If you think that you are being punished by God, you may beg for mercy or perhaps even try to strike some sort of bargain with God. For help, you would turn to a priest.

Midwives were the first healthcare professionals, but the first physicians were priests. Hippocrates, the ancient Greek who is considered the father of medicine, was probably a priest in a pagan temple. Hippocrates was born around 460 BC on the island of Kos, the site of an important asclepion, or temple to the Greek god Asclepius. People who were concerned about their health would make a pilgrimage to an asclepeion. Thus, the asclepeia came to serve as health spas and hospitals.

The ancient Greeks believed that Asclepius was the son of their sun god, Apollo. Both Apollo and Asclepius were called "the Healer." The rod of Asclepius was a stick with a snake wound around it (Figure 1). It is used as a symbol of medicine to this day. Originally, the rod of Asclepius probably represented the treatment for a horrible disease called Guinea worm or dracunculiasis. Guinea worms are long parasitic worms that cause agonizingly painful sores on the legs. The worms have to be pulled slowly out of the skin by being wound around a stick. (As I'll explain in chapter 19, these worms are on the verge of extinction as I write this book).

The caduceus, or herald's staff, which has two snakes wrapped around a winged staff, has also been used to represent medicine (Figure 1). It originally represented the messenger god, Hermes (Mercury), who was the messenger of the Gods, as well as the god of commerce and thieves. Perhaps the staff of Asclepius should be used to symbolize the humanitarian aspects of healthcare, while the staff of Hermes should represent the profit motive of the healthcare industry!

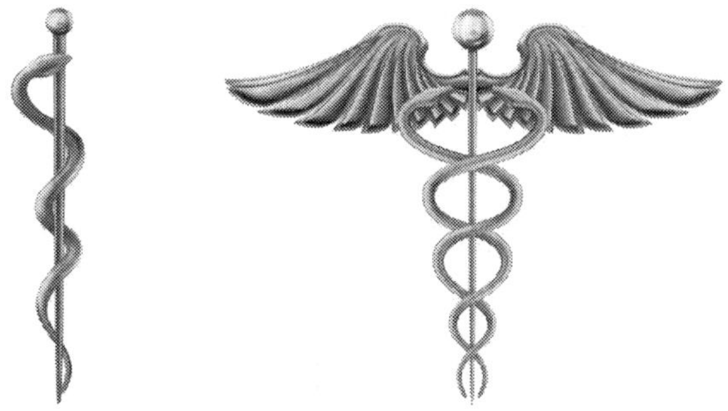

Figure 1. The Rod of Asclepius (left) was the original symbol of medicine. The caduceus or Staff of Hermes (right) was the symbol of Hermes (Mercury), who was the messenger of the gods and the god of commerce and thieves.

In a military setting, the caduceus was carried by the messengers who were sent to negotiate peace terms. Thus, soldiers were taught that they should not kill anyone who was carrying the caduceus. Eventually, military doctors also started using the caduceus symbol, for protection. Today, the Red Cross or Red Crescent emblem is used to mark humanitarian and medical buildings and vehicles in battle zones.

The ancient Greeks believed that Asclepius had several daughters. One was Hygieia, the goddess of good health and cleanliness. Her name was the source of our word *hygiene*. Another of his daughters was Panacea, the goddess of universal remedy. Even today, the word *panacea* means a cure-all.

Eventually, some of the ancient Greek philosophers started to doubt the power and even the existence of their gods. Thus, many educated Greeks turned away from supernatural explanations for disease. Instead, they started to look for ordinary physical causes and practical cures. The people who took that approach to providing healthcare stopped being priests and started being physicians. One particular man, named Hippocrates, came to represent that approach to medicine. Thus, he is considered the Father of Medicine.

Hippocrates probably came from a priestly family, but his ideas about medicine were strictly nonreligious. He explained illness in terms of ordinary physical causes, such as environment, diet, and lifestyle. According to legend, Hippocrates traveled all over the ancient Greek world teaching that idea to other physicians.

The idea that illness is the result of natural causes, as opposed to supernatural causes, would probably have made Hippocrates unpopular with some other priests, as well as with some of the secular authorities. If patients stopped believing that illness was the work of the gods, then priests would lose power and prestige. So would the secular authorities because religion would no longer serve the purpose of social control. Legend has it that the authorities were so angry with Hippocrates that they sent him to prison for 20 years.

While in prison, Hippocrates would have had a lot of time on his hands. According to legend, he used that time to write down his ideas about medicine. Many writings attributed to Hippocrates have survived to the present day. Many modern historians believe that Hippocrates was a real person, as opposed to a mythical character. However, nobody really knows which of the Hippocratic writings were really written by Hippocrates and which were written by his followers and their students. When modern-day people say that Hippocrates wrote something, they really mean that some anonymous Hippocratic author wrote it, not necessarily Hippocrates himself.

The Hippocratic writings make fascinating reading, especially for anyone with modern medical training. Hippocrates believed in careful, detailed observation of the patient's condition and the course of the illness. As a result, the Hippocratic writings contain the oldest known descriptions of many disorders, such as migraine headache. (Of course, some of their medical knowledge may have come from older sources, especially from Egypt.)

The Hippocratics thought that all illness should be explained in terms of ordinary physical causes. Nowhere in any of the Hippocratic writings do you find any suggestion that any disease is the result of a magical or supernatural cause. In the discussion of epilepsy, the Hippocratic author even complained that people turn to supernatural explanations out of ignorance.

Hippocrates was on the right track in saying that we should search for the physical causes of illness. Unfortunately, back then nobody knew enough about biology or chemistry to figure out what those physical causes actually were.

Although the ancient Greeks knew about air, oxygen had not yet been discovered. There were no microscopes back then, so nobody knew that the body is made up of cells, and no one had any idea that bacteria or viruses exist. Although people knew that children tend to look like their parents, nobody knew about genes or chromosomes. Although people knew that the heart and blood existed, they had no idea that the heart pushed the blood around a circular path: from the heart out to the rest of the body and then back to the heart. Even some of the ancient Greek ideas about basic human anatomy were incorrect because there was a taboo against doing dissections of human remains. As a result, doctors didn't do autopsies to figure out why a patient died. So even if someone wanted to explain illness in terms of natural phenomena, the explanations they came up with were usually wrong.

Although Hippocrates and his followers stressed observation, they also had theories to help them make sense of what they saw and to guide them in choosing treatments. Their main theory was based on a very primitive theory of chemistry. Like modern chemists, the Hippocratics believed that all matter is made up of invisibly small particles called atoms. However, the Hippocratics thought that there were only four elements, which meant four kinds of atoms: earth, water, air, and fire. To a modern chemist, these "elements" actually represent three phases of matter (solid, liquid, and gas) plus energy. Modern scientists have identified 118 different elements.

Hippocrates believed that his four elements were associated with four basic physical properties: hotness and coldness, wetness and dryness. The four elements gave these properties to four basic bodily fluids, called the humors: blood, yellow bile, black bile, and phlegm. One of the major goals of Hippocratic medicine was to restore the normal balance among these four humors within the body, thus allowing the body to heal itself.

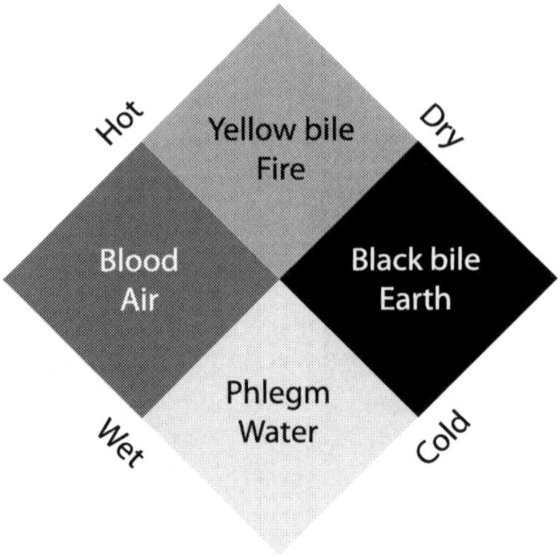

Figure 2. The Hippocratics believed that the body was made up of four elements: air, fire, earth, and water. These elements were represented in the body by four fluids (humors): blood, yellow bile, black bile, and phlegm. Many of the European and Islamic medical treatments from ancient times to the 19th century were attempts to restore the balance of these fluids in the body.

Hippocrates mainly advocated gentle, supportive treatments, with a heavy emphasis on dietary therapies. However, the Hippocratic writings also explain how to intervene in some serious cases, such as how to set broken bones and how to place a tube through the chest wall to drain fluid from inside the chest. Some of these techniques had been handed down from the ancient Egyptians and Babylonians. Some of the medical information recorded in the Hippocratic writings remains important today. Also, some ancient surgical instruments look almost exactly like their modern counterparts.

During the days of the Roman Empire, the Hippocratic ideas about medicine were extended by another Greek physician, Galen of Pergamon. Galen came to fame as a physician to the gladiators. He then served as the personal physician to several Roman emperors at the height of the Roman Empire. Galen's teachings served as the basis of European and Islamic medical training up until modern times.

Besides fire, which represented heat, the Greeks were aware of another kind of energy, one that enabled a body to move. They referred to this kinetic form of energy as *pneuma*, which meant breath or spirit. *Pneuma* represented the breath of life. The ancient Greeks believed that *pneuma* flowed through the arteries and nerves and made the body move. When people die, they stop breathing. Thus, the Greeks believed that *pneuma* had something to do with the soul.

This idea of *pneuma* is strikingly similar to what is called *chi* in traditional Chinese medicine or *prana* in Ayurvedic medicine. In other words, the main concepts of these Eastern medical systems used to be central to Western medicine. However, modern medicine discarded these concepts when science started to give us better explanations of how the body works.

In ancient times, nobody knew the real causes of disease. Thus, they could not explain why some diseases occurred only in certain times and places. An endemic disease is a disease that occurs in some places but not in others. One example is malaria, which tended to occur only in swampy areas. If you drained a swamp, the people who lived in that area stopped getting malaria.

The ancients believed that malaria was caused by the bad smells that come from a swamp. The word *malaria* literally meant bad air. Galen believed that this bad air, or miasma, was a major cause of disease. He believed that when meat or plants rot, they produce a miasma that could make people sick. Sick people, in turn, could generate miasma, which explained how they could pass a disease on to other people.

Epidemic diseases, which were diseases that occurred during some periods of time but not in others, were also a puzzle to ancient medical thinkers. What could cause a major outbreak of disease, such as an epidemic of smallpox or the Black Death? To explain epidemics, many medieval medical thinkers, particularly in the Islamic world, turned to astrology.

It actually made sense that some alignments of the heavenly bodies could produce miasma that caused epidemic diseases. After all, cold and flu season occurs in the fall and winter, when the sun passed through the constellations of Libra through Ares. Today, some epidemiologists think that the sun does matter. They suspect that cold and flu season in Europe and North America results from lots of people having low levels of vitamin D, the sunshine vitamin, during the winter months.

In 1546, an Italian physician named Girolamo Fracastoro came up with a new explanation for why some diseases seem to spread from person to person. He thought that some diseases are caused by particles that are too small to be seen. These particles could be transferred from person to person, either by direct contact or by some object that the sick person had touched. The particles could even spread through the air for a considerable distance. These particles could explain why some diseases seem to be contagious. The best way to prevent the spread of many contagious diseases was to quarantine the sick, which originally meant to separate them from other people for forty days.

Doctors and nurses can accidentally spread disease from one patient to another, especially if they don't wash their hands between patients. One of the first doctors to recognize that problem was Ignaz Semmelweis, who had been put in charge of obstetrics at Vienna General Hospital in 1847.

At that time, the doctors at Vienna General Hospital had just started doing autopsies on patients who died in hospital. At the same time, the death rate from a terrible disease called childbed fever rose dramatically among the women who had just given birth at the hospital. In some months, as many as 30% of the maternity patients died. Semmelweis noticed that the death rate was much higher among the women whose babies had been delivered by doctors, as opposed to midwives. After Semmelweis started making the doctors wash their hands, the death rate among the doctors' maternity patients dropped to about 1%.

Many doctors refused to follow Semmelweis' advice because it did not fit in with any of Galen's theories. Nor did the scientists of the day know what kinds of particles could cause disease. More than 150 years earlier, a Dutch linen merchant named Anthonie van Leeuwenhoek had discovered the existence of bacteria by looking at samples of pond water and scrapings from his own teeth under a powerful homemade lens. Yet nobody knew what bacteria were, or where they came from. It wasn't until the second half of the 19th century that scientists proved that some bacteria cause disease.

The question of where bacteria come from was hard to answer. Do bacteria just appear, all by themselves, whenever the conditions are right? For example, ice crystals will form on a damp windowpane when the film of water freezes. Ice crystals aren't the descendants of other ice crystals. Instead, the water just turns into ice crystals when the temperature drops below the freezing point.

For thousands of years, people thought that certain kinds of living things arose in a similar way. For example, they thought that rotting meat naturally turns into maggots. This theory was called spontaneous generation. Then, in 1668, an Italian physician named Francesco Redi showed that maggots would appear on rotting meat only if flies had laid eggs on it. The maggots would then become flies, which would then mate and lay eggs, and the whole cycle would repeat itself. Eventually, scientists realized that all living plants and animals are descended from parents of the same species. All living things are part of a family tree that stretches back to the dawn of life. This theory is called univocal generation.

In 1859, a young French chemist named Louis Pasteur showed that bacteria also came from other living bacteria. He boiled some beef broth to kill all the bacteria. Then, he found that bacteria grew only in the broth that was exposed to dust from the air, which carried live bacteria with it. Unless the broth contained live bacteria, no bacteria would grow. That's why canned food doesn't start to rot until you open the can.

Pasteur figured that if bacteria could cause meat to rot, they could also cause disease. So did a British surgeon named James Lister. Lister started using carbolic acid as an antiseptic in wounds. He also sprayed a mist of carbolic acid in the air in the operating room. As a result, a lot fewer patients died of infection. This practice was called antiseptic surgery. Back then, many doctors thought that pus and other signs of infection were a natural and even beneficial part of the healing process. Nowadays, doctors and nurses go to great lengths to keep wounds from becoming infected.

The germ theory of disease is the idea that some diseases result from an infection with a particular germ, such as a bacterium or a fungus. (It doesn't mean that all diseases are the result of infection.) In 1867, Pasteur showed that two diseases that were killing silkworms were infectious. These diseases could be prevented by keeping the healthy silkworms separate from anything that had been contaminated by sick ones.

In 1873, a Norwegian physician named Armauer Hansen became the first person to link a particular human disease to a particular bacterium. He showed that leprosy is due to infection with a bacillus (rod-shaped bacterium) called *Mycobacterium leprae*. In 1875, a German physician named Robert Koch proved that anthrax, a disease that can affect humans or animals, is caused by a bacillus called *Bacillus anthracis*. In 1882, Koch proved that tuberculosis is the result of infection with the tubercle bacillus: *Mycobacterium tuberculosis*.

Pasteur knew that rabies is contagious. Rabid animals can spread the disease to other animals and to human beings by biting them. Pasteur guessed correctly that rabies is due to some germ in the rabid animal's saliva. In the 1880s, Pasteur developed an effective vaccine to prevent rabies. However, he couldn't isolate the rabies germ. So he concluded that it is simply too small to be seen through his microscope. Later on, other researchers found that several other infectious diseases, including yellow fever, smallpox, and polio, also had to be the result of germs that are too small to be seen through an ordinary microscope. Today, those germs are called viruses.

Although bacteria are living things, viruses are not. As I'll explain in more detail in chapter 12, a virus is not a living thing. A virus is a thing that was made by a living cell. A virus is just a set of genes wrapped up in a delivery system. If those viral genes are brought into a living cell, the cell may follow the instructions encoded in those genes. Those viral genes tell the cell to make new copies of that virus, just as a computer virus tells a computer to copy and spread the computer virus.

There are millions and millions of species of bacteria, and who knows how many different kinds of viruses. However, most bacteria and viruses pose no threat whatsoever to human health. The inner and outer surfaces of healthy people's bodies are simply teeming with bacteria. To figure out whether a particular bacterium is responsible for causing a particular disease, Robert Koch worked out four rules of thumb, which are called Koch's postulates:

- The bacterium must be found in all organisms suffering from the disease but not in healthy organisms.
- The bacterium must be isolated from a diseased organism and grown in pure culture.
- The cultured bacterium should cause disease when introduced into a healthy organism.
- The same bacterium should be isolated again from the organism that became diseased after the bacterium was introduced.

To understand how and when to use Koch's postulates, imagine that a particular germ is being tried for murder. Koch's first and fourth postulates show that the germ was present at the scene of the crime. The second and third postulates help to rule out other suspects. If all four of Koch's postulates are met, you can be sure, beyond a reasonable doubt, that the germ is guilty of causing that disease.

Unfortunately, you cannot always get all of the evidence that you would like to have, whether in science or in a criminal case. Nevertheless, you might still have enough evidence to convict a suspect. Thus, you can sometimes still be confident that a particular germ causes a particular disease, even if one of Koch's postulates hasn't been met. Many people, especially antivaccination zealots and HIV denialists, misunderstand that point.

Each of Koch's postulates poses some sort of technical or ethical problem. The biggest problem with the first postulate is diagnosis. How can you tell one disease from another? Many diseases that are caused by different germs have similar symptoms. For example, many different germs can cause an illness that looks like the common cold. Also, a particular germ can sometimes cause different symptoms in different patients. The classic example is the plague, which is caused by a bacterium called *Yersinia pestis*. This bacterium can cause three seemingly different diseases. If the infection is mainly in the lymph nodes, the result is bubonic plague. If the lungs are infected, the result is pneumonic plague. If the infection is running rampant throughout the bloodstream, the result is septicemic plague. Sometimes, the disease will progress from one form to another as the infection spreads in the body.

Another problem with Koch's first postulate is that some people can carry an infection without getting sick from it. In the early 20th century, an Irish immigrant named Mary Mallon worked as a cook for wealthy families in New York City and Long Island. Mallon seemed healthy, but typhoid fever kept breaking out in households where she worked. She infected more than 50 people, three of whom died. When "Typhoid Mary" refused to stop working as a cook, she was arrested and was held in quarantine for the rest of her life.

You can also run into difficulty with Koch's second postulate. As I will explain in chapter 9, some bacteria are hard to grow in a laboratory. They may need special nutrients or simply a long time to grow. Some disease-causing bacteria have become so highly adapted to a parasitic lifestyle that they cannot grow and divide unless they are inside another living cell. Because these obligate intracellular parasites can be grown only inside other living cells, they cannot be grown in pure culture. As I will explain in chapter 12, viruses cannot be grown in pure culture, either. They can be produced only inside living cells. However, viruses can be produced in cell cultures and then purified through crystallization.

Even if you cannot fulfill Koch's second postulate, you can sometimes build a convincing case that a particular germ is responsible for causing a particular disease. As I mentioned above, *Mycobacterium leprae*, which causes leprosy, was the first bacterium that was shown to cause a disease in human beings. However, *Mycobacterium leprae* has become so adapted to a parasitic lifestyle that it cannot reproduce outside of another living cell. As a result, scientists cannot grow a pure culture of *Mycobacterium leprae*. Even the attempts to produce the bacteria in cell cultures have failed. Even today, *Mycobacterium leprae* can be grown only in a living animal, such as an armadillo or a mouse with a genetic immune disorder.

There are two problems with Koch's third postulate—one practical, the other moral. The practical problem is that it's sometimes impossible to cause a particular disease in an experimental subject. Either the germ has become too weak to cause the disease, or the subject is already immune to it. For example, Pasteur had found that when he inoculated chickens with *Pasteurella multocida*, the bacillus that causes fowl cholera, the chickens always died within 48 hours. But after one of the cultures had been weakened by the summer heat, it no longer made the chickens sick. Instead, it made the chickens immune to fowl cholera. Thus, Pasteur discovered that dead or weakened bacteria could be used to make an effective vaccine. This discovery was a major advance in the development of vaccines.

The moral problem with Koch's third postulate is that it would be not only morally wrong but illegal to give a human being a potentially deadly infection, just to see if he or she gets sick. Some people argue that Koch's third postulate was never fulfilled in the case of HIV and AIDS. Thus, they claim that we therefore don't really know whether HIV causes AIDS. But when you cannot do an experiment, you can sometimes find natural experiments—situations where a treated group and a reasonably well-matched control group arose by accident—that provide the evidence you need.

The accidental contamination of blood products with HIV set up a natural experiment. After HIV testing became available, scientists tested the stored samples of blood products that had been given to patients. This testing showed that patients got AIDS from blood products only if those blood products had been contaminated with HIV.

Many nonscientists and even a few cranks within the scientific community have insisted that HIV does not cause AIDS. They may admit that AIDS patients are often infected with HIV, but they insist that the HIV itself is harmless. Instead, they believe that AIDS is due to other cofactors. In reality, there are always numerous factors that affect whether exposure to a particular germ will make someone sick.

Some people are naturally resistant to some infections. Sometimes, this natural resistance is genetic. Other people become immune to an infectious disease because they have already had it or a similar infection. On the other hand, some people have poor resistance for one reason or another. For example, people with cystic fibrosis have thick, sticky mucus that is hard to clear from the lungs. As a result, they are at high risk for lung infections. Some infectious diseases, such as measles and AIDS, attack the immune system. Thus, they make a person more susceptible to other infections.

In other words, a germ is not always able to make a person sick. In those cases, exposure to that germ would not be a *sufficient* cause of that disease. Nevertheless, exposure to a particular germ is a *necessary* cause of some diseases. The smallpox virus is a necessary cause of smallpox. If you are never exposed to the smallpox virus, you will never get smallpox. Likewise, if you are never exposed to poliovirus, you will never get polio. The same goes for the viruses that cause measles, mumps, and rubella. The same goes for the bacterium that causes whooping cough. If you can eradicate those germs, you can achieve permanent 100% success in preventing those diseases.

The smallpox virus has something important in common with the measles, mumps, and rubella viruses. Each of those viruses causes infections only in human beings. There is no wild reservoir of these viruses to reinfect the human population. Once we stop the polio, measles, mumps, and rubella viruses from being transmitted from person to person, those viruses will become extinct. Thus, those diseases will never happen to anyone ever again. As a result, we can eliminate the diseases themselves and then avoid even the small risk associated with the vaccines to prevent them.

A worldwide vaccination campaign drove smallpox into extinction. Likewise, rinderpest, which was a measles-like disease of cattle, has been driven into extinction through a campaign to vaccinate cattle. As I write this, the Global Polio Eradication Initiative is about to eradicate polio from the face of the earth. Worldwide vaccination campaigns could drive measles, mumps, and rubella into extinction. Once those viruses have gone the way of the dodo bird, then nobody will have to be vaccinated against those diseases ever again.

Some bacterial diseases occur only in human beings. Vaccination has practically eliminated some of these diseases, at least in some geographic areas. For example, diphtheria was a major cause of death in the United States in 1900, but now it is practically nonexistent in the United States. Thus, the diphtheria vaccine has provided a great deal of protection for the entire population, even for the people who were never vaccinated. Unfortunately, major outbreaks of diphtheria occurred in the former Soviet Union in the 1990s, after vaccination coverage dropped. In the United States today, we are seeing outbreaks of whooping cough, especially in areas where many people are refusing to have their children vaccinated.

For thousands of years, human beings have been praying for deliverance from terrible plagues like smallpox and cholera. Over the past 200 years, the medical profession has learned how to provide this deliverance. People are still praying for an end to the AIDS epidemic.

When the AIDS epidemic broke out, it took scientists only a few years to prove that AIDS is caused by the human immunodeficiency virus (HIV), which is a retrovirus. HIV is similar to the feline leukemia virus (FeLV), which is a retrovirus that causes immune suppression in cats. Tragically, efforts to develop an effective vaccine against HIV have failed so far. Nevertheless, scientists have found ways for people to prevent the spread of the disease and have developed medications that dramatically improve the health and life expectancy of infected people.

Inexplicably, many influential people refused to accept that HIV causes AIDS or that the anti-AIDS medications save lives. Public health experts estimate that the South African government's refusal to accept grants and free anti-AIDS drugs led to the avoidable deaths of a third of a million people. We live in an age when the biggest threat to our health is not germs per se but foolishness.

3

How Governments Fight Infectious Disease

In high school biology, I learned that my skin is my first line of defense against dangerous germs. Then, from studying economic geography in college and editing medical textbooks and journals for a living, I learned that the U.S. Centers for Disease Control and Prevention and the state and local boards of health in the United States were my real first line of defense against dangerous germs.

Thanks to federal, state, and local public health efforts, some deadly germs including the smallpox virus never got anywhere near me. The last reported case of smallpox in the United States occurred more than 10 years before I was born. I have never even met anyone who has had smallpox. Meanwhile, smallpox continued to kill people in some poor countries until I was in high school. I was among the first children to be vaccinated against measles. Today, measles is no longer endemic in the United States, although we still have outbreaks that can be traced to imported cases of measles. But in 2011, measles killed 158,000 people worldwide; 95% of these deaths were in poor countries with weak public health systems.

Many people in the United States have such a strong antigovernment bias that they find it hard to imagine government as being good for their health. We in the United States have also been programmed into thinking that health is a purely personal matter and that healthcare should be a for-profit business. This attitude may explain why the United States is the only industrialized country that lacks a not-for-profit national health insurance plan that covers everyone. That fact, in turn, probably explains why life expectancy is shorter in the United States than in Western Europe and Canada.

In the United States, the people on the political right tend to think of government as the enemy of freedom and a threat to capitalism. In contrast, many people on the left believe that government and the scientific community have been entirely corrupted by the capitalists who own the major corporations. Both the right-wingers and the left-wingers are suspicious of scientists and view government as the problem, not as a mechanism for solving problems. As a result, many of our problems go unsolved.

The governments in the rich countries have had stunning success in solving the problem of infectious disease. As a result, the average person lives a much longer, healthier life. In 1776, life expectancy at birth in the United States was only about 37. By 1900, it had risen to about 47, thanks largely to the widespread and often mandatory use of smallpox vaccination.

The United States government started keeping official statistics on causes of death in 1900 (Table 1). By then, smallpox was no longer a major cause of death in the United States. In 1900, the number 1 killer was "influenza and pneumonia," which could be due to viral or bacterial infections. Tuberculosis, which by then was known to be a bacterial infection, was number 2. Gastrointestinal infections, such as cholera and typhoid fever, were number 3. Heart disease, including the heart problems that could result from a bad case of strep throat, was number 4. Diphtheria, which is another bacterial infection, was number 10. Notice that today, "influenza and pneumonia" is the only one of our top 10 killers that is infectious.

Table 1. Causes of death in the United States in 1900 and 2010

1900	2010
1. Influenza and pneumonia	1. Heart disease
2. Tuberculosis	2. Cancer
3. Gastrointestinal infections	3. Chronic lung disease
4. Heart disease	4. Cerebrovascular disease (stroke)
5. Cerebrovascular disease (mainly strokes)	5. Accidents
6. Kidney disease	6. Alzheimer disease (senility)
7. Accidents	7. Diabetes
8. Cancer	8. Kidney disease
9. Senility	9. Influenza and pneumonia
10. Diphtheria	10. Suicide

Notice that tuberculosis, gastrointestinal disease, and diphtheria have dropped off the list. Tuberculosis is now rare in the United States. In many recent years, we haven't had even a single reported case of diphtheria. The only infectious disease that's still among our top ten causes of death is influenza and pneumonia, which has fallen to ninth place. Although pneumonia once killed many people of all ages, most deaths from pneumonia nowadays are among the elderly. Today, our main killers are not infectious diseases but the chronic degenerative diseases that result from our lifestyle: our rich, fatty diet as well as cigarette smoking and alcohol abuse.

Today, life expectancy in the United States and other rich countries is in the late 70s. Yet in many poor countries, life expectancy is still in the 30s and 40s. The difference is that the rich countries do a great job of preventing and treating infectious disease. However, even the people in a poor country can have a long life expectancy if their government does a good job of preventing and treating infectious disease.

The dramatic increase in life expectancy in the United States and other industrialized countries was due largely to improvements in public health. Public health is the science and art of preventing disease, prolonging life, and promoting health through organized efforts and informed choices of government, public and private organizations, and individuals. Public health is one of the most important functions of government. Public health measures fall into four general categories: sanitation, vaccination, education, and medication. Many antivaccination zealots claim that the other measures make vaccination unnecessary. They are wrong.

Sanitation helps to prevent infectious diseases from being spread through contaminated water and food. Vaccination helps to prevent the transmission of diseases that spread easily from person to person, especially by airborne droplets. Education helps people learn how to prevent the transmission of sexually transmitted infections and blood-borne infections and to avoid the noninfectious diseases that result from lifestyle. Medication can help to reduce the spread of some infections, in addition to reducing suffering and death from infectious disease and some noninfectious diseases.

Sometimes, a government can stop a deadly epidemic by taking some simple action. In 1854, an epidemic of cholera broke out in the Soho neighborhood of London, England. At the time, the London sewer system had not yet reached Soho, so the raw sewage from leaking or overflowing cesspools sometimes contaminated the drinking water. Dr. John Snow suspected that cholera was being spread by this contaminated water.

Snow found that practically everyone who got sick in the epidemic had drunk water from a particular well on Broad Street (Figure 3). After Snow persuaded the local authorities that the well had been contaminated, they had the handle removed from the pump. After that, people stopped getting cholera. However, Snow himself was not entirely sure that removing the handle stopped the epidemic. He thought it was possible that the epidemic had simply run its natural course. That same year, an Italian physician named Filippo Paccini found a comma-shaped bacterium (now called *Vibrio cholerae*) that he believed was the cause of cholera. In 1884, Robert Koch showed that Paccini's bacteria were always found in people with cholera but never found in people with other diarrheal diseases.

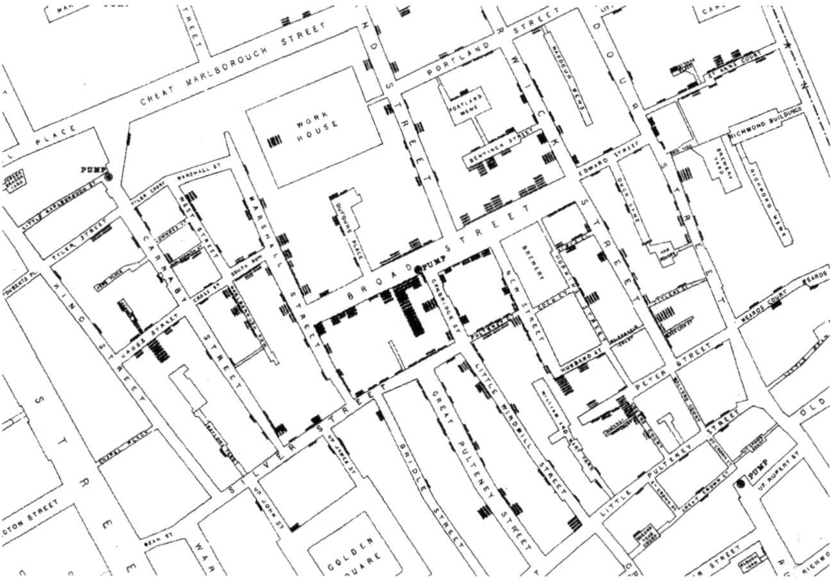

Figure 3. Most of the deaths in the 1854 cholera epidemic in London were clustered around a single water pump on Broad Street. Map drawn and lithographed by Charles Cheffins. From Snow J. *On the Mode of Communication of Cholera*, 2nd Ed, London, UK: John Churchill; 1855.

In the United States, the death rate from infectious disease dropped sharply in the late 19th and early 20th century. Much of this decrease was due to the installation of modern sewerage systems and water treatment plants. Some of it was due to regulation of the food industry. For example, the federal government started inspecting meat and requiring pasteurization of milk. Also, state and local boards of health started inspecting restaurants and tracing the sources of disease outbreaks. For example, when the New York City Health Department found that Mary "Typhoid Mary" Mallon was responsible for spreading typhoid fever, they put her in quarantine.

Today, we know that cholera is caused by Paccini's *Vibrio cholerae* bacteria. Typhoid fever is caused by another bacterium, *Salmonella typhi*. These bacteria infect the lining of the intestine. People catch these diseases by swallowing something that has been contaminated by an infected person's poop (feces). Scientists call this the fecal-oral route of transmission. Diseases can spread by the fecal-oral route when raw sewage contaminates drinking water, when animal droppings contaminate food, or when food handlers fail to wash their hands after going to the bathroom.

Other bacteria that can be spread by the fecal-oral route include other *Salmonella* species as well as *Shigella*. Viruses can also spread by the fecal-oral route. The virus that causes polio is one example. Another is the virus that causes hepatitis A, which was originally called infectious hepatitis. Some parasites, including protozoa such as *Giardia* and worms such as *Ascaris*, are also spread by the fecal-oral route.

Sanitation and hygiene help to prevent the fecal-oral transmission of infectious disease. Sanitation refers mainly to the control of human and animal feces. Hygiene refers to personal cleanliness, such as hand washing. That's why state and local boards of health require restaurants to post signs in their restrooms, reminding employees to wash their hands after using the restroom.

Thanks to improvements in sanitation, we stopped having epidemics of cholera and typhoid fever in the United States. That's why we do not vaccinate children against cholera and typhoid fever in the United States. People in the U.S. generally do not get those vaccines unless they join the military or plan to visit a country with poor sanitation.

The United States stopped having cholera epidemics by the early 20th century. But at around the same time, it started having epidemics of paralytic polio. Sanitation reduced but did not completely stop the spread of the virus that causes polio. Although fewer people were catching poliovirus, they tended to catch it at a later age, when they were more likely to end up paralyzed by the infection.

In societies with poor sanitation, nearly everyone was repeatedly exposed to poliovirus. The first infection usually occurred during infancy, while they were still being protected by the antibodies from their mother's milk. Those maternal antibodies usually protected the baby against paralysis while the baby's immune system learned to make its own antibodies against poliovirus. Even though poliovirus infection was common, only a few babies ended up paralyzed, and those cases were often spread out over time. With the improvements in sanitation, people started catching the poliovirus later in childhood, when they were no longer protected by maternal antibodies. As a result, they were at much higher risk of becoming paralyzed from a poliovirus infection. Also, the cases of paralysis tended to occur in big clusters, rather than being spread out over time. The outbreaks of paralysis and death among school-age children created widespread terror.

Sanitation was able to reduce but not eliminate the spread of poliovirus. Poliovirus mainly infects the intestines. Thus, it spreads mainly by the fecal-oral route. However, poliovirus can also infect the lining of the nasal passages, just like the viruses that cause the common cold. As a result, you could catch polio from touching something that an infected person had touched after wiping his nose, or perhaps even by being in the same room as an infected person. That's why improved sanitation was not enough to wipe out polio, and why we needed the polio vaccine.

Vaccination is the only reliable way to prevent diseases that are easily spread from person to person by casual contact or by airborne droplets. Today, vaccination is a key part of strategies for preventing diseases such as measles. Surveillance and quarantine can help to limit the spread of an epidemic, but those strategies can be used only after a person is known to be infected. Many germs, especially poliovirus and the measles virus, can be spread by people who do not even look particularly sick. People with measles are highly contagious for a day or two before the obvious signs of measles appear. Some people with poliovirus infections seem to have only a minor flu-like illness or never look sick at all. Thus, surveillance and quarantine are not a substitute for vaccination against polio and measles.

Vaccination helps to protect the person who got the vaccine. It also helps to protect everyone else. If you have become immune to measles, you cannot catch the measles. Nor can you spread it to anyone else. If enough of the people within a community are immune to measles, then the measles virus will have a hard time finding its next victim. That's why epidemics tend to die out on their own. The protective effect of having many immunized people within a community is called community immunity or herd immunity. I'll explain the mathematics of herd immunity in chapter 15.

Governments' role in vaccination goes beyond requiring that people receive certain vaccinations. In the United States, the federal government has long played an important role in helping to develop new vaccines and in ensuring that the vaccines that are given to the public are safe and effective. In chapter 16, I'll discuss how and why vaccines are regulated.

Some antivaccination zealots point out that the death rate from measles and some other vaccine-preventable diseases started to decrease even before the vaccines came out. Yet from that fact, they conclude that the introduction of vaccines made no difference and that vaccines are therefore unnecessary. They are wrong. Death rates did start to decrease because of improvements in nutrition and medical care. In particular, antibiotics helped keep children from dying of bacterial pneumonia that often occurred in the wake of a measles infection. Yet even after these advances in medical care, there were still tens of thousands of children every year who ended up hospitalized with measles, thousands who ended up with permanent disabilities such as blindness and mental retardation, and about 500 deaths per year. Even today, there is no effective treatment for measles virus infection. The only way to prevent those deaths was to prevent the measles virus infection to begin with.

Measles vaccination has saved lives. It has also prevented many cases of blindness, deafness, and mental retardation. The purpose of vaccination is not just to prevent death. It is also to prevent illness, hospitalizations, and lifelong disability.

Education is important for limiting the spread of sexually transmitted and blood-borne infections. Those diseases are caused by germs that cannot survive for long outside the human body. Thus, you must have intimate contact with an infected person in order to catch those diseases. Examples include bacterial diseases such as syphilis and gonorrhea and viral diseases such as AIDS and hepatitis B and C. The sexually transmitted diseases can also be spread by sharing razors or hypodermic needles or by transfusion of contaminated blood. That's why hepatitis B was once called serum hepatitis.

Most of the sexually transmitted and blood-borne diseases are chronic infections. Chronic means that they last a long time. To cause a chronic infection, a germ has to be good at surviving and multiplying despite the activity of the human immune system. It's hard to make an effective vaccine against a disease that can do that. Thus, it is not surprising that there is no vaccine against syphilis or gonorrhea. We have effective vaccines against only two of the sexually transmitted infections: hepatitis B and some strains of human papillomavirus (HPV).

Education can help to reduce the risk of some diseases that can spread through somewhat less intimate contact. For example, an antibiotic-resistant bacterium called MRSA (methicillin-resistant *Staphylococcus aureus*) can be easily spread by people sharing athletic equipment in gyms. Ordinary cleanliness can help to reduce the spread of MRSA.

It often takes a combination of sanitation and education to control the diseases that are spread by pests, such as rodents and mosquitos. Sanitation would involve attempts to clean up the environment and the food supply. Education would involve attempts to teach people how to protect themselves.

Every so often, the U.S. Food and Drug Administration demands a recall of potentially contaminated processed food, such as peanut butter that has been contaminated by *Salmonella*. The *Salmonella* bacteria do not infect peanuts. *Salmonella* bacteria live inside the intestines of animals. They get into the peanut butter when rats or pigeons poop on the peanuts at the factory. Intestinal bacteria can also get onto vegetables that have been fertilized with fresh manure.

The U.S. Department of Agriculture and the FDA make and enforce regulations to protect the public from food-borne infections. Some organic farmers were outraged when the FDA suggested that farmers should not use fresh manure to fertilize vegetables that will be eaten raw. Yet this rule would help keep our salads free from the bacteria that are spread by the fecal-oral route, especially the antibiotic-resistant bacteria in the manure from factory farms.

Mosquito control is perhaps the oldest public health measure. The ancient Romans knew that malaria occurred in swampy areas, and that draining a swamp eliminated the malaria. In the 19th century, scientists discovered that malaria is due to a parasite that is carried by mosquitos, rather than being caused by the odor of the swamp.

Malaria used to be common in much of the southern United States. It started to become less common in the 1880s, thanks to the invention of window screens. After World War II, malaria was largely eliminated from the United States through an aggressive campaign of mosquito control.

Malaria is a vector-borne disease. A vector is any organism that carries an infectious agent and transmits it to another living organism. Mosquitos are the vector that transmits the single-celled parasite that causes malaria. Mosquitoes can serve as vectors for many viral or parasitic diseases. However, mosquitoes never seem to transmit bacterial diseases. However, other kinds of blood-sucking parasites can transmit bacterial diseases. Fleas can spread the plague bacteria. Ticks are responsible for transmitting many bacterial diseases, including Lyme disease and Rocky Mountain spotted fever.

For a vector to transmit a disease, three things must happen. First, the vector must pick up the infectious agent from an infected host. Second, the infectious agent must survive and possibly mature or even reproduce in the vector, but without killing the vector. Third, the vector must then deliver the infectious agent to a new host. Several species of mosquito are efficient at transmitting yellow fever because the yellow fever virus can infect the mosquito without killing it. In contrast, mosquitos cannot transmit AIDS because mosquitos digest HIV along with their blood meal. To a mosquito, HIV is food.

Many disease-causing organisms have become highly dependent on a particular species of vector. Thus, the best way to control the spread of those diseases is to control the vector. Sometimes, governments can do that directly, by spraying the areas where the mosquitos breed. In other situations, they educate the public about how to control or avoid the vector. For example, governmental and nongovernmental organizations have been handing out insecticide-treated bed nets to keep mosquitos from biting sleeping children.

Medication can relieve suffering and can often save lives. It can sometimes even limit the spread of some infectious diseases. For example, if you cure a case of tuberculosis, the patient will no longer be able to spread the disease to other people. People who have been exposed to whooping cough or diphtheria are often treated with antibiotics, even if they don't look sick. The antibiotics can kill the bacteria that cause whooping cough and diphtheria. However, antibiotics cannot destroy the toxins that the bacteria have made. By the time it is clear that someone with whooping cough or diphtheria has more than a common cold, the bacteria have already released huge amounts of dangerous toxins in the body. Thus, it is best to prevent diphtheria and whooping cough by vaccination.

Government plays an important role in regulating medicine. In the United States, the FDA ensures that the drugs and vaccines that are sold in the United States are effective and safe when used as directed for their intended purpose (see chapter 16). The recommendations for who should get what vaccine, and when, are made by an independent committee, the Advisory Committee on Immunization Practices (ACIP), which submits its recommendations to the Centers for Disease Control and Prevention for approval (see chapter 17). However, the federal government has no authority to force vaccination on anyone, except for people in the military. Laws about vaccination are the responsibility of state governments.

State governments have police power, which means a basic right to make and enforce laws and regulations for the benefit of their communities. The state governments delegate some of this power to county and local governments. We have mandatory vaccination laws for the same reason we have traffic laws: to protect public safety.

The states' police power includes the authority to grant licenses to doctors and other healthcare professionals, as well as to take the license away from any professional who endangers public health. In 1905, the Supreme Court decided (*Jacobson v. Massachusetts*) that state governments do have the authority to make laws that require vaccination and to fine the people who break those laws. Theoretically, people who refuse to vaccinate their children could also be sued for damages in state courts if their unvaccinated children spread a vaccine-preventable disease to other children.

Although states cannot regulate religion, they do have the power to protect children from being abused or neglected by their parents, even for religious reasons. According to a 1944 Supreme Court decision in *Prince v. Massachusetts,*

> Parents may be free to become martyrs themselves. But it does not follow they are free, in identical circumstances, to make martyrs of their children before they have reached the age of full and legal discretion when they can make that choice for themselves.

States have used their police power to refuse to allow unvaccinated children to go to public school. Exemptions can be granted for children who cannot, for medical reasons, be vaccinated. Most states also allow religious exemptions. Some also allow exemptions for "philosophical" reasons. As more parents take advantage of these loopholes, we are seeing more outbreaks of vaccine-preventable disease. Not only are the unvaccinated children unprotected against disease, they pose a threat to other children, including the children who were too sick to be vaccinated and those whose vaccinations did not lead to protective immunity.

Lately, many people have been telling me that the government and the pharmaceutical industry are involved in some huge conspiracy. They claim that vaccination is just a racket. They insist that vaccines do nothing but harm children and line the pockets of the pharmaceutical industry. The truth is that the vaccine business is small potatoes, compared to the rest of the pharmaceutical industry. That's why Big Pharma does not bother to use its influence to persuade the commercial media to educate the public about measles, tetanus, and diphtheria.

Although practically everyone is supposed to be vaccinated, each patient gets at most a few doses of a vaccine over the course of his or her lifetime. Also, the profit margins on vaccines can be slim. Vaccines are expensive to produce, but the price that governments and insurance companies are willing to pay for a vaccine is often quite low. Because of the slim profit margin and modest sales, the profits are relatively small. The real money has been in the blockbuster drugs. A blockbuster drug is one that generates $1 billion or more per year in sales until its patent expires. Many blockbuster drugs are based on a simple chemical compound that is cheap to produce. As a result, the profit margin is high. A huge sales volume combined with a high profit margin results in huge profits.

Although vaccines are a small sideline for Big Pharma, vaccinations are a mainstay of public health efforts. Thus, vaccines are central to the services that pediatricians, family doctors, and nurse practitioners provide. Children have to come in for "well-child" visits to get their shots. In contrast, "alternative" practitioners cannot give vaccinations. Much of the opposition to vaccination comes from chiropractors and other "alternative" practitioners. To understand why, you need to understand what alternative medicine is.

4

How Alternative Medicine Arose

As I explained in chapter 2, ancient Greek physicians struggled to find natural explanations for why people get sick. The ancient Greek physicians also tried to develop a theory that explained what they saw and that would help them choose the best treatment for each patient. Unfortunately, the ancient Greeks knew little about anatomy, less about chemistry, and nothing at all about microbiology. As a result, most of their medical theories were wrong. Nevertheless, those theories were accepted largely without question throughout the middle ages and up to the 19th century.

Hippocratics and Galen argued that medical theories should not be like religious dogma. They emphasized that theories should be tested and confirmed through observation. Galen had set a particularly good example as a physician engaged in a quest for truth. He argued that both reason and observation should be used to confirm whether a theory is true.

Unfortunately, physicians during the Middle Ages and up through the early 19th century ignored that example. Instead, they often regarded

Galen's writings as holy scripture. They ignored Galen's obvious mistakes, and they were slow to embrace ideas, such as hand washing and vaccination, that Galen never mentioned.

During the 18th and early 19th century, medical students in even the best universities were taught many theories that have since been rejected by the scientific community. They were also taught to use many treatments that are rarely if ever used anymore.

Up until the late 19th century, European and North American physicians were taught that disease resulted mainly from imbalance of the humors but could also result from a bad alignment of the planets. They were taught that to restore health, they should draw blood until the patient turned pale or give the patient drugs to induce vomiting or diarrhea until the patient was severely dehydrated.

Sometimes, doctors used dangerous drugs that contained large doses of mercury. Mercury was used because of unscientific ideas from alchemy and astrology. Of course, if mercury poisoning really were a cause of autism, then autism would have become extremely common among the children of people who could afford medical care in the 18th and early 19th century. It would have remained common in the early 20th century because of the widespread use of calomel (mercuric chloride) as a laxative. If autism really were due to mercury poisoning, it would have become less common as the population's overall exposure to mercury decreased.

During the 18th and early 19th century, medical doctors often used "heroic" treatments that were often more dangerous and more unpleasant than the diseases that the doctors were trying to cure. As you might imagine, many patients started to look for alternatives to the kind of medicine that was being taught in the universities of those days. In response to that demand, several schools of alternative medicine arose. Some of them are still popular today.

By *school*, I don't necessarily mean a brick-and-mortar institution. I mean a group of people who follow a common doctrine or who revere a particular teacher. Several of the schools of alternative medicine that arose in those days are still popular today. Hypnosis was derived from mesmerism or animal magnetism, which was created in the 1770s by a German physician and astrologer named Anton Mesmer. Homeopathy was invented in 1796 by a German physician named Samuel Hahnemann. Chiropractic was invented in 1895 by an American layman, D. D. Palmer. Osteopathy started as an alternative school of medicine in the 1870s. Today, however, doctors of osteopathy get training that is practically identical to what medical doctors receive.

All of these alternative schools of medicine promoted theories that were never accepted by scientists. When Mesmerism became popular in Paris in the 1780s, King Louis XVI appointed a commission to investigate it. Some of the most famous scientists of the day, including Antoine Lavoisier and Benjamin Franklin, served on the commission. The commission found no evidence that Mesmer's magnetic fluid existed. Nevertheless, various forms of magnetic healing and magnet therapy remain popular today, even though their rationale has no scientific basis and no research has ever shown them to be effective.

Perhaps the biggest opponent of heroic medicine was Samuel Hahnemann. He urged that doctors should abandon heroic medicine. However, he went too far in the other direction. He created a system of medical treatment that has no effect at all. Hahnemann claimed that when he took a huge dose of an antimalarial drug, he found that it gave him the symptoms of malaria. From that, he developed the concept of "like treats like." So he taught that patients should be given drugs that would theoretically make their symptoms worse. The secret was to use tiny doses. Homeopathy involves doses that are so small that they are no dose at all.

Hahnemann didn't measure his doses in milligrams or even micrograms, as most drugs are measured today. Instead, he created a centesimal scale. To make a 1C solution, you would dilute something a hundred-fold. To make a 2C solution, you would dilute a 1C formulation a hundred-fold. That works out to a 1:10,000 dilution. A 3C solution was 1:1,000,000. A 6C solution would be one part in 10 trillion. Hahnemann routinely recommended 30C solutions, which work out to one part in 1,000,000,000,000,000,000,000,000,000,000,000,000,000,000,000,000,000,000,000,000. That's literally an astronomical figure. To make a 30C dilution, you would have to dilute 1 cubic centimeter of drug (about one fifth of a teaspoonful) in 106 cubic light-years of water.

Hahnemann actually claimed that the more he diluted a solution, the stronger its effects would be. Why? Because he shook the solution really hard in three different directions each time he diluted it. Really, really hard.

Hahnemann's theory had two basic problems: one is practical, the other theoretical. The practical problem is that homeopathic remedies have never been shown to work. That problem is hardly surprising, given the theoretical problem: Hahnemann's theory makes no sense in terms of what we know about chemistry.

For Hahnemann's theory to work, solutions would have to have some amazing properties that have never shown up in a chemistry laboratory. For one thing, a drug preparation would have to get more powerful as the concentration decreases to zero. Once you get to a dilution of 12C, you probably don't have even a single molecule of the original drug left in the solution. That fact springs from something that chemists call the Avogadro limit, which results from the size of molecules.

Why do homeopaths insist that the "essence" of a drug remains in a solution, even after the solution has become so dilute that the drug itself has gone missing? They claim that it's because they shake the solution really hard every time they dilute it. Really, really hard. The shaking supposedly releases a "spirit-like" healing force that imprints itself upon the water. But how do the things that are dissolved in the water know which one of them is supposed to release a "spirit-like" healing force while the rest of them are not? The whole idea is absurd.

Of course, back in Hahnemann's day, you would be better off getting a drop of pure water from a homeopath than being bled to death by a university-trained physician. In that context, giving someone an ineffective but harmless treatment is definitely the lesser of two evils. But it's still an evil because it is dishonest.

Medicine should be based on the best available scientific understanding, and a doctor-patient relationship should be based on honesty. Thus, it would be far better to give the patient no treatment at all than to mislead the patient into thinking that a worthless treatment (placebo) might be effective. Placebos can be used in medical research. However, research subjects are told from the beginning that they might get a placebo. But even in a research setting, patients deserve the best possible treatment. Thus, placebos should not be used unless nobody knows whether giving the experimental treatment is better than doing nothing.

Homeopaths have been divided in their opinions about vaccination. Some homeopaths have wanted to appeal to the public's faith in vaccination in their campaign to promote homeopathy. Thus, some homeopaths have claimed that homeopathy is based on the same principle as vaccination: small doses of a noxious substance would produce beneficial effects on the body. However, vaccines contain a measurable amount of active ingredient, and they have a measurable effect on the body. Homeopathic preparations do not.

Other homeopaths oppose conventional vaccines, offering homeopathic versions which they claim are equally effective but safer. Unfortunately, homeopathic treatments have never been shown to provide any medical benefits. In particular, they have never been shown to make anyone immune to any disease. The people who use homeopathic treatments instead of vaccination can be lulled into a false sense of security. They may believe that their homeopathic treatments are strengthening their immune system. In reality, these people are being protected by the immunity of the vaccinated people all around them.

As I explained in chapter 3, a disease cannot spread within a herd of animals or within a human population if most of those animals or people are already immune to it. That phenomenon is called herd immunity. If an individual has a medical problem that would make vaccination needlessly risky, that individual might nevertheless be protected by herd immunity. Herd immunity also protects the people whose immune systems failed to mount an immune response to vaccination. This protection is important because no vaccine is 100% effective.

One of the other misleading things that Hahnemann did was to coin the term *allopathic medicine* to refer to the standard medical practices of his day. Today, many advocates of alternative medicine still use the term *allopathic medicine* to refer to what's currently being taught in medical schools. Yet there never was any medical philosophy called allopathy. Nor did any physicians refer to themselves as allopaths.

According to Hahnemann, allopathy means using drugs that oppose the symptoms of a disease, instead of working to restore the body's natural balance. Yet the purpose of the heroic medical treatments that the medical doctors of Hahnemann's day performed was not to oppose the patient's symptoms. It was to correct the balance of the bodily humors. Thus, when advocates of alternative medicine criticize allopathic medicine, they are attacking something that never existed.

Of course, the doctors of Hahnemann's day often did use drugs that relieved patients' symptoms. To this day, many drugs are used purely to relieve symptoms. A treatment that is intended to relieve symptoms without addressing the underlying cause of the symptoms is called palliative. The relief of symptoms ought to be an important goal in medicine. Ideally, a drug would relieve the patient's symptoms by solving the underlying problem. For example, an antibiotic can relieve the symptoms of a bacterial infection by curing the infection. However, patients often benefit from treatments to relieve such symptoms as pain and itching, even if the underlying cause is not cured.

I'm always suspicious of people who dismiss the importance of symptoms. Symptoms not only represent suffering, they provide evidence that the patient is sick. Medical care should address the patient's underlying disease whenever possible, but the ultimate outcome should include the relief of symptoms, should it not? Doctors should try to do more than provide short-term relief of symptoms, but relief of symptoms is still an important goal in medicine.

Unlike the founders of Mesmerism and homeopathy, the founder of chiropractic had no medical training of any kind. D. D. Palmer started as a schoolteacher and then became a grocer. Although the world's leading scientists had rejected Anton Mesmer's theory about an invisible magnetic fluid more than 100 years earlier, Palmer set up a magnetic healing practice in Iowa.

Palmer believed that vital energy flowed around the body through the nervous system. (This idea was basically the same as the obsolete theory of *pneuma*). Palmer argued that this flow could be blocked by small misalignments, which he called subluxations, of the bones of the spine. Palmer argued that by correcting subluxations, he was influencing a life force that he called innate intelligence. He later argued that this innate intelligence was a personified part of the universal intelligence (God). Thus, he turned his healing system into a form of religion.

Palmer claimed that 95% of all illnesses resulted from subluxations of the spine. The other 5% resulted from displacements of other joints. He claimed that if these subluxations are corrected, the body will heal itself. Palmer coined the term *chiropractic*, which means "hand practice," to describe his methods.

Scientists took a dim view of Palmer's theory. It was based on the traditional concept of *pneuma*, which they had already rejected in favor of better theories of how the body works. Also, Palmer was trying to explain all disease in terms of a single cause, at a time when scientists were finding many different disease-causing organisms, each of which caused a unique disease. The chiropractors who still adhere closely to Palmer's theories are called "straight" chiropractors.

The invention of x-ray imaging made things even worse for Palmer's theory. The subluxations that chiropractors were supposedly treating didn't necessarily show up on x-ray images. The subluxations that could be seen on x-ray images generally had nothing to do with disease of the internal organs.

Today, it does not matter whether the founder of chiropractic advocated an unscientific theory in the 1890s. Many ideas that were being taught in even the best medical schools back then haven't stood the test of time. All that should matter now is whether today's chiropractors are providing services that have been scientifically proven to be safe and effective.

With the rise of evidence-based medicine and managed care, the chiropractic profession has been under increasing pressure from the federal government, state regulatory agencies, and the health insurance industry to prove that the treatments that chiropractors are providing are not only safe and effective but also worth the expense. This challenge has created a lot of discussion about the future of the chiropractic profession. In response, some chiropractors are promoting evidence-based chiropractic, which is an attempt to establish the efficacy, safety, and cost-effectiveness of services that could fall within the chiropractor's scope of practice.

Palmer taught his students that spinal adjustment was all that was needed to prevent or treat disease. As a result, the first few generations of chiropractors were vocal opponents of the germ theory of disease and thus of vaccination as well. The chiropractic profession's opposition to germ theory and vaccination peaked in the 1940s. It weakened after that, probably because of the widespread public popularity of penicillin and then the polio vaccine. Nevertheless, many chiropractors are still actively spreading antivaccination propaganda.

Some chiropractic organizations tread carefully around the issue of vaccination. Rather than claiming that vaccination doesn't work, they focus on the supposed risks of vaccination. They portray vaccination as a personal choice, as opposed to a social obligation as well as a means of self-defense. In contrast, the College of Chiropractors of Ontario's Standards of Practice states, "Chiropractors may not, in their professional capacity, treat or advise patients/others with respect to immunization/vaccination as it is outside their scope of practice."

In the United States, the state governments regulate medical practice. The state legislatures define each healthcare profession's scope of practice. A state legislature could decide that advice about immunization/vaccination is outside the scope of chiropractic practice. Thus, chiropractors who continue to urge people not to vaccinate their children could theoretically end up losing their chiropractic license in that state. Meanwhile, the state legislatures could also make sure that chiropractors have adequate training to provide the kinds of services that would best serve their patients.

Vaccination is outside a chiropractor's scope of practice. Nevertheless, some health-promoting and perhaps ultimately life-saving services could fall within a chiropractor's scope of practice. Today, our major causes of death and disability in the United States are the chronic degenerative diseases that result from improper diet and a sedentary lifestyle. Drugs and surgery do not prevent or cure those diseases. These diseases can be prevented or cured only by teaching people what to eat and how to exercise. This kind of lifestyle education could fall within the chiropractor's scope of practice. State licensing boards can demand that chiropractors be adequately trained to provide such education.

Osteopathy is another profession that arose in the 19th century. Andrew Taylor Still, MD, founded the first osteopathic medical college in 1892. Dr. Still had become dissatisfied with medicine as it was practiced in his day. He had served as a surgeon in the Union Army during the Civil War, and three of his children died of meningitis in 1864. (As I explain in chapters 32, 33, and 35, we now have vaccines against the three most common bacterial causes of meningitis.) Those horrible experiences brought Dr. Still to the conclusion that medicine, as it was being practiced then, was often ineffective and sometimes harmful.

Like Palmer, Still believed that using manual adjustment (osteopathic manipulative treatment) to correct structural problems could improve the body's ability to heal itself. Osteopathy has traditionally placed a high emphasis on primary and preventive care.

Unlike chiropractors, doctors of osteopathy (DOs) went on to embrace the new developments in medical science. As medical science has advanced, the differences between medical training and osteopathic training have eroded. Nowadays, some MDs are on the faculty at colleges of osteopathy, and some DOs are on the faculty of medical schools. Many graduates of a college of osteopathy go on to train in medical residencies. Also, the use of osteopathic manipulative treatment has declined. Meanwhile, the discipline of physical therapy has developed.

Naturopathy is another school of alternative medicine that arose in the United States at around the turn of the 20th century. However, it arose largely out of the Nature Cure movement that was popular in Germany. Naturopathy was pioneered by a German immigrant named Benedict Lust. Lust bought the rights to the name *Naturopathy* from a colleague, Dr. John Scheel. Lust had training in homeopathy and osteopathy. He marketed health foods and published material on hydrotherapy, physical fitness, and natural healing in German and in English. He eventually started popularizing elements of traditional Hindu medicine, such as Ayurveda and yoga. In 1900, he founded the American School of Naturopathy in New York City. By the mid 1920s, at least 20 schools of naturopathy existed in the United States.

The luck of the naturopathic profession started to run out in 1908, when the American Medical Association's Council on Medical Education (CME) asked the Carnegie Foundation for the Advancement of Teaching to survey medical education in the United States. The report on the survey was authored by Abraham Flexner. Flexner had just published a critical assessment of college and university education in the United States and Canada. In 1910, Flexner published his report on medical education. It was called the Flexner Report (Carnegie Foundation Bulletin Number 4). In it, Flexner revealed that many of the nation's medical schools were for-profit diploma mills that provided a dangerously substandard education. Flexner recommended that all but 31 of the nation's 155 medical schools should be closed.

Flexner's parents were German immigrants, and Flexner himself had traveled and studied in Europe. Flexner wanted to raise the standards of medical education in the United States to match those that prevailed in Germany and France. The Flexner Report established a new model for medical education in the United States. Medical students were to have at least two years of college-level instruction in science before admission to medical school. The medical school curriculum itself was to consist of two years of training in anatomy and physiology and two years of clinical training in a teaching hospital. The report also recommended that states should strengthen their regulation of medical licensure. Flexner also recommended that the medical schools should appoint full-time clinical professors who would be "true university teachers, barred from all but charity practice, in the interest of teaching." Of course, that recommendation was not followed.

The schools that had been teaching alternative medical theories such as homeopathy and naturopathy could not meet the tough new standards. Many of them closed, and the others lost their ability to grant doctor of medicine (MD) degrees. Osteopaths responded to Flexner's challenge by raising the standards of education in the osteopathic colleges. However, the naturopathic schools could not make such changes without abandoning the philosophy of the Natural Cure movement, which rejected drug and surgical treatment as a matter of principle. Most of the naturopathy schools closed, and the remainder could not grant MD degrees. Instead, they granted ND degrees (naturopathic doctor), which did not qualify the holder for a medical license. However, naturopathy was embraced by many chiropractors. Several schools of chiropractic started offering ND degrees as well as doctor of chiropractic (DC) degrees.

In the 1940s and 1950s, the popularity of naturopathy declined because of the development of "miracle drugs" such as penicillin. As chiropractors succeeded in lobbying state legislatures to expand the chiropractic scope of practice, many chiropractic schools stopped offering ND degrees. In 1968, the U.S. Department of Health, Education and Welfare issued a report on naturopathy. The report concluded that naturopathy was not grounded in science and that naturopathic education did not adequately prepare graduates to diagnose and treat illness. The report recommended against expanding Medicare to cover naturopathic services. As of 2015, only 19 states and the territories of Puerto Rico and the U.S. Virgin Islands have licensing laws for naturopaths.

Today, naturopaths and chiropractors are considered to be alternative practitioners, while osteopaths now have equal standing with medical doctors. This raises the question of how to define alternative medicine. How do you draw the line between what is conventional medicine and what is alternative medicine? Medical doctors and scientists draw the line one way. Sociologists would draw it in yet another way. Economists would draw it in a different way. As I'll explain in the next chapter, healthcare reformers need to understand how these different lines are drawn.

5

What Is Quackery?

Some proponents of alternative medicine insist that vaccination is quackery. At the same time, many critics of alternative medicine insist that alternative medicine is quackery. Is it fair to say that either vaccination or alternative medicine is quackery? Before you answer that question, you must define what you mean by *quackery* and what you mean by *alternative medicine.*

The words *quack* and *quackery* came originally from the word *quacksalver,* which meant someone who sold salves or healing lotions. Thus, the word *quacksalver* came to mean someone who aggressively promotes a medicinal product of questionable value. Many of the quacksalvers of the traveling medicine shows in the United States during the 19th century sold products that supposedly contained snake oil. As a result, quacksalvers are often called snake oil salesmen.

A quack or snake oil salesman can be defined as someone who sells or promotes one or more health-related products or services that are unproven and that lack a scientific rationale. If a health-related product or service is effective and reasonably safe for a given purpose, then it is not quackery to promote it for that purpose. Nor is it quackery for a doctor to offer a treatment that has only a small chance of success, as long as the doctor is honest about the poor odds. In contrast, if a product or treatment is clearly ineffective or simply makes no sense scientifically, then promoting it would be quackery.

Quackery is not the only form of bad medicine. Quackery is a form of fraud. However, other kinds of bad doctoring can also result from ignorance, negligence, or incompetence. Ignorance means a lack of knowledge. For example, doctors can spread infection by failing to wash their hands between patients. Before germ theory was understood, doctors were ignorant of the importance of hand washing. But if doctors fail to wash their hands today, it is considered negligence. Incompetence means lack of skill. A doctor whose skills are poor would best be described as an incompetent, as opposed to a quack.

Quackery is easy to define. It's much harder to define alternative medicine. How you define alternative medicine will depend on your perspective. Scientists, medical doctors, sociologists, economists, and consumers would draw the line between alternative and conventional medicine differently because they are trying to answer different kinds of questions. If you care about your own health and public health, you will pay careful attention to how these lines are drawn.

Scientists and regulatory authorities tend to draw the line between what has been supported by scientific evidence and what has not. In the November 11, 1998, issue of the *Journal of the American Medical Association*, Phil B. Fontarosa, MD, and George Lundberg, MD, wrote, "There is no alternative medicine. There is only scientifically proven, evidence-based medicine supported by solid data or unproven medicine, for which scientific evidence is lacking. Whether a therapeutic practice is 'Eastern' or 'Western,' is unconventional or mainstream, or involves mind-body techniques or molecular genetics is largely irrelevant except for historical purposes and cultural interest." To scientists and members of the Skeptics movement, alternative medicine is a collection of theories and techniques that do not have a scientific basis—that is, they are unproven or have been disproven.

Sociologists might draw the line between conventional medicine and alternative medicine differently because they study social behavior. The term *conventional medicine* implies a social convention. Sociologists ask such questions as who decides what is conventional? What are the conventions? Who defines and enforces them? A sociologist would define conventional medicine as the theories and practices that represent the consensus of the medical profession. However, that is a far different definition than medical scientists use.

Not everything that is conventional is scientifically sound, and not everything that is scientifically sound is conventional. Many of the theories and treatments that were central to medical theory and practice for hundreds or thousands of years were eventually rejected as unscientific. Anyone who promoted 18th-century-style medical treatments would be dismissed as a quack.

Unfortunately, it is easy to mistake unconventional ideas for unscientific ideas. For example, the germ theory of disease was once dismissed as unscientific because it did not emerge from the teachings of Hippocrates and Galen. Even today, some physicians dismiss some ideas as unscientific when they are merely unconventional. The clearest example is the hostility that many physicians express toward purely plant-based (vegan) diets.

While Denis Parsons Burkitt was serving as the Surgeon General of the British colonial government of Uganda, he realized that heart attacks, diabetes, and other degenerative diseases that were common in Britain were practically nonexistent among Africans who were eating a low-fat diet based on unrefined starches and vegetables. Large epidemiologic studies showed similar results in other parts of the world. The evidence from epidemiologic studies, laboratory studies, and clinical studies converges on a simple conclusion: these "Western" diseases are the result of eating an overly rich diet based on animal-source foods and processed foods. Clinical research confirms that these diseases can often be successfully managed by changing to a low-fat, plant-based diet.

Unfortunately, most physicians who were trained in the United States have had little training in nutrition or in epidemiologic research methodology. As a result, many of them quibble about the supposed flaws of the individual studies, rather than looking at the evidence as a whole. Note that the tobacco industry's hirelings used make precisely the same complaints about the supposed flaws of the studies that showed that cigarette smoking causes lung cancer. Fortunately, wisdom eventually prevailed and doctors started urging their patients to quit smoking.

Many medical doctors and medical organizations have discouraged people from adopting a vegan diet, out of fear that plant-based diets would lead to protein or calcium deficiency. Yet that fear is unfounded. In practice, people do not get sick from protein or calcium deficiency on a plant-based diet. It is practically impossible even to design a plant-based diet that would fail to provide enough protein to anyone who is getting enough calories. True dietary deficiencies of calcium are also extremely rare. They happen only among children who are so poor that they are eating practically nothing but unfermented cereal grains. Grains are low in calcium, and unfermented grains contain phytates that bind calcium and prevent it from being absorbed.

The failure of the medical profession to provide adequate dietary counseling is a serious threat to public health. Doctors are missing opportunities to prevent, manage, or even cure diseases that respond well to dietary interventions but respond poorly to any medical or surgical treatment. Because of books such as *The China Study* and documentaries such as *Forks Over Knives*, the public is becoming aware of this problem. This awareness is causing many people to lose faith in doctors. It is also eroding people's faith in their government.

Every five years, the U.S. Department of Agriculture and the Department of Health and Human Services issue dietary guidelines for people in the United States. These guidelines have consistently urged people to eat large amounts of animal-source foods (i.e., meat, fish, eggs, and dairy products). These guidelines are designed to help people avoid the nonexistent problem of protein or calcium deficiency. Unfortunately, those animal-source foods are the major underlying cause of our major causes of death and disability, including heart disease and arthritis. Thus, the recommendations seem to be serving the interests of agribusiness and the food industry, rather than the interests of public health. People who are aware of these flaws in the dietary guidelines may suspect that the vaccine recommendations might be similarly flawed. Yet the vaccination recommendations, like any recommendations, must be evaluated on their own merits. (In chapter 17, I explain how the vaccine recommendations are made).

Antivaccination activists typically claim that the recommended vaccine schedule is designed to line the pockets of the pharmaceutical industry. However, the people who are making those claims generally have no training in infectious disease or public health and no background in history or political science. Thus, they are poorly equipped to answer questions about how or why government policy is made. Nor do they have any background in health economics.

Economists study questions of value, buying, selling, and consuming. Thus, economists are interested in the question of who can sell what to whom. Economists would draw a distinction between the things that you could buy from a supermarket or health food store and the things you can buy only from a pharmacist, and then only with a doctor's prescription. Economists distinguish between the kinds of services that can be provided by absolutely anyone and those that can be provided only by a licensed provider, such as a doctor or surgeon or dentist. To an economist, alternative medicine would be goods and services that you could buy over the counter or from unlicensed vendors or that you could simply do for yourself.

Economists recognize that there are high barriers to entry to the healthcare professions. If you want to practice medicine or dentistry or become a nurse in the United States, you must first get the appropriate license from your state government. However, the state governments will not give you a license unless you have completed a long, difficult, and expensive education and passed some tough examinations.

On the other hand, you might be able to set up some kind of alternative healthcare practice, such as some form of "energy healing," without having any training or license at all. You just have to be careful about how you advertise your services. Otherwise, you could be prosecuted for practicing medicine without a license or for consumer fraud. Thus, to an economist, alternative medicine consists of ways to get around the barriers to entry to the trade in healthcare services.

There are also high barriers to entry to the drug trade in the United States. These barriers serve two purposes. Some barriers are intended to keep people from selling dangerous drugs, such as narcotics, to people who do not need them. Many medications are available only by prescription, while some drugs such as LSD cannot legally be sold at all. Other barriers protect the intellectual property rights of the people who invent new drugs. If other people own the patent for a drug, you have to get their permission before you can sell it.

If you invent a new drug or a new vaccine, the FDA makes you conduct a long and expensive research program to prove that your product is safe and effective for a particular use, before doctors can begin prescribing it in the United States. (The European Medicines Agency has similar requirements for medicines to be marketed in the European Union.) As I'll explain in more detail in chapter 16, this process has become more rigorous over time. Today, the research program to develop a new drug may end up costing hundreds of millions of dollars. Even after all that, the FDA can refuse to approve the drug, if the studies produce disappointing results.

Alternative medicine can also represent ways for quacksalvers to get around the barriers to entry to the drug trade. Since the passage of the Dietary Supplement Health and Education Act of 1994, the FDA has had only limited ability to regulate herbal products and vitamin and mineral products. The result has been an explosion in the marketing of herbal and nutritional products of unproven value and questionable safety.

Of course, there's more to economics than the supply side of the equation. There is also a demand side. For consumers, conventional medicine is what they can get from someone with a license to prescribe drugs and possibly perform some sort of surgery. Examples include medical doctors, nurse practitioners, physician assistants, dentists, podiatrists, optometrists, etc. Alternative medicine is what they could get from some provider who cannot prescribe drugs or perform surgery (a chiropractor, an acupuncturist, a naturopath, etc.) or what they can buy over the counter or do for themselves.

Sometimes, a consumer's belief system influences the consumer's choice of practitioner, such as when Christian Scientists choose a Christian Science practitioner instead of a medical doctor. Other times, the choice of practitioner is driven by personal concerns, such as the reputation or bedside manner of a particular practitioner.

People who have a deep distrust of authority or of established social institutions may prefer alternative health practitioners, including "drugless practitioners," such as naturopaths. Naturopaths say that their "drugless" methods are natural and nontoxic and are therefore safer. Yet their practice is "drugless" and nonsurgical because state laws bar them from using prescription drugs or performing surgery and sometimes even from ordering blood tests. (That's why so many "alternative" practitioners order tests on hair or saliva samples.) So when the "drugless practitioners" say that drugs and vaccines are worthless, it may just be a case of sour grapes. (In one of Aesop's fables, a hungry fox was frustrated that he could not jump high enough to reach some grapes that were hanging on a grapevine. As he walked away, he said to the grapes, "You aren't even ripe yet. I don't need any sour grapes.")

Many practitioners of alternative medicine use or sell products that supposedly have some medicinal effect. However, they have an incentive to bad-mouth the products and services that only their competitors can sell. For that reason, many prominent naturopaths are also prominent in the antivaccine movement.

The word *alternative* suggests substitution. Economists often talk about whether one kind of product or service can be considered a substitute for another. Medical doctors often have to choose from among several available alternatives, each of which is more or less a substitute for the others. For example, if a child has a strep throat, the doctor would have to decide whether to prescribe penicillin or some other antibiotic. In other words, the doctor chooses from among several alternatives. But since all of those alternatives are prescription drugs, none of them would be considered alternative medicine.

Of course, medical doctors often use or recommend something other than a drug or a surgical procedure to deal with a medical problem. Yet by doing so, the doctor is practicing *conservative* medicine, not *alternative* medicine. The choice of whether to use some conservative approach or a more aggressive treatment is based on many considerations, including the likely outcome of each possible approach and the patient's preferences.

The term *alternative medicine* originally meant some substitute for the kind of care that can come only from a medical doctor. The term *complementary medicine* was coined to refer to treatments that were to be used in addition to care from a medical doctor. The term *integrative medicine* was coined to refer to a medical doctor's use of unconventional conservative treatments, in addition to standard medical treatments.

The word *holistic* has also been used to refer to alternative medicine. The word *holistic* is supposed to mean relating to a whole, integrated system instead of dealing with only parts of a system. Sometimes, the word *holistic* is used to describe therapies that deal with the mind or spirit as well as the body. Unfortunately, it has often been used as an excuse for sneaking *pneuma* and other outmoded theories and unproved treatments into medical practice.

As I explained in chapter 4, some of the schools of alternative medicine that are still popular today were created in the 18th or 19th century. Others, such as Ayurvedic medicine and traditional Chinese medicine, purport to be even older. A few systems, such as Reiki, are recent inventions but are supposedly based on some ancient teachings. All of these schools have one important thing in common. They include theories that have not been validated scientifically. The medical profession is not alone in rejecting these theories. The alternative medical theories are also rejected by scientists who do not care about the turf wars between medical doctors and alternative practitioners.

The alternative theories may be unscientific, but they are generally simple to understand. They are far simpler to learn than the organic chemistry, cell biology, statistics, and so on that premed and medical students must learn. Like the ancient and medieval medical theories, the alternative theories fail to provide an accurate picture of what is going on in the human body. The medical profession, to its credit, has generally embraced scientific progress, especially with regard to infectious disease. The alternative practitioners have not.

If a treatment has been shown to be safe and effective, it is likely to be incorporated into conventional medicine, regardless of who came up with the treatment or why. That's how traditional herbal remedies like opium and digitalis were transformed into prescription medicines. Conversely, many treatments that were once the standard of care in medicine were discarded after they were shown to be ineffective, needlessly risky, or simply inferior to some new treatment. So the things that work should get absorbed into conventional medicine. The things that don't work tend to be driven to the fringes.

Since the early 1990s, the U.S. National Center for Complementary and Integrative Health (NCCIH; formerly the National Center for Complementary and Alternative Medicine, NCCAM) has spent more than $1.4 billion on researching and promoting alternative medicine. From the beginning, skeptics complained that the money was being badly spent. They pointed out that if a research study was worth doing, it could get funding from some other part of the National Institutes of Health. They also complained that many of the studies that NCCAM was planning to fund were simply preposterous.

The President of the American Physical Society complained that the Office of Alternative Medicine, which was the forerunner of NCCAM, "has emerged as an undiscriminating advocate of unconventional medicine. It has bestowed the considerable prestige of the NIH on a variety of highly dubious practices, some of which clearly violate basic laws of physics and more clearly resemble witchcraft." Skeptics correctly predicted that practically none of the NCCAM-funded research would prove to be of any real value.

NCCIH could be funding research that would fill in an important gap. NIH funds a lot of research on pure science. The drug companies fund a lot of research on drugs. Unfortunately, we don't have nearly enough clinical research on diet and other conservative approaches to preventing and treating important diseases.

Anyone who has read the epidemiologic literature would know to take a dietary approach to preventing and managing chronic degenerative diseases, such as coronary artery disease, type 2 diabetes, and autoimmune disease. Yet we don't have enough clinical research to persuade medical doctors to focus on nutrition. So they end up using expensive and dangerous drugs and surgery to treat conditions that would actually respond better to proper dietary management.

The NCCIH should be funding the research on dietary management and physical therapy and so on. The results of such research could guide public health efforts and improve the value of the services provided by dietitians and other health professionals, including chiropractors. Thus, NCCIH's funding could be helping us find ways to improve our health while saving money on health care.

Although some advocates of alternative medicine claim that vaccination is quackery, there is actually a large body of research that shows that vaccines are effective and surprisingly safe. Vaccines can even be used to drive some diseases into extinction. Yet you don't need to review the scientific literature to know that vaccines are beneficial. All you need are some history lessons and your own personal observation.

Smallpox was once a major cause of death in the United States. It is now extinct. Polio used to cause epidemics of paralysis among children and young adults. Today, we no longer have pediatric wards filled with children in iron lungs. Diphtheria ranked number 10 among the top causes of death in the United States in 1900, but only a handful of cases have been reported in the United States since 2000. Practically everyone who was born before 1957 has had the measles. Measles is now no longer circulating in the United States. These are facts that should be obvious to the casual observer. So should the role of vaccines in fighting these diseases. Thus, vaccination is not quackery. In contrast, the $1.4 billion that the U.S. government has spent on research into alternative medicine has failed to show that alternative medicine has much of value to offer.

6

Logic, Feelings, and Decisions

The controversy over immunization has been going on in North America since the early 18th century. Benjamin Franklin, who was not only one of the Founding Fathers of the United States but a highly respected scientist, weighed in with this opinion:

> In 1736 I lost one of my sons, a fine boy of four years old, by the smallpox taken in the common way. I long regretted bitterly and still regret that I had not given it to him by inoculation. This I mention for the sake of the parents who omit that operation, on the supposition that they should never forgive themselves if a child died under it; my example showing that the regret may be the same either way, and that, therefore, the safer should be chosen.

Franklin spoke as both a scientist and a grieving father. His argument was based on reason as well as emotion. Unfortunately, few people today succeed in making an appeal to both. The antivaccination activists appeal to people's fears. In contrast, the infectious disease specialists and public health authorities generally make purely rational arguments that are hard for anyone but another scientist to understand. Few scientists know how to talk to the rest of us. Also, few nonscientists have enough training in science to understand what the scientists are saying to each other or how scientists make decisions.

What we have is a failure to communicate. This failure of communication results from a serious problem in education, a problem that I explained in my book *Not Trivial: How Studying the Traditional Liberal Arts Can Set You Free.* In the United States, our educational "experts" have developed teaching methods that slow down the rate at which children learn. Even after 13 years of free public education, most people "don't know much about history, don't know much biology." Many of them cannot even read well enough to understand a newspaper article. The result is widespread ignorance about matters of life and death.

The educational "experts" claim that they want children to develop "higher-order thinking skills." Yet they have deliberately suppressed the kinds of lessons that help children learn to think rationally. The ancient Greeks had worked out a system of education that promotes rational thinking. It consisted of seven subjects: three verbal arts (grammar, logic, and rhetoric) and four arts of number, space, and time (mathematics, geometry, music, and astronomy). Many people are aware of the problems that resulted from the introduction of New Math during the 1960s. However, few people understand the importance of another major change in education policy from the 1960s: the removal of grammar from grammar school.

Grammar is the study of how words are altered and combined to form meaningful sentences. Grammar lessons teach the student to parse, which means to break a sentence down into its parts and to describe what each word is doing in that sentence. After children learn to parse, their reading comprehension improves. Learning a foreign language becomes easier. Children must learn to parse before they can learn to reason. That's why the ancient Greeks taught their sons grammar, then logic. Logic is the study of arguments. Arguments are made up of statements of fact that support a particular conclusion. The study of logic teaches you how to use evidence to draw reasonable conclusions.

To understand scientific arguments, you need to be able to think logically. You must be able to recognize good and bad arguments. A logical argument uses a set of statements of fact (premises) to support a particular conclusion. The premises are like a series of stepping stones that take you to some destination.

There are two basic kinds of logical argument: deductive and inductive. A deductive argument, such as a mathematical proof, is intended to lead you to a conclusion that is unquestionably true. In a valid argument, the conclusion has to be true if the premises are true. A sound argument is a valid argument that has true premises. If an argument is sound, you can be certain that its conclusion is true. Unfortunately, we seldom get that kind of certainty in the life sciences. Often, we have to rely on inductive arguments.

The best that an inductive argument can do is to show that its conclusion is unlikely to be false. For example, a prosecuting attorney's arguments in a criminal case are inductive arguments. The prosecution doesn't have to prove that the defendant is definitely guilty. The prosecution merely has to show that it is unreasonable to believe that the defendant is innocent.

Even the best inductive argument is never valid or sound because the conclusion could still be false. Instead, a good inductive argument is described as strong. We can never know for sure whether Franklin's son would have lived if he'd been inoculated against smallpox. However, one can make a strong argument that the boy's odds of survival would have been much greater with the inoculation than without it.

You can run into two basic problems in logic. One is false premises. If one or more of your stepping-stones are missing or are too slippery to step on, then you cannot use them to reach your conclusion. Unless you find some other route, you might not be able to get to your conclusion at all. Also, your stepping-stones might not take you where you want to go. A conclusion that is not supported by a given set of premises is called a non sequitur, which is Latin for "it does not follow." The conclusion itself could still be true, but the premises do not support it.

By studying logic, you can learn to recognize the kinds of bad arguments that can fool people into accepting false conclusions. These kinds of misleading arguments are called logical fallacies. One common fallacy is called *post hoc ergo propter hoc*, which is Latin for "after it therefore because of it." Many parents are convinced that the measles-mumps-rubella vaccine caused their child's autism because they first noticed the signs of autism after the child got the vaccination. However, that timing is just a coincidence. The signs of autism start to become obvious when the child is 18 months to 2 years of age, regardless of whether the child has been vaccinated. Extensive studies have shown that the vaccination does not increase the child's risk of getting autism.

Post hoc ergo propter hoc is just one the fallacies of questionable cause. Another is the fallacy of the single cause. Many alternative medical theories try to explain all disease in terms of one single cause, so that all sick people can be given the same treatment. For example, D. D. Palmer, the creator of chiropractic, argued that all disease was the result of misalignments of the joints, mainly the joints of the spine. He then argued that chiropractic manipulation would be the proper remedy in all cases.

Scientists do like a theory to be simple yet powerful. Osteopaths, in particular, would have embraced Palmer's theory if the evidence really did support the idea that adjusting the spine could cure anything but a backache. But to be scientific, a theory must account for all of the available evidence. Palmer's chiropractic theory did not. Scientists like a theory to be as simple as possible, but no simpler. The theory has to be complicated enough to account for everything we know.

Another logical fallacy that accounts for a lot of the support for alternative medicine is the appeal to tradition (*argumentum ad antiquitatem*). The appeal to tradition is based on the idea that a theory or practice must be good if it is old or traditional. As I explained in chapter 3, many people are interested in ancient medical traditions. Ayurvedic medicine and traditional Chinese medicine appeal to many people because they believe that those healing systems are thousands of years old. Homeopathy is more than 200 years old. Even some of the recently developed alternative medicine approaches, such as Reiki, are portrayed as being inspired by ancient wisdom.

Of course, scientists shouldn't care at all whether an idea is new or old. Thus, they should reject any appeal to tradition. They should also reject the opposite kind of argument, the appeal to novelty (*argumentum ad novitatem*). Whether an idea is old or new shouldn't matter. All that should matter is the quality of the evidence that supports it.

Young people should be learning the basic skills of logical reasoning in middle school and high school. They should be learning how to tell whether premises are true, whether deductive arguments are valid, and whether inductive arguments are strong. They should learn to recognize errors in reasoning. That's what it means to learn to reason. Once you learn to reason, you can begin to study rhetoric, which is the art of persuasive speech.

The basic principles of rhetoric that were taught in ancient Greece are still important today. The ancient Greek philosopher Aristotle taught that there were three means of persuasion: *logos*, *pathos*, and *ethos*. *Logos* means facts and reason. *Pathos* means feelings. *Ethos* means a person's reputation. To understand science or even just to be a reasonable person, you must understand the proper roles of *logos*, *pathos*, and *ethos* in rhetoric.

When many nonscientists think about scientists, they may imagine a mad scientist alone in his laboratory. Yet scientists spend a lot of time reading each other's work and even just talking with one another. Scientists share their observations with each other; then, they discuss what all of that evidence means. Most scientific discussions deal with matters of fact: what are the facts, and what is the simplest logical explanation for all of those facts?

In discussions of that kind, *logos* is the only thing that is supposed to matter. When you are trying to figure out what is true and what is false, it's best to set your feelings aside. The emotional circuits in the human brain are powerful but primitive. They are practically the same as those in a dog or a cat. These emotional circuits are often powerful enough to override common sense. As a result, people often behave irrationally when their emotions get the better of them.

One of the purposes of education is to teach people how to use reason instead of emotion when sorting out matters of fact. Yet an appeal to emotion is still appropriate in one particular kind of discussion. *Logos* is important for figuring out what is true. But to decide what to *do* about those truths, you must also use your feelings. Philosophers discovered that principle centuries ago, and modern brain research shows that they were right. People who have had an injury to the parts of the brain that process emotion find it hard to make even the simplest decisions, even if they can still do math and logic problems.

Franklin's story about his son illustrates a big problem with emotions and decision-making. Franklin failed to have his son inoculated against smallpox because he was afraid of the 3% risk that the child would die from the inoculation. (Back then, patients were inoculated with pus from someone with a case of genuine smallpox, which was dangerous.) Yet without the inoculation, the child ran a 30% risk of dying if he caught smallpox naturally. Like everyone else who lived in Philadelphia at the time, the child eventually caught smallpox.

Clearly, the safest course of action would have been to inoculate the child. Yet that choice would go against a natural human tendency called inaction bias. Most people would rather do nothing than take even a small risk for an uncertain payoff. Now that most parents in the United States have never seen a case of measles or polio, they have no fear of the vaccine-preventable diseases. Thus, even a small fear of the possible side effects of a vaccine, plus inaction bias, could lead them to shun vaccination.

Nobody knows whether Franklin's son would have survived if he had been inoculated. However, the inoculation would have decreased the child's risk of death by 90%. Looking back, Franklin realized that fear had led him to make an irrational decision—one that he regretted for the rest of his life.

Whenever you use statements of fact to support or justify your beliefs, you are making an argument. Two things can go wrong in that process. Your facts could be wrong and/or there could be something wrong with your reasoning. I've seen antivaccination activists make both kinds of mistake. Often, the mistakes are so outrageous that I have a hard time believing that they are mistakes and not deliberate lies.

I have seen many antivaccination activists claim that measles is a harmless disease and that having measles is actually beneficial to the child. Roald Dahl disagreed:

> Olivia, my eldest daughter, caught measles when she was seven years old. As the illness took its usual course I can remember reading to her often in bed and not feeling particularly alarmed about it. Then one morning, when she was well on the road to recovery, I was sitting on her bed showing her how to fashion little animals out of coloured pipe-cleaners, and when it came to her turn to make one herself, I noticed that her fingers and her mind were not working together and she couldn't do anything. "Are you feeling all right?" I asked her. "I feel all sleepy," she said. In an hour, she was unconscious. In twelve hours she was dead. The measles had turned into a terrible thing called measles encephalitis and there was nothing the doctors could do to save her.

Olivia Dahl died in 1962, just a few years before the measles vaccine was introduced. Yet even today, medical doctors have no effective treatment for measles encephalitis. Nor can they prevent a case of measles from causing deafness, seizures, blindness, or mental retardation. In other words, the antivaccination activists' claim that measles is harmless is utterly false.

Sometimes, the antivaccination activists provide some true statements but then use them in a misleading argument to support false conclusions. For example, many antivaccination activists use scare tactics involving the ingredients and contaminants in vaccines. They imply that since vaccines contain tiny amounts of potentially toxic substances, the vaccines themselves must be toxic. (Thus, they are committing the fallacy of composition.)

The people who claim that vaccines are toxic never seem to have any training in toxicology, which is the study of poisons. They don't seem to understand a fundamental toxicological principle that has been known since the middle ages: *Sola dosis facit venenum* (only the dose makes the poison). For example, ethyl alcohol is the alcohol in alcoholic beverages. However, the effects of drinking a small glass of apple cider with only trace amounts of ethyl alcohol are different from the effects of drinking an entire fifth of whiskey.

In particular, many antivaccination activists point out that many vaccines contain formaldehyde. They argue that since formaldehyde is known to be poisonous, the vaccine must therefore be poisonous. Yes, trace amounts of formaldehyde can be found in some vaccines. However, the human body naturally produces tiny amounts of formaldehyde. The tiny dose of formaldehyde that a child would get from a vaccine is insignificant and is broken down quickly.

In general, the antivaccination activists want you to be terrified of vaccines but to have no fear of the diseases that those vaccines are intended to prevent. They want you to act on that unreasoning fear of the vaccines instead of making a rational decision based on facts and logical arguments. Yet when irrational fears lead people to make bad decisions, children end up dying of preventable diseases, as Benjamin Franklin found to his lasting sorrow.

In this chapter, I've discussed two of the three Aristotelian means of persuasion: *logos* and *pathos*. You need *logos* (facts and logic) to figure out truths. Then, you need your emotions to help you figure out what you want to do about those truths. But what about *ethos*? *Ethos* means character or reputation. Ethos should not matter in a purely scientific discussion, but it is important in practical decision-making.

One of the classical logical fallacies deals directly with *ethos*. It's called the argument from authority (*argumentum ad verecundiam*). An argument from authority has the following form:

> A is an authority figure.
> A says that B is true.
> Therefore, B must be true.

This kind of argument is invalid because it is possible for B to be false even if an authority figure says that B is true. Yet if the authority figure is truly trustworthy, you can use this kind of argument to support the idea that B is unlikely to be false. In other words, the strength of this argument depends on the trustworthiness of the authority figure.

In the next chapter, I'll deal with the question of *ethos*. What is a scientific reputation, and what role does a scientific reputation play in science? Are some people more trustworthy than others are? Why does it make sense to pay more attention to the Professor's opinions about scientific issues than to Ginger Grant's?

7

Why Reputation Matters

Ethos (which means character) should not matter in a scientific discussion. Smart and honest people are sometimes wrong, and fools and liars sometimes say things that are true. If you argue that some idea must be true because some famous authority supports it, you commit a logical fallacy called the appeal to authority (in Latin, *argumentum ad verecundiam*). For centuries, progress in medicine stagnated because the professors of medicine in the European universities refused to accept that Galen could have been wrong about anything. Today, the scientific community and the medical profession are far more interested in evidence than in the opinions of authorities. Individual scientists are not always perfectly reasonable. However, the scientific community as a whole does tend to embrace the theory with the strongest scientific basis. Thus, the opinions of scientists should carry a lot of weight in an inductive argument.

Although an appeal to authority should carry no weight in science, scientists do care about their scientific reputation. If you have a good scientific reputation, it means that other scientists think that you are smart and knowledgeable, that you have done a lot of important work, and that you are honest. Taken together, these things mean that you are a reliable source of information, at least on certain topics. A wise person would therefore listen carefully to what you say.

The first step in developing a scientific reputation is to get an advanced degree, such as a doctor of philosophy degree (PhD), in some field of science—preferably at a university where a lot of important research in that field is being done. You could also get a doctor of medicine (MD) or doctor of osteopathy (DO) degree and then go into research. Then, you must do a lot of important research and get the results published in highly respected scientific journals. Writing some textbooks on your subject also helps.

Scientific publishing companies typically use a process of peer review to decide what to publish. They'll send your manuscript to other experts, usually without telling them who wrote it. Those experts will then review the manuscript and help the editor decide whether it is worth publishing. Often, they provide useful advice to the author. As an editor and writer in medical publishing, I have seen this process first-hand. In contrast, the companies that publish books for a consumer audience may publish whatever they think will sell, even if it is complete nonsense. For example, they will publish diet books written by authors who are clearly overweight. Just because a book is labeled "nonfiction" does not mean that it tells the truth.

Scientists work hard to earn a good scientific reputation. Without it, they will never get on the tenure track at a major university. Nor will they be able to get funding to support their research. Scientists with a good reputation might also be paid to serve as expert witnesses in court cases.

When businessmen or -women compile their résumé, their credentials and experience can usually fit on one or two sheets of paper. Instead of compiling a brief résumé, scientists compile an extensive document called a curriculum vitae (CV), which means "course of life" in Latin. A scientist's CV is usually many pages long. It describes the scientist's education and work experience, which often includes teaching jobs at colleges and universities as well as research projects. It also includes a list of all of his or her scientific publications and patents. A CV tells you what kinds of work that scientist has done. That information can be important. Often, even scientists know very little outside of their narrow field of expertise.

Nowadays, I can often find a scientist's CV on the Internet. If I cannot find his or her CV, I can search a citation database such as MEDLINE to see what kinds of publications the person has to his or her credit. MEDLINE is a database maintained by the U.S. National Library of Medicine. It contains many millions of citations of journal articles, mainly about medicine and the related life sciences. You can access MEDLINE yourself for free through Pubmed: www.pubmed.com.

I took some courses on statistics and research design in college. I have worked in medical and veterinary publishing for many years. Thus, I have read or edited a lot of textbooks and journal articles about many different aspects of medicine. I have also written research protocols and clinical study reports. Often, I see or hear someone who claims to have an MD or DO or PhD degree spouting what seems to me to be ridiculous nonsense about some aspect of medicine or nutrition. Many of these people talk about the "protocols" of the research they are supposedly performing. Yet when I look them up in MEDLINE, I invariably find that they have few if any publications to their name and usually no publications on the relevant subject. In other words, none of their "research" has passed muster at any of the journals indexed in MEDLINE. It makes me doubt that they are involved in any real research at all. Even I have a few articles indexed in MEDLINE, and I'm just a science writer, not a researcher.

Researchers normally try to publish their work. If they cannot get their early work published, then they won't be able to get funding for their later work. In other words, people who claim to be scientists but have no publication history are probably phonies. They may fool the public, but they generally cannot fool the scientific community and they shouldn't fool a competent journalist.

Of course, even people who have the highest scientific credentials can sometimes go off the deep end. This happens so often to Nobel laureates that people have started making wry comments about "the

Nobel disease." For example, William Shockley won a Nobel Prize in Physics for inventing the transistor, but his views on genetics were a load of racist nonsense. Nikolaas Tinbergen shared the 1973 Nobel Prize in Physiology or Medicine for his work on animal behavior. Yet even in his Nobel acceptance speech, he said a lot of nonsense about autism.

Luc Montagnier is a virologist who shared the 2008 Nobel Prize in Physiology or Medicine for discovering HIV, the virus that causes AIDS. Since then, Montagnier has been promoting wacky theories about the electromagnetic waves that he thinks are being emitted by DNA. Montagnier has also embraced views that support homeopathy and oppose vaccination. He has gone so far off into left field that a group of 35 Nobel laureates wrote to the government of Cameroon, begging them not to put him in charge of their AIDS research center.

Eccentricity has always been tolerated in the scientific community. In fact, truly brilliant mathematicians and physicists are expected to be a bit peculiar. Although eccentricity is tolerated in the scientific community, dishonesty is not. The fastest way for a scientist to destroy his or her career is to be caught lying about his or her research.

If you get caught submitting false data to the FDA, lying to FDA investigators, paying or accepting bribes, or selling samples of prescription drugs, the FDA can bar you from the pharmaceutical industry for life. Likewise, if you are caught committing crimes or making false claims or otherwise betraying the public trust, the National Institutes of Health can bar you from working on any project that receives NIH funding. When physicians misbehave, the state governments can take away their license to practice medicine.

The need to preserve one's scientific reputation and perhaps one's professional license helps to enforce a code of honesty among scientists and physicians. As a result, scientific mistakes are fairly common but scientific misconduct is rare. For example, only about 3 out of every 10,000 articles published in scientific journals are retracted.

The FDA monitors everything that pharmaceutical companies say about the products they sell. If the company says anything that does not meet the FDA's strict standards for truth and fairness, the company may get a warning letter from the FDA. You can read these warning letters on the FDA's Web site. Pharmaceutical executives take an FDA warning letter seriously. If they do not heed that warning, the product could be recalled or seized, the company may lose its permission to sell the product, the company could be fined, and its executives could even face criminal charges.

In contrast, few of the people who are involved in the antivaccination movement have a scientific reputation or a medical license. Nor does anything bad happen to them if they are caught lying. For example, they can make false claims about their services. The FDA does try to restrict what they say about the dietary supplements they sell. However, the FDA does not punish them for telling lies about drugs or vaccines. (In contrast, the FDA would punish a pharmaceutical company for making false statements about its competitors' products.) Since there are no consequences for lying, antivaccination rhetoric is filled with silly mistakes and outrageous lies. Sometimes, this nonsense is financially motivated, such as when people try to build a phony legal case against vaccine manufacturers or try to sell some sort of alternative treatment (see chapter 18). Yet I think much of the antivaccination rhetoric is sincere, but misguided.

Several years ago, I caught someone in a lie. At first, I felt anger and disgust over what I felt was a betrayal. However, my sister, who is a field biologist, gave me a different perspective on the problem. She pointed out that the person in question had no science education. My scientist sister explained, "People like that sometimes aren't data people. They don't lie, exactly. They just don't think that facts or logic matter."

At that point, I realized something that the ancient Greeks knew 2400 years ago. People who have never been taught how to use facts and logic to solve problems are profoundly disabled socially. They cannot deal with truth. They can deal only in "truthiness," a term coined by comedian and political satirist Stephen Colbert and listed as the Merriam-Webster's #1 word of the year for 2006. With tongue firmly in cheek, Colbert defined truthiness as "truth that comes from the gut, not books." The American Dialect Society defined it as "the quality of preferring concepts or facts one wishes to be true, rather than concepts or facts known to be true."

On his television show, Stephen Colbert played the role of an ignorant and egotistical right-wing pundit. In real life, however, he is wise and thoughtful. In an interview with the Onion's A.V. Club, Colbert explained:

> Truthiness is tearing apart our country, and I don't mean the argument over who came up with the word... It used to be, everyone was entitled to their own opinion, but not their own facts. But that's not the case anymore. Facts matter not at all.... Truthiness is "What I say is right, and [nothing] anyone else says could possibly be true." It's not only that I *feel* it to be true, but that *I* feel it to be true. There's not only an emotional quality, but there's a selfish quality.

If facts and logic do not matter to you, then you cannot be honest. If you feel that whatever you believe must therefore be true, and that anyone who disagrees with you must therefore be an idiot, then you cannot base your interpersonal relationships on mutual respect. Nor will you learn anything from listening to other people. Instead, stubbornness becomes valued as a way to struggle for position within a dominance hierarchy. It's a baboon mentality.

In ancient Greece and Rome, the sons of aristocrats were given an education that was designed to help them become rational human beings and functioning members of civil society. Central to that education were the seven liberal arts: grammar, logic, rhetoric, mathematics, geometry, music, and astronomy. The liberal arts were called the liberal arts because they were considered appropriate for freeborn men, as opposed to slaves. The word *civility*, which we now use to mean politeness, originally meant training in the liberal arts and the humanities, including philosophy. Before one can take part in productive conversations about matters of life and death, one must learn how to use facts and logic to find truth.

In the early 20th century, John Dewey, who was supposedly our foremost philosopher of education, dismissed the importance of learning facts and truths in school. Dewey even thought that it didn't matter if a child failed to learn to read in primary school. Instead, Dewey spoke about "social success." It should therefore come as no surprise that the people whose education was shaped by Dewey's ideas should come to fear and despise the smartest, best-informed, and most honest members of our society, while showering attention and praise upon celebrities, even upon the ones who are fools and charlatans.

It's easy to be biased against scientists if you learned nothing about the scientific method in school. Unfortunately, an extreme form of anti-science bias is being spread by some humanities departments in colleges and graduate schools. As physicist Alan Sokal has explained, the postmodernist movement has spread a bizarre form of extreme skepticism about science. Many postmodernists seem to suggest that all truth is relative to the observer. It's as if they see no difference between what *is* true and what someone *thinks* is true. For example, Samuel Hahnemann presumably believed in homeopathy. So a postmodernist would consider homeopathy to be "true" for Hahnemann. Likewise, Louis Pasteur believed in germ theory, so germ theory would be "true" for Pasteur. Thus, both theories would be equally "true." Many postmodernists pretend that they do not believe that there is any reliable way to decide whether either Hahnemann's theory or Pasteur's actually provides an accurate description of the real world. Yet even a casual observer cannot avoid noticing that Pasteur's theory led to the development of techniques (pasteurization) and products (vaccines and eventually antibiotics and antivirals) that have saved millions of lives, while Hahnemann's homeopathic products have not saved any lives at all.

Many postmodernists assume, quite cynically, that scientists simply choose whatever theory serves their personal needs, without regard to whether the theory makes sense and is supported by evidence. These postmodernists assume that all scientific theories are simply "narratives" intended to serve as ways to oppress other people, rather than being attempts to explain natural phenomena or to solve practical problems. Thus, these postmodernists would tend to be highly critical of any theory or technology that is promoted by any powerful person. At the same time, postmodernists can be overly sympathetic to theories that have been rejected by the scientific community. Thus, pseudoscience and primitive superstitions are given greater weight than the best-supported scientific theories. To use a *Gilligan's Island* metaphor, postmodernists would pay more attention to the witch doctor than to the Professor because they assume that the Professor has no special knowledge and is probably just a servant of Thurston Howell, III. Of course, it is far easier to dismiss the Professor as a tool of capitalism than to understand what the Professor is saying.

Postmodernist ideology poses a serious threat to public health, especially in poor countries. Postmodernist contempt for science and modern medicine provides an excuse for depriving poor people of the benefits of vaccines and antibiotics and even clean drinking water. While the rich can fly to the world's best hospitals to enjoy the best that medical science has to offer, "traditional healing" is presumably good enough for poor people in poor countries. To a postmodernist, the suggestion that the rich countries should lead and finance efforts to vaccinate all the children in poor countries against measles and other deadly diseases would be "imperialist." If there's no reason to believe that scientific medicine has anything of real value to offer, then there's no moral obligation to make those benefits available to everyone. As a result, this disregard for science allows postmodernist leftists to support exactly the same health policies as racist social Darwinists, who actually want to see high death rates among poor nonwhites.

Traditionally, leftists have been the people who want everyone, including poor people's children, to get modern medical care, including vaccination. Shortly after the Cuban Revolution, the Cuban government launched a mass vaccination campaign against polio. Even today, Cuba has an extensive vaccination program and remarkably low rates of vaccine-preventable disease. Since the Cuban Revolution, Cuba has sent tens of thousands of medical doctors to various countries in Latin America, Africa, and Oceania. Cuba's medical missions have used modern medicine to serve an explicitly anti-imperialist political agenda. Yet when I offered the Cuban vaccination campaign and medical missions as evidence that vaccination is not necessarily a capitalist, imperialist plot, one supposedly leftist antivaccination zealot told me that I am an idiot for not realizing that Cuba under Fidel Castro was a capitalist country.

The failure of our education system to teach facts about science and history and to help people develop basic skills in reasoning explains why we are having ugly, pointless debates about vaccination. In the next chapter, I will explain why debates are pointless. I will also describe the kinds of conversations that could actually help us make good decisions.

8

Why Our Debates Are Unproductive

Freedom of speech is guaranteed by the Bill of Rights that was appended to the U.S. Constitution. In fact, the Founding Fathers thought that freedom of speech is so important that they put it at the very top of the Bill of Rights. Most of us in the United States have been indoctrinated with the idea that open debate allows good ideas to outcompete bad ideas in the marketplace of ideas. Yet few of us have ever studied economics. Thus, most Americans have never heard the term *market failure.* Economists know that markets are not always the most practical or ethical way to distribute goods and services. After all, we have outlawed the slave trade, and we don't allow just anyone to buy and sell morphine. Nor is the type of debate that has become commonplace in our society likely to help us solve scientific problems or social conflicts.

I've mentioned that discussions can serve two important purposes: to decide what is true and to decide what to do. To get a better understanding of these discussions, it also helps to understand the different kinds of discourse.

The word *discourse* originally meant the ability to have orderly thought. Today, it can mean either an exchange of ideas, as in a conversation, or a formal and orderly and usually extended expression of thought about a subject. There are several different kinds of discourse. Four of them are important here: polemic, debate, negotiation, and dialectic. Unfortunately, in discussions about vaccination, there's plenty of polemic, debate, and negotiation but practically no dialectic, outside of scientific circles.

A polemic is an attack on someone else's ideas. A polemic is not necessarily unfair, but it is one-sided. Therefore, it should not necessarily be taken at face value. When the person whose ideas are being attacked gets a chance to reply, you have a debate. A debate is a competition in which two or more people attack each other's ideas. The participants in a debate are expected to stick to their starting position from beginning to end. They are not supposed to persuade each other or to learn from each other. They make no attempt to find common ground or to work out their differences. Instead, they are supposed to persuade somebody else to take their side.

Americans are exposed to plenty of polemics, especially in church. They also hear a lot of polemics over the airwaves. Many people are taught, as part of their religious training, that they have miraculously stumbled upon the One True Faith. They have been urged to promote their One True Faith by any means necessary, even by lying. In theology, that sort of lie is called a pious fiction. Thus, many people learn an ugly and unproductive style of conversation in which there are no rules and in which facts do not matter. In particular, impolite people use such ugly debating tactics when they try to dominate people who are better educated than they are. Such conversations are not only ugly, they are pointless.

Court cases are essentially debates. The lawyers for each side are supposed to serve their client's position from beginning to end. The lawyers for the opposing sides do not try to persuade each other. Instead, they try to persuade the jury, while the judge enforces rules that are intended to promote fairness. In high schools and colleges, debate is also a competitive team sport. Each team tries to impress a judge with the quality of their arguments. Political debates are also part of a competition. The candidates compete to win votes in the upcoming election. They do not try to persuade each other. They certainly are not trying to find truth.

Many Americans seem to enjoy "debating." Unfortunately, there is no impartial judge to enforce basic rules of sportsmanship and to decide who wins. As a result, people tend to hammer away at each other with their talking points in the most uncivilized way, until one of the participants gets tired or quits in disgust. Nobody learns anything, and no problems are solved.

Many people have no idea that civilized people follow certain kinds of rules in a discussion. The statements that you offer to support your ideas should be true. Also, these statements should be put together in coherent arguments that obey the rules of logic. When someone else points out your mistakes, you should accept the correction. In other words, you ought to be honest and reasonable. Instead, many people have been trained to stick to their conclusion, regardless of the facts. Rather than adjusting their conclusion to fit the evidence, they may make up whatever "evidence" they need to fit their conclusion.

Even the debates that involve rules and a judge are not much better. Debaters and law students learn to follow certain rules. However, they also learn to twist those rules to serve a particular cause or client. The purpose is advocacy for its own sake, not the pursuit of truth and justice.

The polemicist and the debater are trying to neutralize an opponent. They are not necessarily trying to bring the opponent over to their side, and they are not trying to find areas of agreement. In contrast, the purpose of a negotiation is to reach an agreement about what is to be done. Sometimes, the negotiation is just haggling over a price. Often, more is at stake, such as when representatives from labor and management negotiate about working conditions or when diplomats negotiate a peace treaty.

The goal of a negotiation is to work out a deal that everyone involved will accept. However, the deal might not be ideal for any of the negotiators. As Mick Jagger explained, "You can't always get what you want. But if you try sometime, you'll find, you'll get what you need." Of course, some people feel that they are entitled to get their own way, 100% of the time. If anyone suggests that they give up anything, they react with scorn. To them, compromise is a dirty word. They want to fulfill all of their own desires. To hell with everyone else.

A sales pitch is the opening move in a negotiation. Much of the rhetoric about health care is really just a sales pitch in disguise. The alternative medicine entrepreneurs want to sell goods such as dietary supplements or services such as coffee enemas. The American Medical Association also makes sales pitches. It has worked aggressively to promote the services of medical doctors as opposed to other providers, such as midwives. For years, it tried unsuccessfully to drive chiropractors out of business. Of course, the pharmaceutical companies want you to see your doctor and ask about their products.

At least the pharmaceutical ads are regulated. If a pharmaceutical company says something false or misleading in a drug ad, the FDA may send them a warning letter. The warning is not an empty threat. If the company doesn't mend its ways, the FDA can make it impossible for the company to do business. The executives could even end up in prison.

Pharmaceutical executives live in fear of getting a warning letter. They particularly want to avoid ending up on the debarment list, which is a list of people who are not allowed to work in the pharmaceutical industry in the United States. Each time a drug company applies for approval of a drug, it must give the FDA a signed statement that no debarred people worked on that application. A drug company that illegally hires a debarred person, even as a consultant, can be fined up to $1 million. A debarred person who is caught working for a pharmaceutical company can be fined $250,000.

Many people distrust pharmaceutical companies because they know that pharmaceutical companies make money from selling pharmaceutical products. Yet for many people, this circle of distrust has expanded to include everyone who works at the FDA and the entire medical profession. Some people go so far as to distrust everyone who is related in any way to the scientific community, out of the fear that all scientists have been corrupted by the pharmaceutical industry. Yet the people who fear all scientists never seem to question the motives of the alternative medicine entrepreneurs, some of whom make millions from selling overpriced or even worthless and potentially dangerous goods. It's an oddly selective form of paranoia.

It would be foolish to reject a cure for a deadly disease, simply because someone is selling it in order to make a profit. Many potential new treatments are discovered through research that is funded by government grants or by charities. However, pharmaceutical companies do many of the big clinical trials that must be done before a new drug can be made available to the public. In 2014, the Tufts Center for the Study of Drug Development estimated that the average out-of-pocket costs for developing a new prescription drug averaged $1.4 billion. The time cost of that money (the return that investors could have made if they had invested that money elsewhere) was about $1.2 billion. This average cost per approved drug is so high partly because so many drugs fail to make it to market. The costs for the additional research that the FDA demands as a condition of approval averaged $312 million per drug. Once the drug is approved, the investors want to recoup their investment and make a profit.

Many Americans have been indoctrinated to believe that all of society's problems are likely to be solved by for-profit businesses through the "magic of the marketplace." Because of this indoctrination, many conservatives have come to believe that the government is the enemy of business and by extension the enemy of the people. In contrast, many liberals have developed the fear that the government is the puppet of the corporations and does nothing to protect the public against profit-hungry corporations. For these doctrinaire conservatives and liberals, any discussion about the pharmaceutical industry is as an opportunity to establish how strongly conservative or liberal they are. Thus, they view political discussions as a way of expressing their self-concept, rather than as an opportunity to develop a consensus on practical solutions to real problems, such as what is the best way to preserve health and care for the sick. As a result, they cannot play a productive role in democratic discussions about healthcare policy. What should healthcare cost, and who should pay for it? These are serious questions and should be answered through some political consensus.

Pharmaceutical companies are for-profit businesses. They exist to provide a return on investment for their shareholders. They do that mainly by selling pharmaceuticals. Often, they have to invest a lot of money in research before they can sell a drug. Once that drug is approved, it's understandable that the people who run the corporation would want to make as much money on that drug as possible.

The public often does benefit from the products that pharmaceutical companies bring to market. However, pharmaceutical companies are not public health agencies. Nor are they social welfare agencies. Because the pharmaceutical company's interests sometimes conflict with the public's interests, the pharmaceutical industry has become increasingly regulated. The goal of these regulations is to protect the public. It would be silly to imagine that these rules are unnecessary. It would be equally silly to deny that these rules exist or to insist that they have no real effect. The important question for public health activists to address is how those rules should be written and enforced. How can we protect public safety without stifling innovation or unduly delaying the introduction of important new drugs?

Our system of regulation for the pharmaceutical industry has been built in response to tragedies and scandals. Unfortunately, people often remember the scandal or tragedy, while paying little attention to the reforms that were made in response to it. After a tragedy or scandal comes to light, the FDA and its counterparts in other countries issue new regulations to prevent similar things from happening in the future. As a result of these developments, pharmaceutical companies are now required to report all of the research they conduct, the FDA is getting better at spotting evidence that a drug may be causing a rare but serious side effect, and some of the worst excesses of the pharmaceutical sales force have been reined in. A trade group called the Pharmaceutical Research and Manufacturers of America (PhRMA) has also established a code of conduct for how its member companies may interact with doctors. For example, the PHRMA guidelines now prohibit drug companies from giving doctors tickets to sporting events.

Few people outside of the pharmaceutical industry understand how much stricter the regulatory environment has become since 1990. Nor do most people seem to realize that none of the tragedies and scandals in recent years have involved vaccine safety or the promotion of vaccines. That's because public health concerns, rather than the profit motive, drive vaccine development.

In the United States, the development of vaccines is driven largely by the National Institutes of Health and the Centers for Disease Control and Prevention. Vaccines are intended to solve public health problems, not to generate profits (even though for-profit companies manufacture and distribute the vaccines). As I'll discuss in more detail in chapter 16, vaccines have to meet much higher safety standards than do other medicinal products. That's because vaccines are recommended for nearly everyone, especially children, and because they are intended to keep healthy people healthy.

Even if the idea for a vaccine comes from a government scientist, the government generally has to involve at least one drug company in the development and production of the final product. It is difficult and expensive to follow the FDA's Good Manufacturing Practices for making a vaccine. Thus, it is generally better to have a private concern, whether for-profit or nonprofit, produce the vaccine under government supervision than to have the government produce it, while supervising itself.

Many people distrust any study that was done by a pharmaceutical company. But anyone who has read about the pharmaceutical industry in the business press knows that studies don't necessarily turn out the way a company wants. Nor does the FDA always do what even a big company wants it to do. Sometimes, the FDA even forces companies to take highly profitable drugs off the market.

The FDA decides what drugs can be sold in the United States, and even what sales pitches a drug company can make. To get approval from the FDA to sell a drug product for the treatment of a particular disease, or even to give a new drug to human beings in a clinical trial, you have to do a lot of research and report all of the results to the FDA. The FDA doesn't have enough staff to audit all of the data in every drug application. However, the FDA does punish people who are caught falsifying their reports or leaving out important information.

For many years, the FDA has required drug companies to do clinical studies of the drugs that they hope to sell. However, the companies did not always have to make all of those results available to the medical profession or to the public. As a result, drug companies tended to publish only the studies with positive results. (To be fair, it would be hard to find a journal that would publish negative results.) Now, drug companies have to publish the results of all of their clinical trials. You can read about those trials on a Web site: www.clinicaltrials.gov.

There are still some big problems in how drugs are evaluated in the United States. The main problem is that the research doesn't always make valid comparisons or look at relevant outcomes. Most of our major causes of death and disability in the United States today are related to an overly rich diet, smoking, and alcohol abuse. The solution to those problems is to eat better, stop smoking, and cut way back on the booze. If a disorder such as atherosclerosis or type 2 diabetes can be reversed by diet, why isn't a drug for those conditions being compared to the best possible diet therapy? Why don't all of the subjects have to try proper dietary management first, before receiving a potentially dangerous drug?

How can you decide whom to trust, when so many people are trying to sell you something? The solution to this problem is to follow a basic, commonsense principle that was spelled out in *Robert's Rules of Order*, which is the standard rulebook that Americans have long used when discussing things in public gatherings. Consider this passage from *Robert's Rules*, under the section Decorum in Debate: "It is not allowable to arraign the motives of a member, but the nature or consequences of a measure may be condemned in strong terms. It is not the man, but the measure, that is the subject of debate." In other words, you base your judgments on the facts, not on your suspicions about people's motives. You should apply *logos* and then *pathos*, not *ethos*, in making your decisions.

Many Americans seem to have lost faith in medical researchers. They know that some research is done by for-profit companies who want to sell a product. Thus, the results of their research should be taken with a grain of salt. However, it is often possible to detect when people have faked their research results. The old-fashioned way is have someone else repeat the study and see if they get different results. Thus, the FDA generally requires two independent clinical trials for approval of a new drug or a new indication for an existing drug. Pharmaceutical companies now hire compliance auditors to make sure that the company's investigators are following all of the rules for the conduct of the studies and the reporting of results.

The purpose of polemics and debate is to win in some competition. The purpose of negotiation is to get the best possible deal for yourself or for your client. In contrast, the purpose of dialectic is to search for truth. In dialectic, people share their observations and opinions so that they can work out a better understanding together. It's not about ego, so nobody loses. Dialectic is a teaching and learning experience in which everyone wins. Dialectic enables people to work together to achieve greater understanding than anyone would have achieved independently. The classic example of this process involved the discussions about the nature of light.

The ancient Greek philosopher Aristotle thought that light is a disturbance that travels through the air. Thus, light is a wave phenomenon, like the ripples that travel on the surface of a pond. Another ancient Greek philosopher, Democritus, thought that light is a stream of particles. For nearly two and a half millennia, individual philosophers and scientists took one side or the other in that debate. Then, in the 20th century, scientists learned enough about the behavior of light that they could work out a theory that would explain why light sometimes behaves like a wave and sometimes behaves like a stream of particles. This particle-wave duality is central to modern physics.

The particle-wave duality is important for microbiologists because it led to the development of the electron microscope, which allows for much greater magnification than a light microscope. Thanks to the electron microscope, we can actually see viruses.

I do often see dialectic about vaccines and vaccination, but only within scientific circles. Public health authorities care very much about the safety of vaccines, and they try to design vaccination schedules to bring about the best results in terms of public health. That's why the CDC stopped recommending routine smallpox vaccinations for children in the United States in 1972, several years before smallpox became extinct. At that point, public health experts had stopped trying for universal coverage with the smallpox vaccine. Instead, they were using a "ring vaccination" strategy, which meant vaccinating everyone in the area surrounding a known outbreak. As soon as scientists are certain that polio is extinct, they'll call for an end to polio vaccination. The same goes for vaccines for other eradicable diseases, such as measles, mumps, and rubella.

Nowadays, you'll rarely find real dialectic outside of scientific circles. Most of the discourse that I see about alternative medicine and vaccination is actually either polemics or a form of negotiation. The participants are either attacking their real or imagined enemies or trying to sell you something. Often, people do both at the same time. Neither polemics nor negotiation is inherently bad. I see nothing wrong with criticizing the real shortcomings of our healthcare system. I wrote a book about how the medical profession should be managing diabetes. Nor do I think that it is inherently bad for people to try to sell goods and services, as long as those goods and services have real value and are promoted honestly. What matters is whether you are seeking the truth and serving justice. If your cause is just, truth will serve it.

Part II

The Biology of Infectious Disease

Before I discuss any particular vaccine-preventable diseases, I need to explain some basic facts about germs and the immune system. Some of the vaccine-preventable diseases are caused by bacteria. Others are caused by viruses. In the next few chapters, I'll explain what bacteria and viruses are, how they make you sick, how your immune system tries to fight infections, and what other kinds of treatments can be used against them.

Vaccines are developed against the diseases that pose the biggest threats to public health. A relatively mild disease can be a public health problem if it is common. A rare disease can be a public health concern if it is severe. Vaccines are used to prevent the diseases that are likely to cause suffering, disability, disfigurement, and even death to people within a given population and that typically respond poorly to any available treatment. There is no way to cure the blindness, deafness, or mental retardation that can result from measles. Nor is there any way to regrow the hands and feet that can be lost because of a meningococcal infection. That's why public health authorities become so concerned when people refuse to vaccinate their children against those diseases.

Public health authorities use statistics to express the size of the threat that these diseases pose to public health. In chapter 15, I'll talk about some of the math that you will need to know if you want to get involved in discussions about vaccination policy.

The chapters in this part contain some highly technical information. I won't be offended if you just skim them at first. But if you want to make a productive contribution to discussions about vaccination and public health, you really need to know this material.

9

What Are Bacteria?

Bacteria are the smallest living things. They are also the most adaptable. In the movie *Jurassic Park*, one of the scientist characters explained that "life finds a way." The forms of life that are the most likely to find a way to survive are bacteria. Some species of bacteria have found ways to live inside glaciers. Others have found ways to live in volcanic hot springs that are as caustic as battery acid and are hot enough to blister your skin. Thriving colonies of still other bacteria have been found in high-level nuclear waste. Of course, there are also many bacteria living in much more comfortable places, such as on and in our bodies.

Bacteria are so adaptable because they can evolve far more quickly than we can. Any of the cells of a person's body could get a useful mutation. However, the mutation cannot be handed down to that person's children unless it is in the cells that give rise to the sperm or egg cells. Even then, it would take many years for a baby who inherits that useful mutation to reproduce. In contrast, any bacterium that gets a useful mutation can divide. Some bacteria divide as quickly as once every 20 minutes, if the conditions are right. Thus, you can end up with a huge population of those mutant bacteria within 24 hours.

Some bacteria can even share their genes with other bacteria, even with bacteria from an unrelated species. As a result, bacteria have developed ways to adapt to practically any environment. The human body is one of those environments.

Every human body has trillions of bacteria living on its inner and outer surfaces, especially inside the intestines. Most of those bacteria are harmless to a living person. Some are even useful. Some help us digest our food. Others produce vitamins that we need to survive.

Scientists are starting to discover how important these normal bacteria are to human health. For example, some good bacteria can help to protect us from bad bacteria. People whose gut bacteria have been wiped out by antibiotics can end up with a serious *Clostridium difficile* infection of the intestine. One effective way of treating this problem is to give the person a dose of gut bacteria from a healthy person. This procedure is called a fecal transplant.

To understand what bacteria are, you need to know a little about how biologists classify living things. This kind of classification is called taxonomy. For most of human history, no one had any idea that bacteria even existed. They could study only those living things that were large enough to be seen with the naked eye. When scientists first started classifying things, they started out by sorting everything into two categories: living and nonliving. Living things can grow, develop, and reproduce themselves. Nonliving things cannot.

Early scientists divided all living things into two categories: animals and plants. Animals were animated. They could move around under their own power. Plants stayed planted. Seaweeds might get tossed around by the waves, but they do not swim. After the invention of the microscope, scientists also tried to classify all microscopic living things as either animals or plants. The most obvious difference was in the structure of their cells.

In the 1830s, German scientists realized that all living things are made up of small units called cells. A bacterium, which is the smallest living thing, consists of one single tiny cell. The plants and animals and fungi that are big enough to be seen with the naked eye are made up of collections of many large cells.

By the 1850s, scientists realized that all cells are the descendants of other living cells, which reproduce by splitting in two. For example, all of the cells in your body are the direct descendants of a single fertilized egg, which then split numerous times. Likewise, all bacteria are the descendants of other bacteria.

In a plant, each cell is surrounded by a fibrous shell called a cell wall. In contrast, no animal cells have a cell wall (Figure 4). Fungi and bacteria also have cell walls, so at first it made sense to classify fungi and bacteria as plants. Yet when you look at the structure and chemistry of the cell walls, it becomes clear that plant cell walls are completely different from fungal cell walls, and both the plant and fungal cell walls are completely different from bacterial cell walls.

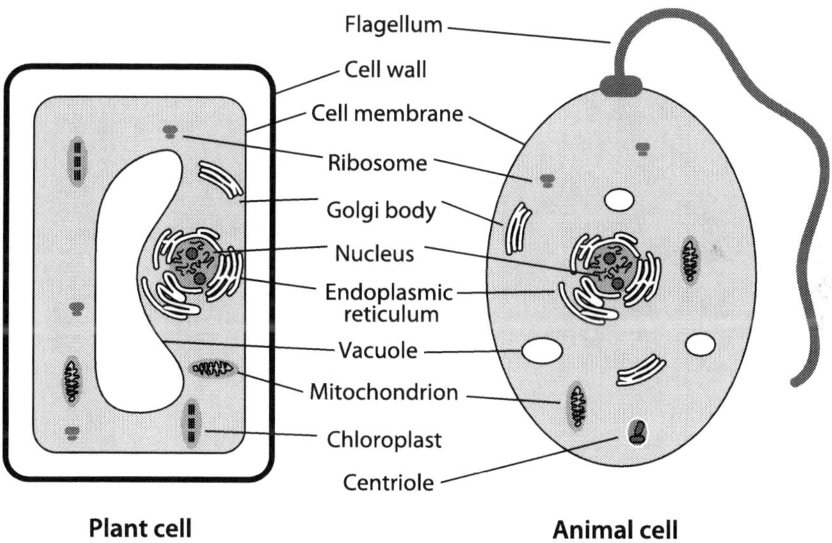

Figure 4. The cells of plants, animals, and fungi are relatively large and complex. Note that animal cells do not have a cell wall or chloroplasts. The cells of bacteria are small and simple. The flagella that are found on some animal cells and on the reproductive cells of plants are structurally different from the flagella found on bacteria.

The cells of animals, plants, and fungi differ from bacteria in an important way. When you look at the cells of an animal, plant, or fungus through an ordinary microscope, you can usually see a single big dot inside. That dot is called the nucleus, which is the Latin word for kernel. The nucleus contains chromosomes, which contain the cell's genes. The DNA is a long molecule. In the chromosomes of plants and animals, the DNA is twisted around spools made out of small proteins called histones.

Most of the cells in your body contain exactly one nucleus. Some kinds of cells, such as liver cells and some cancer cells, have more than one nucleus. Red blood cells start off with a nucleus, but their nucleus disappears as they mature.

All of the organisms that have a proper nucleus in their cells—animals, plants, and fungi, plus lots of single-celled organisms—have now been lumped together in a group called the Eukarya, which comes from the Greek for "having a good kernel." The single-celled organisms that never have a proper nucleus are called prokaryotes ("before having a kernel") because prokaryotes appeared before eukaryotes.

All eukaryotes have some important things in common. Each of their cells has internal membranes that divide its interior into separate compartments. In contrast, the interior of a prokaryote cell is just one open compartment. In other words, a eukaryote cell is like a sprawling mansion with many rooms, while a prokaryote cell is like a small, one-room cabin. Like eukaryotes, the prokaryotes have genes in the form of DNA. However, the prokaryote DNA is not packaged in chromosomes.

Prokaryotes may look simple, but they are incredibly diverse. As you can see from Figure 5, most of the varieties of living things are really prokaryotes. As microbiology advanced, many scientists started to believe that the most important division among living things was not between animals and plants. It was between two different kinds of prokaryote. The eukaryotes—animals, plants, fungi, etc.—are really just an offshoot of a strange group of prokaryotes called archaea.

The archaea have something important in common with the eukaryotes: the histones associated with their DNA. Although the archaea don't really have proper chromosomes like those you'd find in an animal cell or plant cell, they do have some histones bound to their DNA.

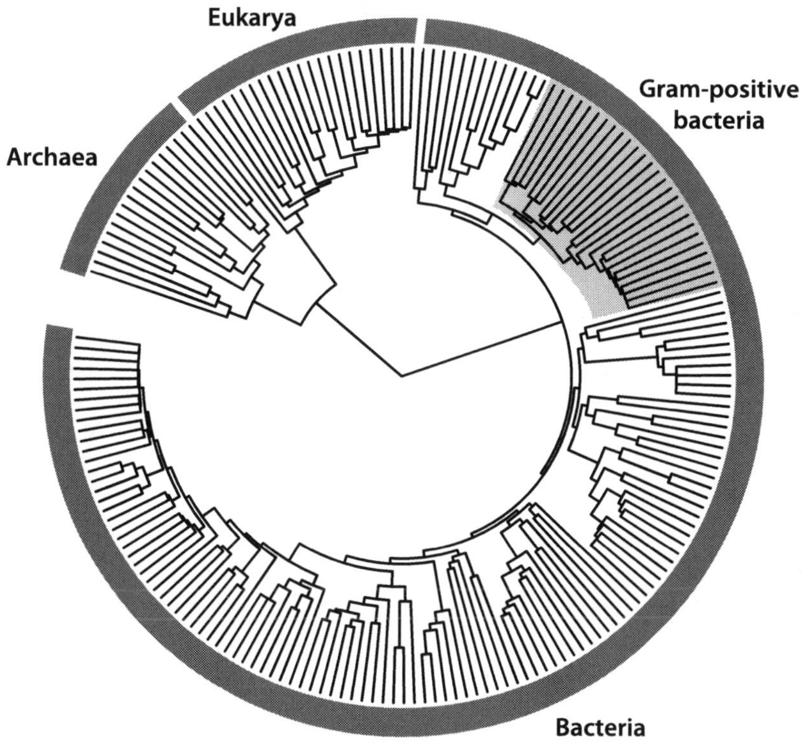

Figure 5. All of the plants, animals, and fungi that we can see around us are members of the Eukarya, which make up only a tiny portion of the tree of life. Most of the living things on planet Earth are actually bacteria. Note that the gram-positive bacteria are all related to each other. Data from Letunic and Bork (2006) Bioinformatics 23(1):127-128.

Bacteria have genes made of DNA, but they don't have histones. Instead, most of their DNA is in a big, naked, tangled circle called a nucleoid. Bacteria can also have smaller rings of DNA called plasmids. Bacteria can pass these plasmids to other bacteria, even to unrelated bacteria. That's how the genes for antibiotic resistance can jump from one strain of bacteria to another, and even from one species of bacteria to an unrelated species.

Of course, not all of a eukaryote's DNA is found in the nuclei of its cells. All eukaryotic cells contain tiny structures called mitochondria. Each mitochondrion has its own DNA. Plant cells have mitochondria. Plant cells also have chloroplasts, which also have their own DNA. Mitochondria and chloroplasts look a lot like bacteria, but without cell walls (Figure 6).

Like bacterial DNA, mitochondrial DNA is in a naked ring, without histones. In fact, most microbiologists are now convinced that mitochondria and chloroplasts are descended from ancient bacteria that learned how to live inside an archaeon. These ancient bacteria and their archeon host developed a symbiotic relationship, which means a relationship that is good for both parties. Mitochondria allow a cell to use oxygen to burn fuel. Chloroplasts enable plants to do photosynthesis.

As you can see from Figure 5, bacteria are really the most diverse and plentiful form of life on Earth. They are everywhere, and they do many important things. We could not survive without them. There are also many bacteria on your body. You have more bacteria in your mouth than there are human beings on the planet. You have more bacteria on your body's outer and inner surfaces—mainly inside your intestines—than you have cells in your body. This idea might be frightening to someone who is afraid of germs. However, it helps to explain a puzzling fact about the history of medicine.

Scientists got their first glimpse of bacteria in the 1670s, when Anthonie van Leeuwenhoek used his powerful handmade lenses to look at things like pond water or the scrapings from his own teeth. As I explained in chapter 2, it took nearly 200 years for doctors to realize that some bacteria cause disease.

Why did it take so long for scientists to come up with the germ theory of disease? I think that it's because the vast majority of bacteria are harmless. Only a few species of bacteria are likely to cause disease. Before scientists could prove that certain bacteria could make you sick, they had to figure out ways to tell one kind of bacterium from another. The problem is that most bacteria look pretty much alike. Under a microscope, they look like little dots or squiggles, if you can see them at all.

Figure 6. Bacterial cells are much smaller and simpler than the cells of a plant or an animal. The chloroplasts inside plant cells and the mitochondria inside plant and animal cells are probably the descendants of ancient bacteria.

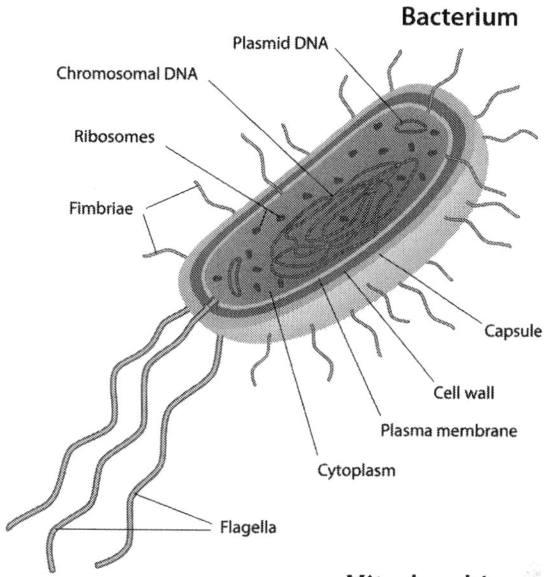

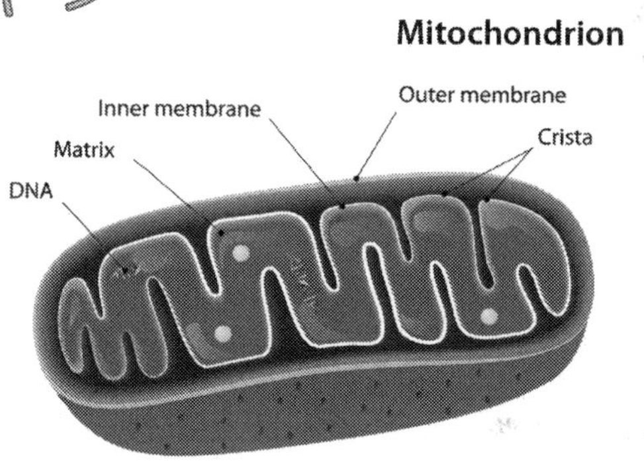

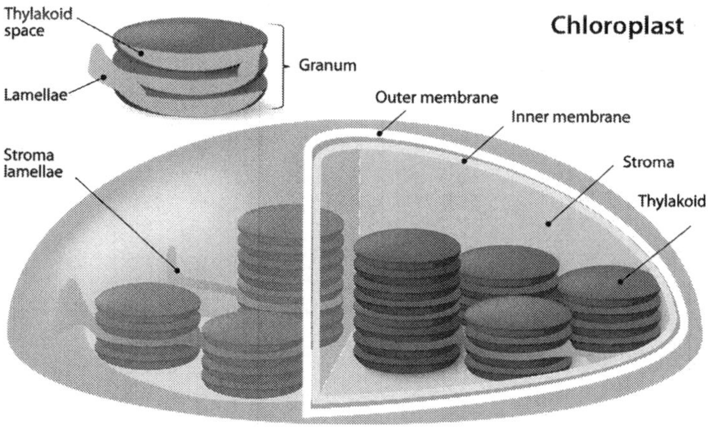

10

Telling One Bacterium From Another

We human beings tend to be highly visual creatures. We mainly use visual clues—such as size, shape, and color—to tell one kind of plant or animal from another. But we cannot see bacteria at all. They are simply too small to be seen with the naked eye. To see them, you need a microscope. Even so, you may need to use special stains to make them visible.

Staining

Stains can also help you tell different kinds of bacteria apart. The stains reveal not only the bacterium's shape but also its chemical makeup. Often, the first step in identifying a bacterium is to use a multistep staining procedure called Gram staining (Figure 7).

Some bacteria have a thick, porous cell wall that takes up lots of crystal violet stain, which turns them dark purple. Treating these stained cells with iodine traps the crystal violet in those thick cell walls. Thus, they remain dark purple even after being washed with a mixture of alcohol and acetone. The bacteria that remain dark purple after being washed with alcohol and acetone are called gram-positive (Figure 8). DNA studies eventually showed that the gram-positive organisms make up an important branch of the bacterial family tree (Figure 5).

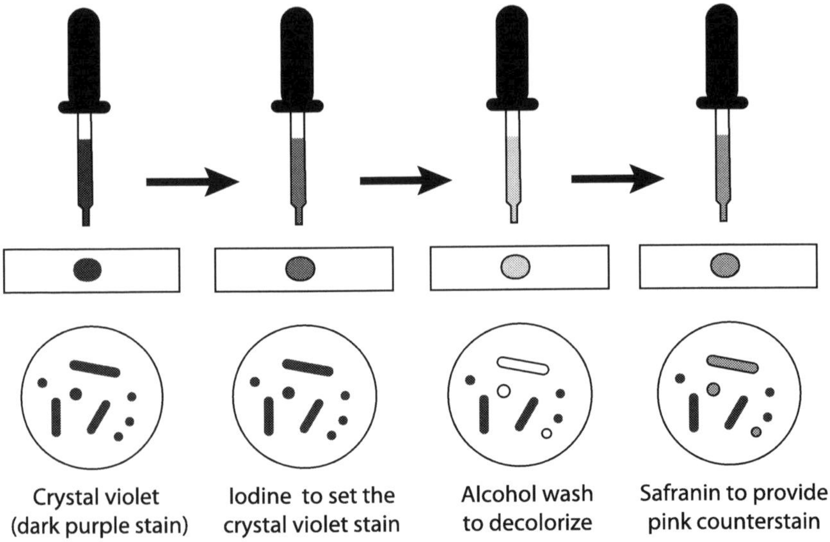

Figure 7. A Gram staining procedure involves five steps: (1) Heat is used to make the bacteria stick to a microscope slide. (2) The bacteria are treated with a dark purple or blue dye. (3) Iodine is used to fix the dye. (4) The dye is rinsed off with a mixture of alcohol and acetone, but the dark purple stain stays in the gram-positive organisms because of the way their cell walls are built. (5) A pink counterstain is used to make the decolorized gram-negative bacteria show up.

Other bacteria are surrounded by an outer membrane that protects the cell wall from the crystal violet. (This membrane is in addition to the regular cell membrane that is inside the cell wall.) However, this outer membrane would be washed away by the mixture of alcohol and acetone. Then, they can be counterstained pink with safranin. They are called gram-negative bacteria (Figure 8).

Some bacteria have a fatty substance called mycolic acid in their cell wall. As a result, they are hard to stain with crystal violet but also hard to decolorize with an acid-alcohol solution. Thus, these bacteria are described as acid-fast. They turn a light purple color from the Gram staining procedure. To get a better look at them, you need to use some other staining technique, such as a Ziehl-Neelsen stain, which turns them bright red.

Members of the genus *Mycobacteria* are acid-fast. Many mycobacterial species are important causes of disease in humans and animals. *Mycobacterium leprae* causes leprosy. *Mycobacterium tuberculosis* and other members of the *Mycobacterium tuberculosis* complex cause tuberculosis. Members of the *Mycobacterium avium* complex are important causes of death in AIDS patients. *Mycobacterium avium paratuberculosis* causes an intestinal disease in cattle. It might also cause Crohn's disease in human beings.

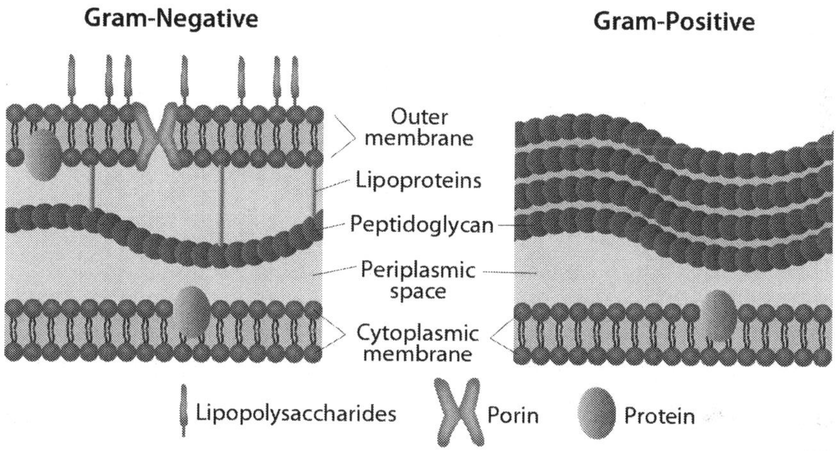

Figure 8. Gram-positive bacteria have a thick layer of peptidoglycan in their cell walls. Gram-negative bacteria have a thinner cell wall that is surrounded by an outer membrane.

Bacterial Shape (Morphology)

Stains make it easier to see a bacterium's shape, which is called its morphology (Figure 9). Most bacteria look like punctuation marks. A bacterium that looks like a period is called a coccus, which means berry. A bacterium that looks like a hyphen or dash is called a bacillus or a rod. Some rods look a bit twisted. The ones that have a slight twist look like commas. The comma-shaped bacteria are called vibrios. The long spiral bacteria that look like corkscrews are called spirochetes.

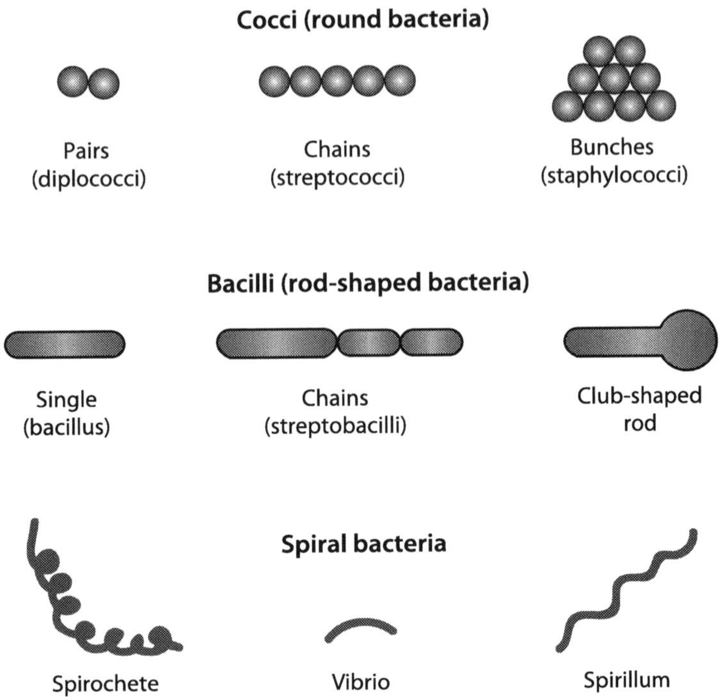

Figure 9. The common shapes of bacteria. A coccus is a round bacterium. Some species of round bacteria can often be found in pairs (diplococci), others in bunches (staphylococci), and still others in chains (streptococci). A rod-shaped bacterium is called a bacillus. Bacilli are sometimes found in chains. Some bacteria are spiral.

Some kinds of bacteria always seem to have a consistent shape, no matter what. In other words, they are monomorphic, which means one shape. Other kinds of bacteria can take on a different shape under different environmental conditions. Sometimes, they vary in shape even within the same culture. The bacteria that can take on more than one overall shape are called pleomorphic (sometimes spelled pleiomorphic) or polymorphic.

Sometimes, the way that bacteria divide gives you a clue to their identity. The cocci that are found in pairs are commonly called diplococci. Bacteria from the genus *Streptococcus* tend to divide along one axis. As a result, they tend to form long chains. In contrast, bacteria from the genus *Staphylococcus* can split along different axes. Thus, they tend to form disorderly clusters that look like bunches of grapes. When the rod-shaped bacteria (bacilli) divide, they never split lengthwise. That's why they can form end-to-end pairs (diplobacilli) and chains (streptobacilli), but never divide to form side-by-side stacks.

Motility

Another clue to a bacterium's identity is its motility, which means whether it can move around by itself. Some bacteria have a whip-like extension called a flagellum that acts like a tiny propeller (Figure 10). Some bacteria have one flagellum. Others have exactly two flagella—one flagellum at either end. Still others have many flagella. Some of those bacteria have all of their flagella in a single tuft. Others have flagella scattered all over their surface. When the flagella rotate counterclockwise, the flagella bunch together and the bacterium "runs" in a particular direction. When the flagella rotate clockwise, the bacterium tumbles around and changes direction.

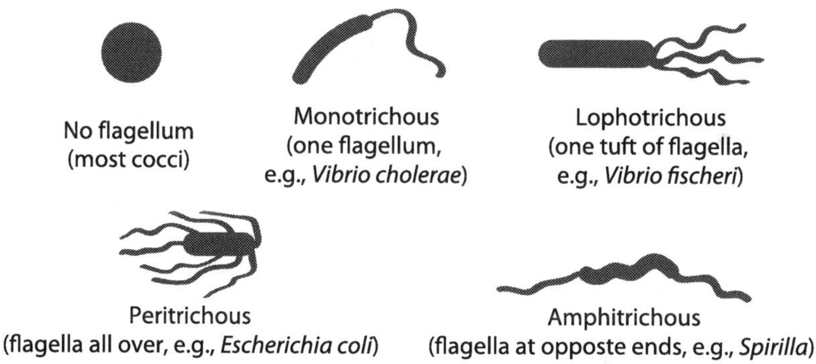

Figure 10. Some bacteria have flagella that serve as propellers.

Of course, some bacteria can move without flagella. Spirochetes have flagella inside their periplasmic space, which propel the spirochete in a corkscrew-like motion. There are also some bacteria that glide along a surface on a slime trail, like a snail.

Spore Formation

Another important clue to a bacterium's identity is how it reacts to conditions that it doesn't like. Some bacteria, like the one that causes anthrax, can convert themselves into tough, dried-up spores that can survive for many years until conditions improve. Spores can be extremely hard to kill because they resist most ordinary household cleaning products.

Response to Culture Conditions

One of the most important clues to the identity of a bacterium is what it takes to get that bacterium to grow in the laboratory, and what the colonies look like when they do grow in the laboratory. Bacteria that are hard to grow in a laboratory are called fastidious. They may need special nutrients, a low-oxygen environment, or just a long time to grow.

As I explained in chapter 10, bacteria have found ways to adapt to many different habitats. Some of these habitats are rich in oxygen, but others have practically no oxygen. Aerobic bacteria need oxygen in the form of O_2, just as the cells of our own body do. Anaerobic bacteria do not need O_2. For energy, many of them simply split glucose molecules into lactic acid, which is a reaction that does not consume oxygen. Bacteria that can switch back and forth between an aerobic or anaerobic lifestyle are called facultative aerobes or facultative anaerobes, depending on which lifestyle they prefer.

Microaerophilic bacteria need oxygen in the form of O_2, but they need O_2 levels that are far lower than what is found in the atmosphere. Some microaerophilic bacteria are capnophiles, which means that they need a high concentration of carbon dioxide. Even fairly low O_2 levels are toxic to some anaerobic bacteria.

If you grow bacteria in a test tube full of liquid, aerobes would end up clustered at the top, where there's plenty of oxygen. The anaerobes would be found at the bottom, as far away from the atmosphere as possible. The facultative aerobes and facultative anaerobes would be found all through the liquid.

In your body, the aerobic bacteria tend to be found in places where there is plenty of oxygen, such as on your skin or in your upper respiratory tract and lungs. Facultative anaerobes, on the other hand, can live on the skin but can then invade deeper structures. Anaerobic bacteria tend to thrive in places where there isn't much oxygen. Some anaerobic bacteria are normal residents of the insides of your intestines. Some of these bacteria provide useful services, such as helping you digest your food and producing important nutrients, such as vitamin K.

Another clue to the identity of a bacterium is the kind of nutrients it needs to survive. Some bacteria live independently like green plants. They make their own fuel by using the energy from sunlight to make sugar out of carbon dioxide and water. Then, they make everything else they need from the sugar, some ammonia, and some minerals. In contrast, most of the bacteria that are likely to cause disease in a human being or other animal are so highly adapted to a parasitic lifestyle that they need to get some complicated nutrients from an animal host. One way to tell different species and strains of bacteria apart is to see what they can and cannot digest, and what they can and cannot do without. For that purpose, you can use special culture media.

Some bacteria have become so highly adapted to a parasitic lifestyle that they cannot reproduce outside of some other living cell. These bacteria are called obligate intracellular parasites. One example is the syphilis spirochete. Until scientists figured out how to grow human cells in cell culture, there was no way to grow syphilis spirochetes in a laboratory. Yet to keep a culture of human cells alive, you may have to treat it with serum from animal blood, thus raising the risk that the culture will become contaminated with some other bacteria or virus. *Mycobacterium leprae,* which is the cause of leprosy, is even more finicky. Scientists cannot yet grow it even in cell culture. It can be grown only in armadillos or in specially bred mice.

When bacteria do grow in a laboratory, the colonies tend to take on a particular appearance, which helps in identifying them. Alexander Fleming used to create pictures by using bacteria as paints. He'd smear the various bacteria on the surface of the culture medium in a Petri dish and then watch the picture emerge as the bacteria grew. Fleming eventually noticed that some of his bacterial cultures would not grow anywhere near a mold called *Penicillium*. The mold was making something that killed bacteria. That's how he discovered penicillin.

Some bacterial strains are susceptible to penicillin or other antibiotics. Others are resistant to various antibiotics. The standard way to test their susceptibility is to put a disk of filter paper soaked with the antibiotic in the Petri dish with the bacteria. If there's a clear zone around the disk, then the bacteria are susceptible to that antibiotic. If the bacteria can grow right up to the disk, they are resistant to the antibiotic. That finding usually means that the antibiotic will be useless in treating infections caused by that germ.

Streptococci all look practically the same under a microscope. When stained by the Gram staining technique, they show up as dark purple dots, often in pairs or chains. Yet some streptococci are dangerous, while others are part of the normal flora found in the mouth and throat of healthy people. To tell the different kinds of streptococci apart, scientists started by sorting them into three groups, according to how they look when grown on blood agar.

Streptococci are so adapted to living a parasitic lifestyle that they need some nutrients that come from some other living thing. As a result, they are generally grown in culture media that contain extracts from meat, plant materials, or yeast. In laboratories, they are generally grown on blood agar, which is a gel that contains red blood cells. Some streptococci release hydrogen peroxide, which turns the hemoglobin in the red blood cells green (alpha hemolysis). Thus, you'll see a green area around and underneath the colonies of alpha-hemolytic streptococci that are grown on blood agar. Other streptococci produce enzymes that attack the cell membrane of the red blood cells, causing them to burst (beta-hemolysis). Thus, you'll see a clear area in the blood agar around and under the colonies of beta-hemolytic streptococci. Still other streptococci have no effect on the red blood cells in the blood agar. They are called gamma-hemolytic streptococci.

There are several ways to identify the individual strains of a species of bacteria. One approach is to use an antibody-based test. Antibodies bind specifically to certain antigens. If you add something that contains that antigen to serum that contains those antibodies, the antibody-antigen complexes will stick together in clumps. The strains of bacteria that have a positive result from a particular antibody test make up a serotype.

Typing

Sometimes, antibody-based tests are useful for telling one species of bacteria from another. An American microbiologist named Rebecca Lancefield developed this method for sorting the beta-hemolytic species of streptococci into several groups, each of which contained one or more species. For example, group A were responsible for strep throat and rheumatic fever. Group B can cause pneumonia and meningitis in newborns. Group C cause a disease called strangles in horses. Antibody-based tests can also be used to identify particular strains of a single species of bacteria.

Some antibody-based tests use an antibody that has been bound to some fluorescent dye. This approach, which is called immunofluorescence, can show how a particular antigen is distributed in tissue. But since antibodies are too big to pass through cell membranes, this method cannot show what antigens are present inside a living cell.

Lately, researchers and even medical practitioners have been able to use DNA tests to figure out whether a particular bacterium is present, and to figure out how various species and strains of DNA are related to each other. The results of these studies are sometimes confusing because bacteria can swap genes with other, unrelated bacteria.

When microbiologists are trying to identify particular strains of some bacteria, such as *Haemophilus influenzae*, they look to see if the bacteria have a capsule. Some bacteria secrete a slimy substance that forms a protective capsule surrounding the cell. Some strains of *Haemophilus influenzae* produce a capsule, while others do not. This capsule generally does not take up stain very well. Thus, it appears as a pale halo around a stained cell.

Bacterial capsules are made up mainly of a polysaccharide, which is a chain of molecules of simple sugars. (In contrast, a protein is made up of a chain of amino acids.) A capsule helps a bacterium stick to surfaces, and it protects the bacterium from drying out. Thus, it helps the bacterium survive in the environment. The capsule can also serve as a shield that protects the bacterium from the immune system. That's why the *Haemophilus influenzae* strains that have a capsule are far more dangerous than the strains that do not have a capsule.

The capsule hides the bacterial proteins from the host's immune system and makes the bacterium too slippery for white blood cells to swallow. This fact explains why the encapsulated strains of *Haemophilus influenzae* can succeed in invading deep into the body, even to the bones and the brain. In contrast, the unencapsulated strains are generally found only on the surfaces of the respiratory tract, where they can cause earaches and sinus infections.

It's easy for the immune system to make antibodies to foreign proteins. It is much harder for the immune system to make antibodies to a polysaccharide. But once the immune system does make antibodies to the polysaccharide in a bacterial capsule, those antibodies can stick to the capsule. Thus, the antibodies enable white blood cells to grab the bacterium and swallow it.

The polysaccharide in the capsule of a bacterium is usually made up of repeating units of one to six simple sugars. That sounds simple. But even that simple system can generate a huge number of possible polysaccharides. More than 90 different serotypes of *Streptococcus pneumoniae* have been identified. Each one has a different polysaccharide in its capsule. Because the immune system can see nothing but the capsule, each of these 90 serotypes looks like a different kind of thing. Antibodies to one of these strains may provide little or no protection against the other strains of the same species.

Once your immune system makes antibodies to the polysaccharide in a bacterium's capsule, those antibodies can fight the bacteria from that particular serotype. However, those antibodies may not provide much protection against other serotypes of the same species. The vaccine against *Haemophilus influenzae* type b is highly effective against that strain, which is the one that has caused the most serious problems. However, that vaccine has no effect on any other strain of *Haemophilus influenzae*. The vaccines against *Streptococcus pneumoniae* were designed to provide protection against the strains that have been causing the most trouble.

11

How Bacteria Cause Disease

Many species of bacteria have found ways to survive on the inner or outer surfaces of the human body. Most of them cause no harm. Some of them are even beneficial. The bacteria that cause no harm are described as commensal. The word *commensal* comes from the Latin for "sharing a table." The bacteria that actually provide some benefit to their host are called symbiotic, which came from the Greek for "living together." The bacteria that cause disease are called pathogens, which literally means that they generate disease.

There are several different ways in which a bacterial infection can harm the body. Some bacteria directly attack the cells of the body, just as they would digest a piece of meat. Others release some harmful substance. For example, tooth decay is the result of acid produced mainly by a bacterium called *Streptococcus mutans* when it digests sugars in the mouth. That's why it's important to clean the sugars and starches from your teeth after you eat.

Some bacteria produce particularly dangerous substances called toxins. There are two basic kinds: exotoxins and endotoxins. Exotoxins (i.e., "outside toxins") are proteins that the bacteria release into their environment as they go about their normal activities. These toxins can be carried around the body by the bloodstream. Thus, even if an infection is limited to the upper respiratory tract, the toxins produced by the bacteria can damage the heart and brain. Sometimes, bacterial toxins can cause serious problems, such as brain damage and death. Some vaccines, such as the ones for diphtheria, tetanus, and whooping cough, are really directed at the toxins produced by the bacteria.

In contrast, endotoxins (which means inside toxins) are part of the structure of the bacteria. Bacteria release endotoxins only after they die. The term *endotoxin* is sometimes used loosely to refer to anything nasty that can be released from a dead bacterium. However, it mainly means a lipopolysaccharide (a fat bound to a chain of sugars) that is found in the membrane that is outside the cell wall of some gram-negative organisms. Endotoxins can trigger an inflammatory response. Huge amounts of endotoxin can cause a potentially deadly problem called endotoxic shock.

Live bacteria can release small amounts of endotoxin as they grow and divide. Dead bacteria can release large amounts as they die. As a result, people may feel worse right after they start taking an antibiotic than they felt before. A particularly severe reaction called the Herxheimer reaction occurs in patients receiving antibiotic treatment for syphilis. The Herxheimer reaction can also result from antibiotic treatment of several other diseases, including Lyme disease, Q fever, or cat scratch disease. The patient may need anti-inflammatory drugs to control the inflammation and intravenous fluids to keep blood pressure from dropping too low.

Most of the bacteria and fungi that live on us or in us are easily held in check by the immune system, at least until we die. At that point, the bacteria and fungi rapidly start to digest the body. Remarkably few species of bacteria are likely to cause problems while we are still alive. To do that, they must find some way to sneak past the immune system, at least for a while, as I will describe in more detail in chapter 14.

Some bacteria can sneak past the immune system long enough to sicken or even kill their host. But if their host dies, they die, too. That could be a dead end for their family tree. To keep from going extinct, any parasite, including pathogenic bacteria, must find some way to get from one host to the next.

The most efficient way for a germ to get from one human host to the next is to make their host spew them out into the environment. For a respiratory infection, the most efficient way to do that is to make the person cough or sneeze. For a gastrointestinal infection, the most efficient way to do that is to cause vomiting and diarrhea.

The bacteria that are targeted by vaccines can all live on or in the body and can get past our immune defenses long enough to cause serious trouble. Some of them have a capsule that allows them to hide from the immune system.

Many bacteria can colonize the body, which means living quietly on the body's surface without causing any noticeable problems. However, if bacteria start causing trouble, the problem is called an infection. Mild infections just cause minor inflammation. Severe infections can cause major problems, such as tissue damage or even death.

Although it's normal to have bacteria on the inner and outer surfaces of the body, it is not normal to have bacteria inside the tissues or in the bloodstream. If the infection is more than skin-deep, it is called an invasive infection. The presence of live bacteria in the bloodstream is called bacteremia. A serious, invasive infection can to a widespread inflammatory response called sepsis, which can lead to multiple organ failure and death.

If the bacteria are so invasive that they infect the bones and bone marrow, the problem is called osteomyelitis. If the bacteria enter the fluid surrounding the brain and spinal cord, the problem is called bacterial meningitis. Even with antibiotic treatment, the death rate from bacterial meningitis is over 10%. Roughly 20% of the survivors are left with permanent disabilities, such as brain damage, hearing loss, and kidney problems. Some patients need extensive skin grafting and may even lose their hands and feet. *Haemophilus influenzae* type b (Hib) was once the main cause of bacterial meningitis in children under 5. Fortunately, the incidence of Hib meningitis in the United States has gone down by more than 99% since the introduction of the Hib vaccine.

Vaccinations against the meningococcus and the pneumococcus have also led to decreases in cases of bacterial meningitis caused by those bacteria.

12

Antibiotics and Antibiotic Resistance

We have antibiotics, so why bother to vaccinate people against bacterial diseases? The answer is simple. An ounce of prevention is sometimes worth far more than a pound of cure. Some bacterial infections can cause so much damage so fast that the patient could die or end up with serious, lifelong disabilities even if the germ that causes the problem is susceptible to antibiotics. For example, bacterial meningitis can cause serious problems (permanent brain damage, loss of hands and feet, or even death) within hours after the first symptoms arise.

Vaccination can also help us deal with the emerging problem of antibiotic resistance. Not only do vaccine-makers target the most antibiotic-resistant strains of bacteria, but the use of vaccines can decrease the general population's need for antibiotic therapy.

There are many different kinds of antibiotics . They all have one thing in common: they take advantage of some difference between bacterial cells and animal cells. One of the key differences is the overall structure of the cells.

Bacteria have cell walls. Animal cells do not. Several antibiotics, including penicillin, work by making it hard for the bacteria to build a new cell wall as the organism grows and divides. Others, such as vancomycin, work by disrupting the existing cell wall.

Like animal cells, bacteria have ribosomes, which are structures that assemble new proteins. However, the bacterial ribosomes are slightly different from animal ribosomes. Some antibiotics target a subunit of the bacterial ribosomes. Thus, these antibiotics prevent bacteria from making new proteins, which the bacteria need in order to grow and divide. However, these antibiotics do not interfere with an animal cell's ability to make new proteins.

The sulfa drugs make it impossible for bacteria to make their own supply of a vitamin called folate. This disruption of folate synthesis is not a problem in a human cell because human cells cannot make their own folate to begin with. We need to get folate ready-made from our diet. Sulfa drugs don't kill the bacteria. They just keep the bacteria from growing and dividing. In other words, they are bacteriostatic, as opposed to bacteriocidal.

Some antibiotics, such as the quinolones, attack the enzymes that are involved in processing bacterial DNA. Still others disrupt the bacterial cell membrane, which is slightly different from an animal cell membrane.

Unfortunately, bacteria have figured out ways to get around these antibiotics. Long before the discovery of penicillin, some bacteria had figured out how to make an enzyme that breaks down penicillin. Others have a mutated version of the site where penicillin would normally bind. These bacteria can survive and divide even if they come into contact with penicillin.

The purpose of antibiotic therapy is to kill all of the dangerous germs. Unfortunately, antibiotics also kill many harmless or even helpful bacteria, without necessarily killing all of the dangerous ones. The bacteria that survive a course of antibiotic tend to be the ones that are most resistant to that antibiotic. They can then thrive because their competition has been killed off. That's why the overuse of antibiotics has led to the development of antibiotic-resistant strains of bacteria. To make matters worse, bacteria can swap genes with other bacteria, even with bacteria from other species. Thus, the genes for antibiotic resistance can spread from one species to another.

Bacteria can develop antibiotic resistance really fast, often faster than scientists can develop new antibiotics. Fortunately, we can develop vaccines against some of the most dangerous strains of antibiotic-resistant bacteria. These vaccines can then help to prevent these antibiotic-resistant bacteria from spreading in the population. For example, before the development of the Hib vaccine, roughly 30% of the *Haemophilus influenzae* type b infections were resistant to amoxicillin. Since the introduction of the vaccines, *Haemophilus influenzae* type b has practically disappeared from children in the United States.

13

Viruses, Genes, and Proteins

In chapter 9, I explained that early scientists tried to classify everything as either living or nonliving. Although you will sometimes hear people talk about vaccines made out of "live" viruses, viruses are never truly alive.

All living things are made up of one or more cells. A bacterium is a single cell. An adult human body is made of about 40 trillion cells. A virus is not a cell. It is a thing that was made by a cell.

All living things grow and reproduce themselves, and all living things use energy to do work. Viruses do not grow. Nor do they reproduce themselves. Instead, the virus's host cell makes new copies of the virus. (This process of making new copies of the virus is called amplification.) Nor does the virus use energy to do any work. The living cells do all the work.

A virus is just a set of genes wrapped in a delivery system that enables those genes to get passed from one cell to the next. The virus's host cell uses its own energy and other resources to make new copies of the virus. The host cell then sheds those new copies of the virus, which may then be picked up by another cell.

Genes are just recipes for proteins. Some viral genes are recipes for the proteins that make up the virus's protein coat. Other viral genes are for enzymes that control chemical reactions inside the host cell.

Cells reproduce themselves by splitting in two. Viruses do not reproduce themselves. Instead, the host cell copies the viral genes. The host cell also makes all the other parts of the virus. The viral genes and the other parts of the virus then automatically fit together to form new copies of that virus. It's a process called molecular self-assembly.

A cell may take in one copy of the virus but release thousands of new copies of that virus. Thus, the host cell amplifies the message that is carried by that virus.

When we talk about a virus, we sometimes mean a virion, which is a single infectious viral particle. Each virion is merely a set of genes wrapped up in some sort of delivery system. The genes can be encoded in DNA or RNA. This genetic material is then packaged in a protein coat, which is called a capsid (Figure 11). In some kinds of virus, the capsid is surrounded by a fatty envelope.

For a virus to get into a cell, the virus must have something on its outer surface that binds to something on the outer surface of the cell. For this binding to occur, there often has to be a very specific lock-and-key type of fit between something on the outside of the virus and something on the outside of the cell (Figure 12).

If a cell is not displaying the right sort of protein on its outer surface, the virus cannot attach itself and therefore cannot enter. That fact explains why viral infections can be limited to a particular type of cell in a particular species of host. Thus, viral infections can affect some species but not others, some individuals within a species but not others, and even some cell types within the body but not others. It all depends on whether the virus has the key that it needs to enter the cell.

If the virus has an envelope, that envelope can fuse with the cell's cell membrane, allowing the viral contents to enter the cell. Some nonenveloped viruses can inject their genes into the cell, leaving their protein coat outside. Still other viruses fool the cell into thinking that they are food. As a result, the cell engulfs the virus.

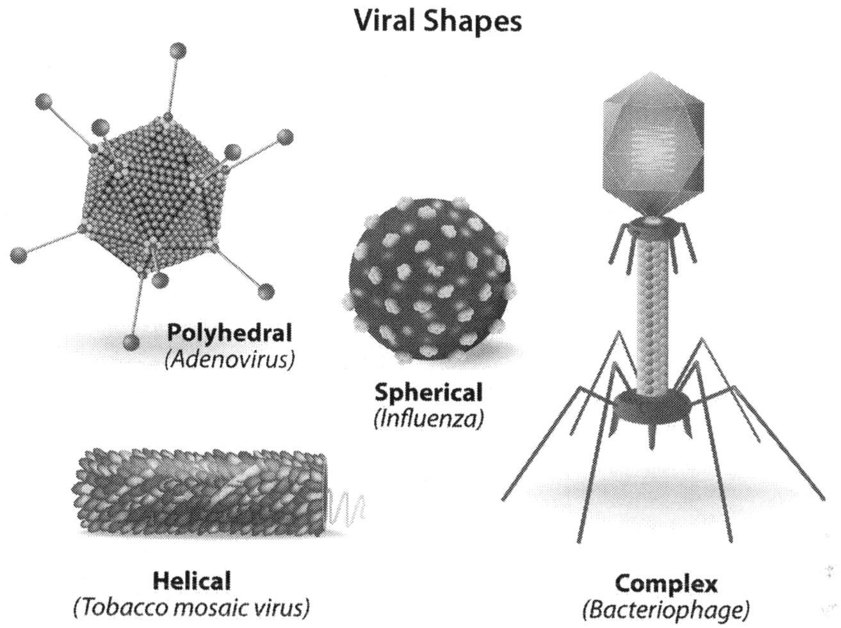

Figure 11. Viruses consist of a set of genes wrapped in a protein coat called a capsid. Capsids come in many different shapes. In some viruses, the capsid is surrounded by a fatty envelope.

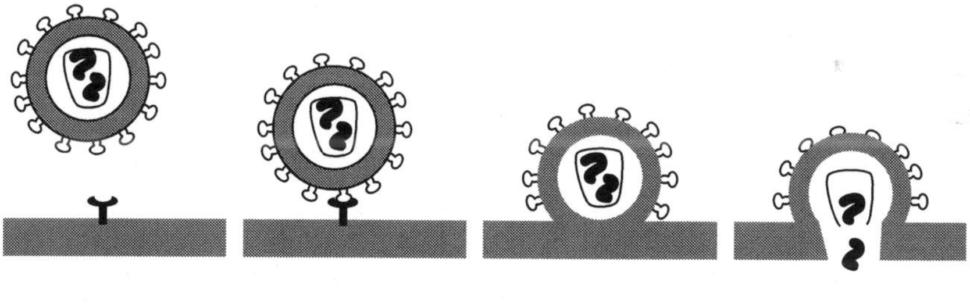

Figure 12. To enter a cell, HIV must first attach to the CD4+ receptor on the outside of the cell. The viral envelope then fuses with the cell membrane, allowing the contents of the virus to enter the cell. Some nonenveloped viruses inject their genes into the cell, leaving the protein coat outside. Other viruses are engulfed by the host cell.

Having an envelope is sometimes an advantage and sometimes a disadvantage for the virus. The envelope makes it easier for viruses to enter a cell. Since the envelope is typically made from the host cell's cell membrane, maybe with the addition of a few glycoproteins from the virus itself, the envelope makes it easier for the virus to hide from the body's immune system, which is why so many enveloped viruses can cause chronic infections.

Fortunately, however, the virus's fatty envelope can easily be destroyed by heat, drying, or detergents. As a result, the enveloped viruses can generally be spread only by fairly close contact. HIV is spread only by sexual contact, by contaminated blood products, or by contaminated hypodermic syringes. The herpesviruses can be spread by kissing or by sharing a drinking glass. The hepatitis B virus is easier to catch than HIV but harder to catch than a typical herpesvirus.

Although measles virus is also an enveloped virus, it is much tougher than HIV. The measles virus can survive in the environment outside of its host for a few hours. In contrast, the parvovirus that is so dangerous to young puppies doesn't have an envelope. As a result, it can remain infectious for months in the environment, if conditions are right.

Once a virus gets inside a cell, the cell may then follow the instructions in the viral DNA. Thus, the cell will end up using its resources to make new copies of the virus, which can then be spread to other cells.

The viruses that we talk about in medicine are a lot like computer viruses. A computer virus is a computer program: a set of instructions. If the computer runs that program, the program can tell the computer to do unproductive or even harmful things, such as damaging its own data files or program files. Some computer viruses can even cause the computer to damage its own hardware. Computer viruses also tell the computer to make new copies of the virus, which may then be passed along to other computers.

There are several different ways for a virus to leave its host cell (Figure 13). Some infected cells spit the viruses out. Other infected cells burst, thus spilling the viruses into the environment. The release of virions from the host cell is called viral shedding. Once the new virions have left their host cell, they can go on to infect new host cells.

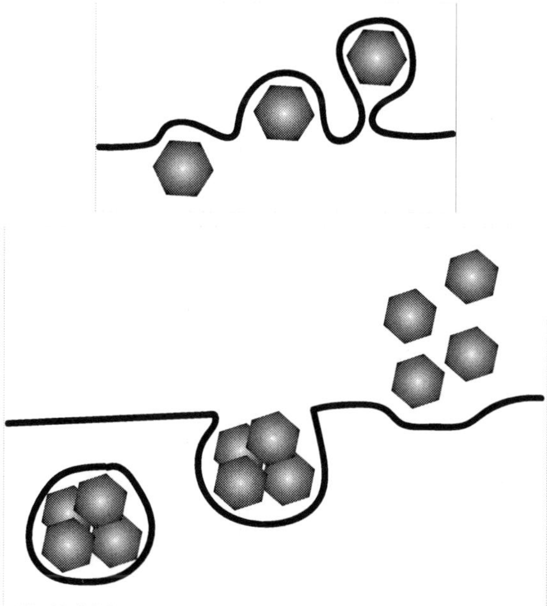

Figure 13. Some viruses leave the cell through budding. These viruses wrap themselves in a fatty envelope made out of the cell membrane. Many nonenveloped viruses leave the cell through a process called reverse endocytosis. Some viruses simply cause their host cell to burst.

The viruses that produce severe acute illnesses tend to get produced very quickly. The viruses that produce chronic illnesses, especially those that are hard to spread, may be produced much more slowly but over a longer period of time.

As I mentioned in chapter 9, some species of bacteria have become so highly adapted to a parasitic lifestyle that they cannot grow and divide unless they are inside another cell. Such bacteria are called obligate intracellular parasites. Similarly, viruses can be produced only inside living cells. Thus, you cannot grow a pure culture of viruses in a laboratory. However, if you can get some cultured cells to produce the virus for you, you might be able to purify the viruses through crystallization, as if the virus were an ordinary chemical.

If a virus is never truly alive, then what does it mean for a vaccine to be made from a "killed" virus? A "killed" or "inactivated" virus is one that has been damaged so that living cells can no longer make new copies of it. Thus, it cannot cause an infection. To make a "killed" vaccine, you need to damage the virus badly enough that it cannot cause infection. However, the virus must still look more or less like the wild virus to the immune system. The goal is to get the immune system to make antibodies that will protect the vaccinated person or animal against the wild virus. Note that the term "inactivated" refers to the virus, not to the vaccine itself. An "inactivated" vaccine can still be effective.

Sometimes, you'll hear about vaccines that contain "live" or "modified-live" viruses. Of course, viruses are never truly alive, in a biological sense. The terms "live," "modified-live," and "attenuated" mean that the virus can be picked up by a cell and copied. In other words, a "live" virus can infect a cell. These viruses have been altered so that they will produce an infection that is so mild that it may produce no symptoms at all. Yet these mild infections teach the immune system how to recognize the wild virus, so that the immune system is prepared to defend the body against the disease.

The usual method of producing a "live" virus vaccine is to have the virus infect cells from a series of several different species of animals. This process is called serial passage. To adapt to each new host, the virus must mutate. As a result, it may lose some of its ability to create problems for a human being (or for some species of domestic animal, in the case of a veterinary vaccine). Ideally, you will eventually end up with a viral strain that won't make you sick but that will enable your body to develop an immune response that will protect you against the wild virus.

On the plus side, the "live" virus vaccines can produce a strong, long-lasting immune response. The more closely the vaccine infection resembles a natural infection, the better the immune response is likely to be. That's why the "live" vaccines for some gastrointestinal infections are given by mouth, while the vaccines for some respiratory infections are dripped or sprayed into the nose. On the minus side, people with a weakened immune system sometimes find it hard to fight even the weakened strain of virus used in the vaccine. For that reason, pregnant women and people with a compromised immune system should not receive "live" vaccines.

The other concern is that the vaccine virus might mutate back to a dangerous form, as has happened with the poliovirus used in the "live" polio vaccine. The "live" polio vaccine has been instrumental in stopping the circulation of polio. Unfortunately, the vaccine itself caused a dozen or so cases of paralytic polio per year in the United States. Today, children in the United States receive a killed polio virus, but one with broader coverage than the original Salk vaccine had.

In a laboratory setting, scientists use serial passage to make a virus weaker. Unfortunately, a natural form of serial passage that occurs on farms can make the influenza virus more dangerous. There are many different strains of influenza virus. Each has become adapted to a particular species, such as chickens, pigs, and human beings. Unfortunately, those different strains can be passed from one species to another, especially when poultry and swine are grown on the same farm. When virions of two different strains of influenza virus infect the same host, those viruses can end up swapping genes. The resulting hybrid form of influenza virus can be particularly dangerous. The Great Pandemic of 1918-1919 was due to an influenza virus that probably came from pigs. Influenza viruses that come from birds are also potentially dangerous. That's why virologists and public health authorities are so worried about new strains of "bird flu" and "swine flu."

Louis Pasteur was the first person to suspect that viruses exist. He knew that rabies was caused by some sort of germ that was carried by the saliva of rabid animals. Yet he could not associate any bacterium with the disease. He concluded that the rabies germ was simply too small to be visible under his microscope. Later research showed that several other diseases, including yellow fever and a plant disease called tobacco mosaic disease, had to be caused by some infectious agent that was too small to be seen under a conventional microscope.

The standard way to figure out whether a disease is viral, as opposed to bacterial, is to see whether fluid from an infected animal or plant can still transmit disease, even after being passed through a filter that is fine enough to trap all bacteria. The germs that are small enough to pass through that kind of filter were called filterable viruses. The word *virus* means poison in Latin. Some people believed that since viruses could pass through such fine filters, they had to be liquid. Later on, the development of filters with even finer pores showed that viruses are tiny solid particles.

Although an ordinary microscope is not powerful enough to let us see individual virions, it can show that infected cells often contain small structures that look like crystals. These structures did turn out to be crystals made up of virions (Figure 14). Once scientists started finding these crystals, they could use X-ray crystallography to get some idea of the structure of the individual virions that made up the crystals. They would aim a beam of X-rays at the crystal and take a picture of how the X-rays bounced off. A similar process had been used to figure out the structure of DNA molecules.

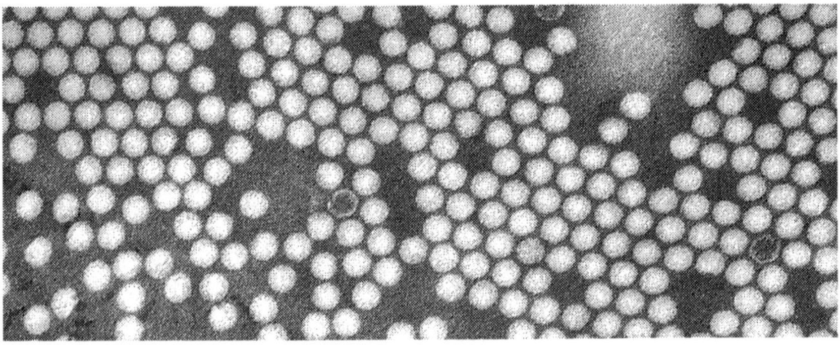

Figure 14. Viruses such as poliovirus can sometimes arrange themselves into a crystal structure, as if they were a mineral.

With a conventional microscope, you can magnify things by only about 1250-fold. But with an electron microscope, which uses a beam of electrons instead of visible light, you can get magnifications of 100,000-fold. Thus, the electron microscope made it possible to see the structure of individual virions.

Today, virologists use many different techniques to study viruses. One especially important technique is to decode the viral genes. In some viruses, the genes are encoded in DNA. In others, the genes are encoded in RNA.

All living things, including all living cells and even the mitochondria and chloroplasts within living cells, have their genes encoded in a double strand of a chemical called DNA. The DNA molecule looks like a twisted rope ladder (Figure 15). The sides of the ladder are made of a sugar called deoxyribose. The rungs of the ladder are made of pairs of nucleobases. Together, a deoxyribose sugar and a nucleobase make up a nucleotide. The pairs of nucleotides are held together by hydrogen bonds, which are far weaker than the covalent bonds that hold everything else within the DNA molecule together. Thus, the two strands of the DNA molecule can split down the middle, sort of like a zipper unzipping.

Figure 15. DNA consists of a twisted ladder made up of smaller units called nucleotides. The sides of the ladder are made of a 5-carbon sugar called deoxyribose, plus at least one phosphate group. The rungs of the ladder are made of pairs of nucleobases. There are four different nucleobases: cytosine (C) can bind with guanine (G), and adenine (A) can bind with thymine (T). These four nucleobases make up a four-letter code that stores genetic information.

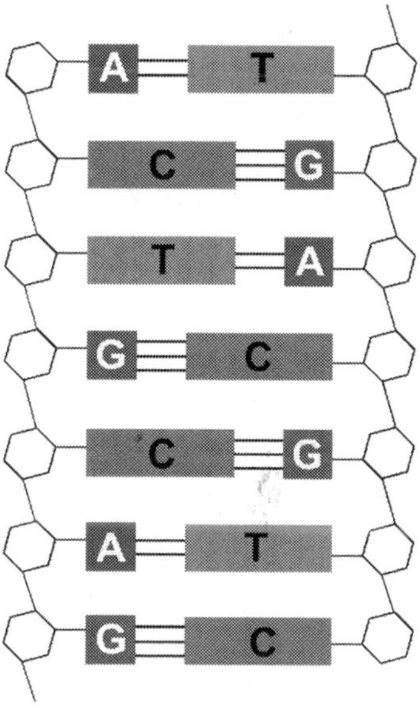

There are only four nucleobases in DNA: guanine, adenine, thymine, and cytosine. Thus, a strand of DNA is like a very long piece of text written with only four letters: G, A, T, and C. Guanine can form a hydrogen bond only with cytosine, and adenine only with thymine. If you have a sequence of GAGCAT on one strand, the opposite strand will have to have the complementary sequence: CTCGTA.

The DNA code involves nucleotides in groups of three, called codons. Some codons stand for a particular amino acid. For example, a string of three thymines (TTT) stands for the amino acid phenylalanine. The DNA code that most living things use can represent 20 different amino acids. (Some bacteria have figured out a trick for encoding two other amino acids.) The DNA code also includes signals for where the genes start and stop. A codon consisting of thymine-adenine-adenine (TAA) is a stop sign.

All living things use this same DNA code, which is why scientists could take a gene from a fish and get it to work inside the cells of a tomato plant. More importantly, they also figured out how to put the genes for human insulin in some bacteria, which then made large amounts of a protein that is identical to natural human insulin. This development allowed diabetics to be treated with insulin that is identical to the insulin their pancreas is supposed to make, as opposed to the slightly different insulin that came from the pancreases of cattle or pigs. (I explain this in detail in my book *Thin Diabetes, Fat Diabetes*).

Each gene is just a stretch of DNA that represents the recipe for a polypeptide, which is a string of amino acids. Some proteins consist of a single polypeptide, which is encoded by a single gene. Other proteins consist of two or more polypeptide subunits, which may be the products of two or more different genes.

Any change in the DNA of an organism is called a mutation. There are many kinds of mutations (Figure 16). Mutations are like typographical errors. Some have no real effect. Others are catastrophically bad. A few can be advantageous. Some are a mixed blessing. For example, if you inherited the gene for sickle-cell anemia from only one of your parents, you will be resistant to malaria. But if you got that mutant gene from both parents, you will end up with sickle-cell anemia, a painful disease that can shorten your life expectancy.

The mutation that causes sickle-cell anemia is an example of a point mutation, which is sometimes called a single-nucleotide polymorphism (SNP). It means that one nucleotide has been swapped for another. Sometimes, the new codon still calls for the same amino acid as the old one did. As a result, the mutated gene still produces exactly the same protein. In contrast, a missense mutation means that the mutated codon calls for a different amino acid. Sometimes, the new amino acid is similar enough to the old one that the new protein is still pretty much like the old one. SNPs that have no significant effect on the function of the protein are called silent. However, not all SNPs are silent. Sickle-cell anemia is the result of a missense mutation that radically alters the properties of the hemoglobin protein. Some cases of Duchenne muscular dystrophy are due to a nonsense mutation that creates a premature stop codon, which shortens the protein.

Original gene	AAA THE RED CAT ATE THE FAT RAT ZZZ	
Point mutation	AAA THE RED CA**R** ATE THE FAT RAT ZZZ	Wrong amino acid
Insertion	AAA THE **BIG** RED CAT ATE THE FAT RAT ZZZ	New amino acid has been inserted
Deletion	AAA **THE CAT** ATE THE FAT RAT ZZZ	Amino acid has been deleted
Frame shift	AAA THE **REC ATA TET HEF ATR AT** ZZZ	Message has been garbled
Premature stop codon	AAA THE RED CAT ZZZ **ATE THE FAT RAT** ZZZ	Protein has been shortened

Figure 16. In this example, I have used letters of the English alphabet to stand for the nucleobases (in the DNA code, there are only four letters). I have used English words to represent amino acids. I used AAA to represent a start codon and ZZZ to represent a stop codon.

Other kinds of mutations involve insertion or deletion of one or more nucleotides. Sometimes, these mutations result from "jumping genes" (transposons), which are DNA sequences that can move around in the genome. An insertion or deletion of one or two nucleotides would shift the reading frame of the gene. Remember that the DNA code is based on three-nucleotide sequences called codons. If you shift the reading frame over by one or two nucleotides, the resulting sequence of amino acids would be completely different. Most cases of the hereditary disease Tay-Sachs disease are due to a frame-shift mutation.

All living cells use DNA to store their recipes for proteins. But before they actually make those proteins, cells copy the information from their DNA into a different kind of molecule, called ribonucleic acid (RNA). RNA is similar to DNA, except that it uses ribose instead of deoxyribose for its sugar backbone and it uses uracil instead of thymine.

To make a protein, the cell must first split the DNA that carries the gene for that protein down the middle. Then, it uses the gene as a template for making a molecule of messenger RNA. The messenger RNA then carries the information from that gene to a structure called a ribosome. There, some smaller RNA molecules called transfer RNA bring the amino acids to the ribosome. There, the amino acids are assembled in the proper order into a long chain (Figure 17).

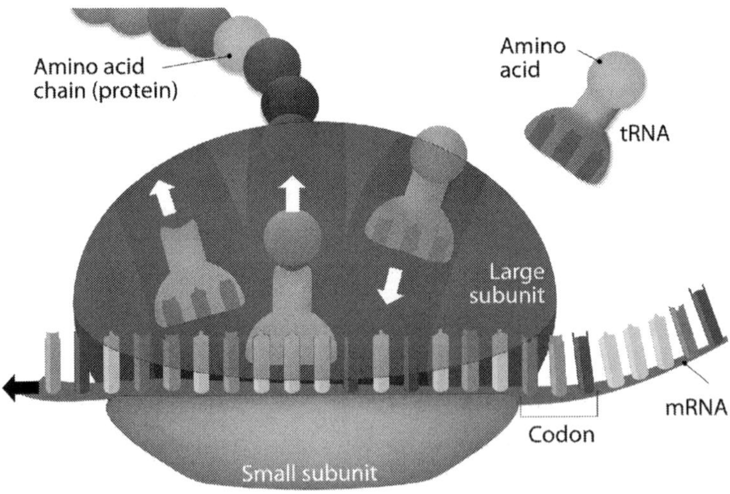

Figure 17. How proteins are made: Messenger RNA (mRNA) copies the genetic information from DNA in the chromosomes of a eukaryote or the nucleoid of a bacterium and carries it to a ribosome, which consists of two subunits. Transport RNA (tRNA) brings amino acids to the ribosome, where they are added to the amino acid chain in the order specified by the mRNA.

As the polypeptide spools off the ribosome, it takes on a particular shape. That shape is determined by its amino acid sequence. Sometimes, the protein undergoes further processing. The cell may use enzymes to add particular sugars to particular spots on the protein. This process is called glycosylation.

Some genes provide the recipe for a whole protein. Other genes provide recipes for subunits that are then combined to form a complex protein. These subunits tend to bind naturally to each other. As a result, the complex proteins tend to assemble themselves. This is a phenomenon called molecular self-assembly.

Each gene says exactly which amino acids should be added, in what order, as its polypeptide is being built. This order, which is called the primary structure, matters a lot because the amino acids differ in their chemical properties. The order of the amino acids determines what shape the polypeptide will have.

Some stretches of polypeptide naturally take on a spiral shape, called an alpha helix. Others end up zigzagged into a sheet called a beta sheet. These basic shapes are called the secondary structure of the protein. Polypeptides can be hundreds or thousands of amino acids long. As a result, they often have stretches of alpha helix plus stretches of beta sheet.

Since the proteins are made in the watery environment inside a cell, the shape of the protein is affected by the fact that some amino acids are attracted to water while others repel water. Some proteins end up in a globular tangle, with the stretches of water-loving amino acids toward the outside and the water-hating ones tucked in the center. The overall shape that results is called the tertiary structure of the protein.

Many proteins consist of two or more different subunits, which are encoded by separate genes. Some proteins even contain some non-protein portions. For example, the hemoglobin molecule consists of four protein subunits (two alpha-globins plus two beta-globins), plus four molecules of an iron-containing pigment called heme.

Hemoglobin, which is the oxygen-carrying protein that makes our blood red, provides an excellent example of what can go wrong if there is even a single error in a gene. The disease called sickle-cell anemia is the result of a single mistake in the gene for the beta-globin subunit of hemoglobin: the sixth codon is GTG instead of GAG. As a result, the sixth amino acid is valine instead of glutamic acid. The mutant hemoglobin works normally under normal conditions. But if the oxygen levels in the blood drop too low, these abnormal hemoglobin molecules tend to clump together within the red blood cell. As a result, the red blood cells become distorted and lose their elasticity. These stiff, sickle-shaped red blood cells can end up blocking small blood vessels, thus cutting off blood flow and leading to tissue damage. The sickle cells have an abnormally short life span, which is why the person ends up anemic.

Some viruses have their genes in the form of a double strand of DNA, just like the genes of living cells. However, most viruses have their genes in a single strand of RNA. In some single-strand RNA viruses, the information encoded in the RNA is in the positive sense, just as in the messenger RNA of the cell. In other kinds of viruses, the RNA is in the negative sense and must be transcribed into positive-sense RNA, with the help of RNA polymerase. Some viruses have a double strand of RNA, which would thus contain the positive and negative sense.

Retroviruses are a particular kind of RNA virus. The prefix *retro-* means reverse. In normal cell metabolism, DNA is used as a template for making messenger RNA, which then is used to make protein. Thus, the usual order is DNA → RNA → protein. In contrast, a retrovirus uses an enzyme called reverse transcriptase to make DNA from its RNA. That DNA is then permanently incorporated into the cell's DNA. With retroviruses, the sequence goes like this: RNA → DNA → RNA → protein.

If the retrovirus infects a cell that gives rise to sperm or egg cells, the newly incorporated gene, called a provirus, can be passed on to the next generation as part of the genome. Geneticists believe that many of our genes came originally from the retroviruses that infected our ancestors.

Viruses that have their genes in the form of RNA tend to mutate far more quickly than double-stranded DNA viruses. The reason is twofold. First, DNA is more chemically stable than RNA. Second, a double strand of DNA carries two copies of the same information: each strand contains a complement of the information on the other strand. If one strand gets damaged, the damage can sometimes be repaired by a cellular enzyme called DNA polymerase, which uses information from the complementary strand of DNA. Although cells have a proofreading mechanism for finding and fixing some errors in DNA, they are far less effective at finding and fixing errors in RNA. As a result, single-stranded RNA viruses can mutate more quickly.

A mutation can happen in any gene. Yet if you compare the genes of distantly related species, you often find that some genes seem to change remarkably little over thousands or even millions of years. Biologists say that such genes are highly conserved. If a gene is highly conserved, you can be confident that it does something that is important for the survival of the organism and that doesn't allow room for error. Thus, any mutations to that gene would probably be lethal. Organisms carrying such mutations would die. Thus, natural selection would weed out such mutations.

On the other hand, some other kinds of genes seem to mutate very fast. The genes for the outer proteins of a flu virus are a perfect example. The viruses that have last year's versions of those proteins tend to die out because so many people are already immune to them. In contrast, the mutants with proteins that the potential hosts' immune systems have never seen before are the ones most likely to survive.

In summary, single-strand RNA viruses like the influenza virus can mutate faster than double-strand DNA viruses because their genes are less stable. Yet even a single-strand RNA virus can remain stable genetically if any mutants are weeded out by natural selection. That could explain why the measles virus stays so stable, despite being a single-stranded RNA virus. On the other hand, even minor mutations can sometimes give a virus an adaptive advantage by making the virus unrecognizable to a host that was previously infected by that virus's ancestors. It's hard to develop an effective vaccine against a rapidly mutating virus, such as an influenza virus or HIV. That's why the vaccine against last year's predominant strain of flu might be ineffective against this year's predominant strain of flu. It's also why it's so hard to produce an effective vaccine against HIV.

To study viruses, you need to be able to produce them in a laboratory. Of course, you cannot just put some viruses in a dish with nutrients and expect them to divide naturally. Viruses are produced only in living cells. Theoretically, you could infect a living animal with the virus, but that would be inefficient, not to mention pointlessly cruel. A better way would be to get some of the right kinds of cells to grow in culture, and then use the cell culture to produce viruses. The right kinds of cell would have to have the right kind of protein on its surface, so that the virus can enter the cell.

Before a poliovirus virion can enter a cell, it must first attach to a protein called CD155. This protein is found only on the cells of human beings, apes, and some Old World monkeys. For that reason, poliovirus can infect human beings but cannot infect any of our domestic animals. Apes and Old World monkeys can be experimentally infected with polio. However, wild apes don't get polio. They don't live in the kind of dense, settled communities that would allow the virus to keep circulating among them.

To produce poliovirus virions, you must get cells that express CD155 to live in a laboratory. Unfortunately, those cells must come from an animal that could be infected with other viruses. Also, those cells were not designed to live in a laboratory dish. To keep those cells alive, you often need to feed them some sort of blood product from some other living animal. Thus, you run the risk that your viral culture will end up infected by some other virus.

The original polio vaccines were made from viruses that were produced in kidney tissue from rhesus monkeys. Unfortunately, that tissue was sometimes contaminated by a virus called SV40, which causes tumors in rodents. I explain the SV40 problem in detail in chapter 21.

Vaccine makers and public health officials must always be on the lookout for contamination of vaccines. As I will explain in chapter 30, a contaminated yellow fever vaccine that was used during World War II caused an outbreak of hepatitis B. However, that contamination resulted from the use of human blood plasma from infected donors as a stabilizer, not from contamination of the cells that produced the vaccine virus. (Back then, there were no tests for hepatitis B infection.)

Fortunately, the viral contamination of the cell cultures used in vaccine production has not led to significant public health problems. The risk of these problems is low for several reasons. First, the contaminant would have to evade detection. The FDA and its European counterpart require the materials used in making vaccines to be tested for viral contamination. The methods used for this purpose are becoming increasingly sensitive. Second, the vaccine product undergoes processes intended to purify the vaccine virus. As a result, the final product may not contain a big enough dose of the contaminant to outrun the patient's immune system and produce a clinical infection. Third, the contaminant would have to survive the vaccine production process without losing its infectivity. For example, most if not all viruses would be inactivated by the processes used in making "killed" vaccines. Fourth, the virus would have to be able to infect the cells of its new host. (If a virus cannot infect human cells, it cannot cause a disease in human beings). Fifth, even if the virus could infect some human cells, the vaccination would have to deliver the virus to the right kinds of cells within the host. Fortunately, it would be highly unusual for a vaccine to deliver a large enough dose of an undetected contaminant to the right kinds of cells to create a problem. Nevertheless, public health officials need to pay careful attention to vaccine safety. I'll explain more about vaccine safety in general in chapter 16.

Few drugs have any effect on viral infections. The reasons are simple. First, it's hard to "kill" the undead. Second, viruses have no cell wall, no cell membrane, and no metabolic processes. Thus, they provide few obvious targets for drugs to hit. Furthermore, viruses hijack the host cell's metabolic machinery. It's hard to find a drug that would interfere with viral replication without disrupting all of the cells in the host's body.

There are three basic kinds of antiviral drugs. A few work by jamming the molecules that a particular virus uses for attaching to a host cell. Thus, they block the virus from entering a new host cell. Other antiviral drugs work by interfering with the production of new viral DNA within the cell, usually by looking enough like a nucleotide to fool the viral enzymes but not the host cell's enzymes. Still other antiviral drugs work by boosting the host's immune response.

The introduction of highly active antiretroviral therapy (HAART) led to a sharp decrease in death rates among HIV-infected people. Yet the drugs themselves have side effects. Some of those side effects are serious and potentially life-threatening. Thus, it would be far better to prevent HIV infection than to treat it with drugs. Unfortunately, we still have no effective vaccine to prevent HIV infection.

14

Vaccines and the Immune System

Fresh meat starts to spoil within hours. However, living flesh stays fresh for years or decades because living organisms have an immune system that fights the bacteria and fungi that would otherwise cause decomposition. Everything you eat and drink, everything you touch, and even the air you breathe is teeming with germs. Yet remarkably few of them pose any threat to your body. Most bacteria and viruses have simply never figured out how to use the human body as a host. Most of those that can use us as a host have never figured out how to get past our innate immune system, which is our first line of defense. As a result, most bacteria and fungi have no success in attacking us, at least until we die. As soon as we die, bacteria and fungi start to work to break down our tissue. They can do that because the blood stops circulating. At death, the bloodstream stops delivering the oxygen and nutrients that our bodies' cells need and taking away waste products. It also stops delivering antibodies and white blood cells to fight infection. Just like any piece of meat, dead tissue immediately starts to spoil. Yet a living person can go for many years without suffering any serious infections.

Only a small, elite group of bacteria and viruses cause infectious diseases. These bacteria and viruses have inherited the ability to use the human body as a host as well as the ability to get past our innate immune system, at least for a while. Fortunately, we are not completely defenseless against these dangerous germs. Besides our innate immune system, we have an adaptive immune system that learns to recognize particular germs and develop a custom-tailored response to fight each one.

The concept behind vaccination is simple. For centuries, observant people have known that there are some diseases that you can catch only once. For example, if you have already had a case of smallpox, you can never get smallpox again. You will be immune to smallpox for the rest of your life. Unfortunately, that one case of smallpox could kill, disfigure, or blind you. For at least a thousand years, people have been trying to figure out how to give someone the mildest possible case of smallpox: a case that would lead to lifelong immunity but without causing illness, disfigurement, disability, and death. The ultimate goal was to find some way to allow the body to develop protective immunity without ever feeling sick.

About a thousand years ago, people in China and India tried to immunize people against smallpox by having them inhale the powdered, dried scabs from someone with a mild case of smallpox. A few hundred years ago, someone in Asia or Africa realized that it was far safer and probably more effective to take some of the pus from someone with smallpox and scratch it into the skin of the person they wanted to immunize. This procedure was called variolation because it exposed people to genuine smallpox, which was called variola.

Scratching the infectious material into the skin was safer than having people inhale it, which we now know is the natural route of smallpox infection. Introducing the virus through the skin probably gave the person's adaptive immune system a head start. That head start is crucial. It allows the immune system to develop an effective adaptive immune response before the infection gets big enough to cause serious problems.

The innate immune system is a primitive system that responds to any kind of threat, regardless of whether you have encountered that threat before. The simple barrier provided by the skin is part of the innate immune system. So are the mucus and tears that wash the moist surfaces of the body. The innate immune system also includes the white blood cells that patrol the body, looking for anything that doesn't belong. They attack anything that looks foreign.

Some of the defense mechanisms that are part of our innate immune system can be unpleasant. Coughing, sneezing, vomiting, and diarrhea help the body rid itself of dangerous substances. Fever helps to fight certain kinds of infections. So even if your innate immune system is killing the germs, you can feel awful. The inflammatory response, which is produced by the innate immune system, causes unpleasant symptoms such as redness, heat, swelling, and pain. If an inflammatory response gets out of control, it can do more harm than good.

Many drugs have anti-inflammatory effects. They may make you feel better, but they tend to suppress the immune system. People who are taking drugs that suppress the immune system are particularly susceptible to some infections. As a result, they should not be given "live" vaccines. Thus, they must rely on herd immunity.

The human innate immune system does a remarkably good job in protecting the human body against most germs, but it is no match for something like smallpox. The adaptive immune system can deal with smallpox, but it might not be able to do it fast enough to prevent illness, horrible scars, blindness, and death. The purpose of vaccination is to prepare the adaptive immune system so that it will be able to fight off a real infection. Ideally, the adaptive immune system responds so efficiently that you would never know that anything was happening.

The adaptive immune system itself has two components: humoral immunity and cell-mediated immunity. Humoral immunity involves the production of antibodies, which can interact with germs that are in the bodily fluids, outside of the body's cells. (The word *humor* refers to bodily fluids.) Antibodies, which are also called immunoglobulins, are large, Y-shaped proteins that have been specifically designed to bind to a particular substance. For example, an antibody might bind to some protein or to some polysaccharide, such as the polysaccharides in a bacterial capsule.

There are five different classes of antibodies: immunoglobulin A (IgA), IgD, IgE, IgG, and IgM. IgA plays a major role in immunity at the mucous membranes. IgD seems to play a role in fighting respiratory infections. IgE, which is found only in mammals, is important in fighting parasites such as worms and protozoa. It is also responsible for allergic reactions. IgG is a relatively small molecule that can be found in blood and throughout the body's tissues. IgG is the only kind of antibody that passes through the placenta to protect the fetus. Colostrum, which is the type of milk that a mother produces immediately after giving birth, is particularly rich in IgG. IgM is a large molecule found mainly in blood.

Antibodies are made by B lymphocytes, which are also called B cells. Like all white blood cells, B cells are created in the bone marrow. When young, "naïve" B cells are exposed to an antigen, some of them dedicate themselves to producing antibodies to that particular antigen, and only that antigen. Then, they divide to produce a population of B cells that are dedicated to that antigen. Most of those cells will become plasma cells, which then go on to produce lots of antibodies. Plasma cells devote so many of their resources to making antibodies that they don't survive long. A few of the B cells will become B memory cells, which will survive for an average of 10 years. That's why the effects of a vaccination can last for years.

Antibodies can do several things to fight an infection. Sometimes, the antibodies can disable a germ or toxin by sticking to some important protein. Antibodies can even cause the germs and other things to clump together (agglutination). Antibodies can also trigger a set of proteins called the membrane attack complex to punch holes in the cell membrane of a bacterium. Antibodies can also mark a germ for destruction by white blood cells.

Each antibody is designed in response to a particular antigen. However, the antibodies that are made against one antigen can sometimes cross-react with some other, similar antigen. For example, the cowpox virus looks enough like the smallpox virus that antibodies to cowpox protect you against smallpox as well. In contrast, the influenza virus mutates so quickly that the antibodies that you made to last year's strain of influenza virus might not protect you against this year's strain.

However, if the influenza vaccine provides even a partial match, it can give you some protection, partly because of cross-reaction and partly because of a phenomenon called affinity maturation. The genes that a B cell uses for making antibodies are about a million times more prone to mutation than other genes are. This phenomenon is called somatic hypermutation. Because of these mutations, some B cells make antibodies that provide a better fit to a particular antigen. During an immune response, the B cells that produce the best antibodies can outcompete other B cells. This process is called clonal selection. As a result, the B cells evolve to produce better and better antibodies to the antigens the body encounters. This improvement in the antibodies is called affinity maturation.

Unfortunately, some foreign antigens look a lot like proteins from our own bodies. Examples include some proteins from the bacteria that cause strep throat and some proteins that come from our food. The antibodies that your body makes to those proteins could end up attacking your own body. That problem is called an autoimmune disease.

Antibodies are very good at fighting germs that are outside of cells. However, they can do nothing about germs that have entered a cell. To fight the infections that occur within cells, especially the ones that can survive inside white blood cells, you need something called cell-mediated immunity. Cell-mediated immunity also plays an important role in fighting fungal infections, certain parasites, and cancers. It also attacks any foreign tissue, such as transplanted organs.

Cell-mediated immunity does not involve antibodies. Instead, it involves various kinds of white blood cells, including natural killer cells as well as cytotoxic T lymphocytes. These cells seek out and destroy the cells that have antigens that suggest that they are infected or cancerous. Cell-mediated immunity also involves various signaling chemicals called cytokines. Some of them can tell a damaged or abnormal cell to self-destruct.

Cytokines are small proteins that serve as messengers in cell-to-cell communication within the immune system. Cytokines can act on the cells that secrete them (autocrine action). They can also act on nearby cells (paracrine action) or on distant cells (endocrine action). For example, some cytokines attract certain white blood cells to come to the scene of an infection. Some cytokines can also tell certain abnormal cells to self-destruct.

Some cytokines can also trigger other cells within the immune system to release even more cytokines. This positive-feedback loop can greatly amplify the immune system's response to a challenge. The body has ways to regulate this process. Unfortunately, some infectious diseases can cause the process to spiral out of control, thus producing a cytokine storm. Some experts suspect that many of the healthy young adults who died in the Great Pandemic of 1918 actually died because the influenza virus infection triggered a cytokine storm.

Vaccines are generally good at getting the immune system to produce antibodies. However, many of them do not provide cell-mediated immunity. Thus, it would be hard to develop an effective vaccine against germs that infect white blood cells, such as the bacteria that cause tuberculosis and the HIV virus that causes AIDS. Thus, it's not surprising that vaccination against tuberculosis had only a limited effect and that there is not yet an effective vaccine against HIV.

Vaccination has come a long way since the days when doctors scratched some pus from a sick person into a healthy person's skin. Modern vaccines are far cleaner and far safer. Furthermore, modern science has made it possible to make vaccines against a much broader range of diseases. Yet all vaccines are based on the same principle: they expose the body to an antigen from a dangerous germ so that the adaptive immune system will be able to fight the germ in case of a real infection.

Variolation and vaccination did cause an infection, though one that is milder than the natural smallpox infection. In contrast, a vaccine made out of dead bacteria or "killed" (inactivated) viruses does not cause an infection at all. Many modern vaccines contain only selected proteins or carbohydrates from a germ. Many of these proteins are made through genetic engineering and have never been in contact with the dangerous germ itself. Thus, these vaccines can never transmit that germ. Nevertheless, these vaccines give the adaptive immune system an opportunity to prepare to fight the live germs in case of a real infection.

It may seem far safer to use "killed" vaccines than "live" vaccines. In fact, "live" vaccines are too risky for use in pregnant women and people with a suppressed immune system. So why are "live" vaccines used at all? The reason is simple: "live" vaccines can provide a more powerful and longer-lasting immune response. Also, the "live" vaccine may be better at producing an immune response at the mucous membranes, which are the moist surfaces that line the body cavities, such as the gastrointestinal and respiratory tracts. These are the sites where most infections enter the body. Some "live" vaccines are injected. Others are given by mouth or are sprayed or dripped into the nose.

In 1952, Jonas Salk developed a killed polio vaccine. Then in 1957, Albert Sabin introduced a live polio vaccine. As I'll explain in detail in chapter 21, both the "killed" vaccine and the "live" vaccine have their upsides and downsides. The "live" vaccine is useful for stopping the spread of poliovirus. However, the "live" vaccine poses more risk than the "killed" vaccine does.

When I was a child, I thought that the oral polio vaccine was a work of sheer genius. I much preferred eating a sugar cube to having a needle stuck in my arm! I wondered why more vaccines weren't available on sugar cubes. The reason is simple. Most vaccines would be broken down by your stomach acid and digestive enzymes before your immune system ever got a chance to look at them.

The oral polio vaccine worked because poliovirus normally infects the gut. Wild poliovirus normally spreads mainly by the fecal-oral route. It is very good at surviving its trip through the human stomach. If it weren't, then polio would never have been such a threat to public health. The other vaccines that are available for oral administration are also for gut infections, such as rotavirus and cholera.

Some "live" vaccines for respiratory infections, such as some influenza vaccines, can be sprayed or dripped into the nose. Like the oral vaccines for gut infections, the intranasal vaccines for respiratory infections deliver live but harmless germs to the normal site of a natural infection. These oral and intranasal vaccines are all "live" vaccines. They contain live (but weakened) bacteria or attenuated viruses that are intended to create an infection that is harmless but nevertheless leads to long-lasting immunity.

Since the germ from a "live" vaccine is expected to multiply in the body to create a harmless infection, the dose of germs that you get from a "live" vaccine is small. Ideally, the infection will involve the tissues that the wild germ would normally infect. The more closely the vaccine-induced infection mimics a natural infection, the stronger and longer-lasting the resulting immune response is likely to be.

Although the "live" vaccines tend to produce strong, long-lasting immunity, especially at the sites where the dangerous germs are most likely to enter the body, they do have some serious drawbacks. One is that they can cause disease in people who have a suppressed immune system. Thus, they should not be given to people with immune system problems or to pregnant women. They should be used with caution in the household contacts of people with immune system problems. Fortunately, people with immune system problems can receive "killed" vaccines, which are made out of dead bacteria or out of viruses that can no longer be reproduced by a living cell.

During 20th century, advances in scientific knowledge made it possible to create vaccines that do not contain whole germs, not even dead ones. The first of these vaccines were against bacterial toxins. By 1900, scientists understood that some bacterial diseases are not due to the bacterium itself but to some toxin (poison) that the bacterium produces. Examples include diphtheria, tetanus, and whooping cough.

Once scientists isolated those toxins, they found that they could make an animal such as a horse immune to the toxin by giving the horse a dose of toxin that had been damaged by heating. Then, an extract of that horse's blood could be used as a drug to treat people who were suffering from that disease. The antibody-rich horse serum is called an antitoxin. Similar products are made from human blood serum to protect people who have just been exposed to hepatitis A, hepatitis B, chickenpox, or measles. These products are called immune globulin or gamma globulin. They have to be given by injection.

Antitoxins and immune globulin provide passive immunity. Passive immunity means that the individual is being protected by someone else's antibodies. Passive immunity occurs in nature when a baby is protected by its mother's antibodies. Before birth, the fetus receives some antibodies through the placenta. After birth, the infant can receive antibodies in breast milk. Passive immunity can help to protect a young mammal, but it can also interfere with the effectiveness of some vaccines. Puppies cannot mount their own immune response to some vaccinations, especially the parvovirus vaccine, until after their mothers' antibodies have been cleared from their system.

After the antitoxins were developed, someone realized that an antitoxin could be combined with the toxin itself to make a reasonably safe and effective vaccine, called a toxin-antitoxin. The toxin would cause the vaccinated person's immune system to make antibodies to the toxin. The antitoxin would then help protect the person from getting sick from the vaccine itself.

Later on, someone realized that you could denature the toxin by treating it with formaldehyde. The formaldehyde damaged the toxin enough that it could no longer cause damage in the body. In other words, the formaldehyde detoxified the toxin, thus turning it into a toxoid. Antibodies that the body produced in response to the toxoid could neutralize the toxin produced by an infection. Today, the vaccinations against diphtheria, whooping cough, and tetanus are made from toxoids. A toxoid made from rattlesnake venom is used to vaccinate dogs against rattlesnake bite.

During the late 20th century, scientists knew enough about the chemistry of bacteria and viruses that they could pinpoint which particular proteins or carbohydrates in the germ were responsible for causing the body to mount a protective immune response. Thus, they could make vaccines that contain only those proteins or carbohydrates, rather than the whole germ. These vaccines are called subunit vaccines.

Subunit vaccines can be produced by two different methods. One is to take the killed bacteria or viruses and break them down chemically, then extract the particular antigens that you need. The other way is to find the genes that provide the recipe for the antigens that you want. You can then put those genes in a bacterium or yeast and get them to make huge quantities of those antigens, which can then be purified. Vaccines made by that method are called recombinant vaccines.

Lately, there has been a vocal movement against the use of any genetically modified organisms (GMOs). Many people are concerned that GMOs are entering the food supply without having been adequately tested. I share that concern. The very first GMO product to hit the market was a tryptophan supplement that contained an unexpected contaminant that caused a disease called eosinophilia myalgia syndrome, which ended up killing about three dozen people and disabling about 1500 more. It makes sense to test GMO products before they go on the market. Fortunately, the GMOs that are used in pharmaceuticals are heavily tested before they go on the market and are subject to postmarketing surveillance, just like any other prescription drug.

If you make any new vaccine or other new drug, whether it is from a GMO or not, that product has to undergo extensive testing for efficacy and safety. Even after the product goes on the market, the FDA will keep track of any safety complaints against it. In contrast, if someone develops a genetically modified version of an edible plant, such as soybeans, that genetically modified plant will be assumed to be substantially similar to conventional soybeans unless it is known to contain something that would be regulated as a food additive.

In other words, many people are concerned that GMO foods are not being adequately tested before they go on the market. In contrast, all drugs and vaccines—GMO or otherwise—are extensively tested before they go on the market. They are carefully scrutinized afterward, as well.

Subunit vaccines have some upsides and some downsides. One big upside is that they do not contain the whole germ. The recombinant vaccines have never been in contact with the germ at all. That's a major selling point for a vaccine against germs that cause a dangerous chronic infection, such as HPV or HIV. Another upside is that some subunit vaccines do not interfere with testing for the disease itself. Some subunit vaccines produce an antibody profile that is different from that produced by the natural infection. Thus, laboratory testing could show whether a person or animal has ever been infected with the wild germ.

Unfortunately, subunit vaccines have some of the same downsides as any other "killed" vaccine. They may not provide strong or long-lasting immunity, and they may not provide immunity at the mucous membranes. Furthermore, if a subunit vaccine doesn't include the right subunits, or if those subunits lose their shape if they are removed from the whole germ, then the vaccine won't work at all. That's why vaccines must be tested for effectiveness, as I'll explain in chapter 16.

"Killed" vaccines, toxoids, and subunit vaccines tend to produce less of an immune response than "live" vaccines do. To compensate for that weakness, vaccine manufacturers put in additives that are intended to produce a mild inflammatory response. These substances are called adjuvants, which means helpers. Antivaccination zealots make a huge fuss about the adjuvants used in vaccines. I'll explain them in more detail in chapter 16.

Many modern vaccine products are polyvalent, which means that several vaccines are combined into one shot. The measles-mumps-rubella shot immunizes you against three different viruses at once. The Gardasil 9 vaccine is a recombinant vaccine that is supposed to cover nine different strains of human papillomavirus.

Some people are concerned that the recommended vaccination schedule would overload a child's system with so many vaccine antigens. Yet it is extremely rare for the recommended vaccines to cause any problems with the immune system. (In contrast, some of the vaccine-preventable diseases do often cause serious problems with the immune system. It's one of the reasons why they make people so sick.) Nor would you expect to see any such effect from vaccination. The vaccine antigens are only a tiny fraction of the antigens that a baby or young child encounters. After all, there are more bacteria on the inner and outer surfaces of the human body than there are cells in the human body.

Because of the discontinuation of smallpox vaccination and the refinement of vaccine products, children are actually exposed to fewer vaccine antigens today than they were a few decades ago. Today's vaccination schedule would expose a child to a total of 315 vaccine antigens.

In contrast, children were exposed to several thousand vaccine antigens in the 1990s. Thus, the argument that the vaccination schedule is exposing children to too many antigens too soon is simply ridiculous.

When I was a child, I thought that it was good to have several vaccinations combined into one shot. I'd rather get one shot against measles, mumps, and rubella than get three separate shots. However, some antivaccination activists have claimed that these polyvalent vaccines are a bad idea. They insist that if you have to have vaccines, each one should be in a different shot. Yet these polyvalent vaccine products have undergone safety and efficacy testing. We really do have evidence of their safety. We should rely on the results of real clinical studies of these vaccines.

Some people believe that only unhealthy people get sick from vaccine-preventable diseases. There is only a small grain of truth in that argument. People who are in generally poor health often are at increased risk of death from infectious disease. People with a damaged immune system may even be at risk for opportunistic infections, which are infectious diseases that cannot gain a toehold in a healthy person. However, some infections seem to be particularly severe among healthy young adults. The influenza strain that caused the Great Pandemic of 1918-1919 was one example. It did kill the very young and the very old. However, it also cut down a surprisingly large number of healthy young adults. That's why public health authorities seem to be so paranoid about influenza viruses that look like the 1918 strain, as well as influenza virus strains that have never infected humans before.

Some antivaccination activists argue that if you take proper care of the body, such as by eating a healthy diet, your body will be able to fight off all of the vaccine-preventable diseases without help from vaccines. I often hear this argument from mothers who describe themselves as "natural" or even "crunchy." Basically, their argument is this. If they live a healthy, natural lifestyle, breast-feed their children, and then feed their children plenty of homemade food and homegrown organic vegetables, the children will be automatically immune to vaccine-preventable disease. The women who make this argument are generally uneducated in history and biology.

If living a natural lifestyle and eating homemade food and organic homegrown vegetables were enough to prevent epidemic disease, then epidemic disease would simply not have been a problem for people in Colonial America. In particular, it would never have decimated the indigenous people. Yet after the Europeans came, bringing smallpox, measles, and yellow fever with them, epidemic diseases devastated the indigenous populations. English Puritans were able to establish colonies in Massachusetts because so many of the indigenous people had just died because of epidemics of smallpox and measles.

History teaches us that germs can attack healthy people. You can learn that lesson from reading about the early days of the AIDS epidemic, if you aren't old enough to remember it personally. Thousands of previously healthy young men fell ill and died. It was such a tragic loss. We must never forget.

15

Crunching the Numbers

Hippocrates taught us how important it is to learn from careful observation of individual patients. Today, we have the statistical methods and computing power to analyze data about large numbers of people. We can then use the results of those calculations to help us answer questions, including questions about cause and effect. Once you know what is happening to large groups of people, you can use that information to figure out the odds of what is likely to happen to yourself and your children. You can also use that information to make rational arguments to guide public health policy.

This idea of using statistics about disease rates and death rates when making decisions about vaccination is hardly new. Back in 1760, the great French mathematician Daniel Bernoulli crunched the numbers on smallpox. Back then, the smallpox inoculation (variolation) could lead to an actual case of deadly smallpox because it uses pus from a smallpox patient. Yet even that primitive means of immunization was far less dangerous than a natural case of smallpox, which was a major cause of death in France back then. In the United States, General George

Washington came to the same conclusion. In 1777, he issued an order for immediate variolation for everyone in the Continental Army who wasn't already immune to smallpox. It was a risky decision. It meant that many of his men would be incapacitated until they recovered from the immunization. However, some military historians believe that it was the most important strategic decision that Washington made during the Revolutionary War.

In the 1770s, immunization against smallpox involved infectious material from a patient with actual smallpox. In 1796, immunization against smallpox became much safer with the development of vaccination, which involved the cowpox virus, not the smallpox virus. As the vaccinia virus was refined, immunization against smallpox became increasingly safe. Yet it was never perfectly safe because it did involve the use of a "live" virus.

By the 1970s, vaccine policy in the United States shifted. Although the immunization procedure had become much safer, the risk of catching smallpox had dropped to zero. Once smallpox became extinct, there was no point in immunizing anyone against it. Thus, even the small risk associated with vaccination was no longer worthwhile. By the early 1970s, smallpox had not been seen in the United States for decades. It was even being stamped out in its last refuges in Africa and Asia. As a result, in 1971 the public health officials in the United States stopped recommending routine smallpox vaccination for children.

Many antivaccination activists claim that vaccination policy is driven purely by the profit motives of the pharmaceutical industry. Some of them even insist that smallpox was never really eradicated. Thus, they have to hide the fact that the U.S. Public Health Service decided in 1971 that routine smallpox vaccination for children in the United States should be discontinued.

If you want to get involved in discussions about vaccine policy, you ought to learn how to crunch some of the numbers for yourself. To do that, you must understand some basic concepts about health statistics. In this chapter, I'll spell out those basic concepts.

If you are a doctor, you are concerned about the health of your patients, one patient at a time. You want to know if your patient has a particular disease, how sick that patient is likely to get, how long the illness is likely to last, and whether the patient recovers or dies. On the other hand, if you are a public health official, your "patient" is the entire population. You will want to know how many people in the population are getting sick and from what diseases, how sick they get, how long they stay sick, and whether they recover or die. If you want to keep track of how these things are changing over time, or if you want to compare your population with another population, you will have to express those numbers as some sort of proportion or ratio. For a common disease, you would use percentages. For a less common disease, you may express the numbers as cases per 100,000 people.

The first question is how many people are getting sick. There are two ways to approach that question. The first is to figure out the **incidence** of a disease, which means the proportion of the population who get sick with that disease within a certain period of time, usually a year. Incidence is often expressed as the number of affected people per 100,000 people per year. That way, you can see how the risk of getting that disease changes over time or how it varies between countries at any given point in time.

Some diseases come and go within a matter of days or weeks. Other diseases can last for years. When you are studying a disease that can last a long time, you will be interested in the **prevalence** of that disease, which refers to the number of people who have that disease at any point in time. Like incidence, prevalence is also often expressed as the number of affected people per 100,000 people during a given year.

Like incidence, prevalence reflects how many people get sick. If the incidence of new cases of a disease drops to zero, then the prevalence of the disease will also eventually drop to zero, as the people with existing cases of the disease either recover or die. However, prevalence also reflects how long people stay sick. If a disease comes and goes within a week or so, then only a small percentage of the population will have that disease at any given point in time, even if many people will have the disease at some point during that year.

The prevalence of disease can tell you several important things. First of all, it can tell you how many people need some sort of medical care at any given time. For a contagious disease, the prevalence can also help you predict what the incidence of the disease is going to be in the future. For example, if you rapidly find and cure all cases of a potentially long-lasting contagious disease, such as tuberculosis, then the infected people are less likely to pass the disease on to someone else. If, on the other hand, infected people stay sick for a longer time, they can infect a lot more people. If the prevalence of a contagious disease that exists only in humans drops to zero, the incidence of that disease will also be zero, forever. The disease will be extinct.

Smallpox has been driven into extinction by vaccination. So has rinderpest, a viral disease that affected cattle. Polio has been driven to the brink of extinction by vaccination. Measles, mumps, and rubella could also be driven into extinction by vaccination. Once a disease has become extinct, there's no further need to vaccinate anyone against it.

Public health authorities are also concerned about how sick a sick person gets. In medicine, the person's state of illness is called morbidity. In practical terms, morbidity means the suffering that a sick person experiences. The morbidity that any given person experiences from having an infection can vary dramatically. For example, many people who are infected with wild poliovirus have no symptoms at all. Others have a mild "stomach flu" that goes away in a few days. Still others end up with paralysis. The paralysis could be merely a slight limp. Or it could be so severe that the person cannot move his or her arms and legs and needs a ventilator to breathe. It's fairly easy to count up how many people die, but how could you reduce all of that other information to a single number?

It's even harder to calculate the burden of disease for a whole population. Burden of disease is a concept that includes all of the bad things that result from the occurrence of that disease. Besides morbidity and mortality, it includes healthcare costs and lost productivity. All of these things are important but are hard to measure. To measure the burden of disease, public health experts have worked out measures such as disability-adjusted life years (DALY), quality-adjusted life years (QALY), and years lost to disability (YLD).

It's easy to tell when someone is dead. However, it can be hard to figure out why that person died. In the early days of the AIDS epidemic, many AIDS patients died of a rare form of pneumonia. Their death certificates may have said pneumonia, but the real cause of death was AIDS. As a result, many of the first deaths from AIDS were hidden among the deaths from pneumonia. After the HIV test came out and HIV infection became a reportable disease, we started getting much better data on the number of people who were dying as a result of HIV/AIDS.

A reportable disease is one that doctors and laboratories must report to the public health authorities whenever they diagnose it. In the United States, doctors must now report every single case of HIV/AIDS and most of the vaccine-preventable diseases to the Centers for Disease Control and Prevention, as well as to their state and local health departments. As a result, we now have good data on the number of people who get a reportable disease, as well as the number of people who die from a reportable disease.

Unfortunately, even many cases of reportable disease go unreported because many mild cases are never properly diagnosed. This problem is called the iceberg phenomenon. An iceberg is a big chunk of ice that is floating in the ocean. You can easily see the portion of the iceberg that sticks up out of the water. Yet most of the iceberg remains hidden underwater. Likewise, the number of diagnosed cases of any given disease might represent the tip of the iceberg. Many more cases may go unrecognized or at least unreported. For example, many mild cases of pertussis (whooping cough) can be mistaken for a common cold. Most cases of poliovirus infection produce no symptoms at all. About 4% to 8% of cases produce a mild nonspecific illness. Only about 1 in 200 cases result in paralysis. Likewise, foodborne infections generally go unreported unless someone ends up dead or hospitalized.

The iceberg phenomenon is a serious problem when you are trying to estimate morbidity from a disease. It can even be a problem when you are trying to calculate mortality. For example, I once tried to find out how many Americans were dying of pulmonary embolism. No one had reliable data, not even the epidemiologists at the Centers for Disease Control and Prevention. Fatal cases of pulmonary embolism can easily be misdiagnosed as heart attack unless an autopsy is performed, and autopsies are seldom performed if an elderly person seems to have died of natural causes. As a result, many cases of fatal pulmonary embolism are probably mistaken for heart attacks.

Mortality statistics tell you the proportion of a population who die within a given span of time. The disease-specific mortality rate tells you how many people die of a particular disease. All-cause mortality statistics tell you how many people died of any cause. Mortality statistics tell you how many people are dying, but they don't tell you how long people are living. To get an idea of how long people are living, you look at life expectancy data. Life expectancy represents the number of years of life remaining for people at a particular age. We usually calculate life expectancy at birth. In 1850, life expectancy at birth in the United States was only 37 years. It's now in the late 70s. The difference was mainly due to a decrease in deaths from infectious disease in childhood. Right now, Japan has the highest life expectancy in the world. In contrast, the United States ranks 40th.

Another way to look at mortality and life expectancy is to calculate the years of potential life lost from a particular disease. A person who dies of pneumonia at age 98 has not lost many years of potential life. A child who dies of pneumonia at age 2 has lost many decades of potential life.

The mortality statistics for a disease reflect two things: how many people get the disease and how deadly the disease is. Some diseases are far more deadly than others. One way to measure the deadliness of a disease is to calculate the case-fatality rate. You divide the number of fatal cases of a disease by the total number of cases of the disease. The case-fatality rate for the common cold is extremely low. In contrast, the case-fatality rate for Ebola is up to 90%.

The case-fatality rate can be hard to calculate if a disease is hard to diagnose. For example, many poliovirus infections cause no sign of illness at all. People tend to notice only the cases that result in paralysis or death. Sometimes, the estimated case-fatality rates for a new strain of flu are shockingly high. However, that high rate may be incorrect: many of the mild early cases may have been overlooked.

In 1620 (the year that the Pilgrims landed on Plymouth Rock), life expectancy in England was only about 35 years, mainly because about 30% of children died in infancy. Back then, many of the diseases that are now preventable by vaccination were common in childhood. When smallpox was endemic, most of its victims were children under five years old. Most people caught smallpox in early childhood. Many of them died, and the rest became immune to smallpox for life. The same went for other potentially deadly diseases, such as measles. Of course, these vaccine-preventable diseases weren't the only cause of death. Many children died from infections that they caught from drinking unclean water, drinking tainted milk, or eating contaminated food. Other children died from malnutrition, accidents, or abuse and neglect. We've made good progress against all of those causes of death.

After the development of germ theory, scientists and public health officials started working out many ways to prevent people from getting sick from infectious disease. Vaccination prevented people from catching and spreading many infectious diseases. Sewage treatment and chlorination of drinking water helped to stop the spread of cholera and typhoid fever. Meat inspection, pasteurization of milk, and general regulation of the food industry helped to prevent food poisoning such as botulism and food-borne infections such as tuberculosis and salmonella.

Germ theory led to improved treatments that reduced the case-fatality rate for many infectious diseases. For example, the development of antitoxins helped reduce deaths from tetanus and diphtheria, even before there was a vaccine to prevent them. The invention of antibiotics also helped save many lives. Although antibiotics do nothing against viruses, they can be helpful in treating the bacterial infections that often occur in the wake of some viral infections. All of these things combined to reduce death rates.

Some diseases even became a bit less deadly on their own. At the end of the 19th century, a much milder form of smallpox started circulating in the United States. It was called variola minor. It was a much less devastating disease than regular smallpox, or variola major. As a result, people with variola minor were better able to spread the disease. For that reason, variola minor became the predominant form of smallpox in the United States, although variola major was also still circulating.

Variola minor killed only about 1% of the people it infected, but the survivors were immune to variola major. As variola minor became the predominant form of smallpox in the United States, the case-fatality rate from smallpox went down, even before better vaccination coverage wiped out both forms of smallpox.

In pre-industrial societies, death rates were high, particularly among children. However, birth rates were also high. As a result, the size of the population tended to remain stable. However, germ theory provided many ways to save lives, particularly the lives of young children. As a result, there were high birth rates and low death rates. The result was the population explosion. Now, birth rates have been dropping to match. In many industrialized countries, the birth rate is now below replacement level.

If you want to get involved in discussions about public health and vaccination policy, you really ought to learn a lot about history, biology, geography, and math. That knowledge will help you spot the lies and misrepresentations that come from antivaccination zealots. For example, many antivaccination activists point out that the death rate from measles started to decline before the measles vaccine was introduced. Of course it did, mainly as a result of improvements in treating the complications of measles, such as bacterial pneumonia. But from that fact, the antivaccination activists draw the false conclusion that vaccination is ineffective.

The measles can kill you directly because the measles virus can kill cells in vital organs. However, most of the deaths due to measles are really the result of complications of the measles. The measles virus can kill some of the cells that line the airways. Just as a scratch in the skin can lead to infection, this injury to the lining of the respiratory tract can make it easier for bacteria to infect the lungs. Also, the measles virus suppresses the immune system. The effects of this immune suppression can linger for a few years. As a result, many people have died of bacterial pneumonia they would not have had if they had not had measles. These infections are called opportunistic infections. They occur only because a germ took advantage of an opportunity created by the measles. The invention of antibiotics and fluid therapy helped keep measles patients from dying of these complications of measles. That's why the case-fatality rate for measles is lower in a rich country than in a poor country.

Unfortunately, not all of the complications of measles can be treated. Even with the best supportive care, a person can still die or end up blind, deaf, or brain-damaged from a case of measles. From 1989 to 1991, there was a resurgence of measles in North and Central America. During that period, 123 children in the United States died of measles. Ninety percent of those deaths were in people who had never been vaccinated against measles.

Today, measles is still common and deadly in Africa. That's because the case-fatality rate for measles is particularly high among people who are malnourished or suffering from malaria or other parasitic infection. The case-fatality rate for measles is about 30% among immunocompromised people, such as people with HIV infection.

The antivaccination activists occasionally mention death rates, even though such talk undermines their basic argument that measles is harmless. However, they never seem to tell the truth about two important kinds of statistics: the basic reproduction rate of a disease (R_0, pronounced "R naught") and the immunization levels required for herd immunity. These are crucial concepts to understand if you want to talk about preventing any contagious disease.

R_0 represents the average number of people who will catch the disease from an infected person. To calculate R_0, you use the following formula: $R_0 = C \times P \times D$

C = the number of contacts the infected person makes per unit of time (day, week, month, etc.)

P = the probability that a contact would become infected through that exposure to the infected person

D = the duration of time that the infected person is infectious to others

Back in the days before measles vaccination, the R_0 for a case of measles generally ranged from 12 to 18 cases. A person with a case of measles is most infectious in the four days before the rash appears. If an infected child spends those four days at a crowded church camp filled with unvaccinated children, the R_0 could be much higher, simply because of the high number of contacts with unvaccinated people.

For an epidemic to sustain itself, the average R_0 must be at least 1. Unless there is at least one new case to replace each infected person who either recovers or dies, the epidemic dies out. Epidemics generally die out when the proportion of the population that has become immune to the disease is $1 - 1/R_0$. So if the R_0 is somewhere in the range of 12 to 18, then you would need to immunize 92% to 94% of the population to keep the disease from sustaining itself. With that level of immunization, you might still have some small outbreaks, but they will be containable.

The fact that you can establish herd immunity with an immunization rate that is less than 100% provides an important margin of safety. It means that you can still protect the population against epidemics even if a few people are unvaccinated or a few people don't mount an immune response to vaccination.

Antivaccination activists often triumphantly point out that people sometimes catch diseases that they've been vaccinated against. Antivaccination zealots use information like that to argue that vaccinations don't work at all and that the whole vaccine industry is a fraud. Yet epidemiologists have always taken vaccine failure into account. Primary vaccine failure means that the vaccination never took—that the patient never developed a protective immune response. Primary vaccine failure can result from a problem in the vaccine or a problem in the patient. Secondary vaccine failure means that the effects of the vaccination wore off faster than expected. The effects of nearly all vaccinations decrease over time. One of the biggest challenges in epidemiology is to design vaccination schedules that would provide the most protection for the fewest number of jabs.

I am not an epidemiologist. However, I have read and edited many textbook chapters and journal articles about epidemiology. As a result, I can usually tell when someone who is writing about epidemiology is clueless. When the antivaccination activists talk about the death rates from measles, they make some glaring mistakes that nobody with any training in epidemiology would make. First of all, they ignore everything but death, which tells me that they do not care if people suffer. Second, they seem to think that completely preventable death is acceptable. Yet to me, the idea that any people are still dying of a disease that could be eradicated is simply appalling.

A case of measles is a miserable experience, even if it doesn't kill you, blind you, deafen you, or leave you with brain damage. That in itself would be a good reason for measles vaccination. The fact that measles can cause blindness, deafness, or brain damage is even more reason for children to be vaccinated against measles. Modern medicine has found ways to reduce the case-fatality rate from measles. However, it often means that the child will have to be hospitalized. In the United States, where many families have inadequate health insurance or none at all, a hospitalization could lead to bankruptcy. The antivaccination activists, in their zeal to scare people away from vaccination, ignore all that. They also ignore the fact that measles can be driven into extinction. After that, nobody will ever need to be vaccinated against measles. The invention of the measles vaccine made it possible to drive measles into extinction. The eradication of smallpox was humanity's greatest triumph. Humanity should be ashamed that measles still exists.

If you want to understand health policy, you must first learn about the health sciences, especially epidemiology. I've seen a few scientists who were respected for their laboratory work speak out against vaccination. Of those few, none were epidemiologists, and their antivaccination arguments were riddled with obviously false assumptions and silly errors in reasoning. If you read the scientific literature, you can find lively discussions about the risks and benefits of some vaccines, as well as discussions about the pluses and minuses of various vaccination strategies, particularly for influenza vaccination. Yet these discussions are generally based on thoughtful consideration of all of the available evidence. In contrast, the antivaccination activists start with the conclusion that vaccination is bad. Then, they may cherry-pick a few confusing facts from the scientific literature and make up a bunch of others to support that conclusion. However, once you understand the basic facts about infectious disease and epidemiology, you become immune to such nonsense.

Part III

The Politics of Vaccination

Whenever the characters in the television program *Gilligan's Island* faced some sort of problem that affected them all, they would talk openly about how to solve it. Any of the castaways could express an opinion. However, the Professor's opinion carried a lot more weight than anyone else's, at least on scientific issues. That system worked because the other castaways knew that they could trust the Professor. They could trust his knowledge, his scientific judgment, and his honesty.

The glamorous movie star Ginger Grant had a different skill set. She could frame any issue in terms of the plot of some Hollywood movie. However, everyone knew that Ginger was otherwise poorly educated, loved being the center of attention, and could be manipulative. They quickly learned that she could turn her seductive charm on and off like a light switch. The other castaways all loved Ginger, despite her obvious character flaws, but they respected the Professor. Yet in our society today, we are turning to poorly educated celebrities instead of to professors for guidance.

Vaccination is a political issue, precisely because each of us does not live alone on a desert island. We all live within each other's airspace. If someone with a case of measles coughs or even breathes near other people, those other people will be exposed to that virus. If you are unvaccinated against measles, you have a much higher chance of catching the measles from somebody else. If you catch the measles, you can spread it to others.

The measles vaccine is not 100% effective. Yet if a high enough percentage of the population is vaccinated, the measles stops circulating. If we vaccinate enough people around the world, then measles will go extinct. So when people refuse to get their children vaccinated against measles, they are helping to keep measles circulating. Because the measles vaccine is not 100% effective, the vaccine refusers are putting even the vaccinated people at risk.

As with any political issue, decisions about vaccine policy should be made through a transparent democratic process. But because complicated scientific issues are involved, we need to be guided by the professors. We need for our scientific institutions—governmental and nongovernmental—to guide and serve the public.

In my book *Not Trivial: How Studying the Traditional Liberal Arts Can Set You Free,* I devoted an entire chapter to the concept of institutional failure. When I say that some institution (e.g., a school or a foundation or even a for-profit textbook publisher) has failed as an institution, I don't mean that it went bankrupt or has ceased to exist. I mean that it has failed to serve the social purposes that a reasonable person would expect it to serve.

A textbook publisher that produces bad textbooks is a failure as a social institution, even if it is profitable as a business. Likewise, a pharmaceutical company would be a social failure if the products it sells are unsafe and/or ineffective. A public health agency of the government would be a social failure if it allowed a pharmaceutical company to sell unsafe or ineffective products.

All societies need to have some governmental institutions that serve public health. All societies also need citizen activists to serve as watchdogs, to ensure that the governmental institutions are really serving the public. In chapters 16 and 17, I talk about how our public health institutions in the United States deal with questions about vaccinations. In chapter 18, I talk about the history of the antivaccination movement. In chapter 19, I talk about how smallpox was eradicated, and how various governmental and nongovernmental organizations are attempting to eradicate other infectious diseases, so that no one will need to be vaccinated against them in the future.

16

Vaccine Safety

Every decision in medicine involves some sort of tradeoff between benefits and risks. To the scientific community, the benefits of the currently recommended vaccines are clear. (See Part IV for a discussion of how dangerous each of the vaccine-preventable diseases is.) Also, the risks associated with the vaccines themselves are remarkably small, thanks to tight regulation of the vaccine business. The risks are not zero, which is why I advocate eradication of the eradicable diseases. (Once a disease is eradicated, we can stop vaccinating against it.) Meanwhile, we must continue to vaccinate, to protect children against the risks associated with the vaccine-preventable diseases themselves. In this chapter, I explain how the FDA works to ensure that the vaccines that are available for use in the United States are effective and as safe as humanly possible.

Many antivaccination zealots have told me that vaccine makers never bother to test the vaccines that they sell. But in the United States, the FDA requires all vaccines to be extensively tested in human subjects before they go on the market. The testing is overseen by the FDA's

Center for Biologics Evaluation and Research. After the vaccine goes on the market, the FDA keeps track of all reports of adverse events associated with vaccines. The FDA may also require other kinds of studies, to establish whether a reported health problem, such as autism, really has any relationship to any vaccine. Other countries have similar regulatory agencies that demand similar studies of the vaccines to be sold within their borders.

When challenged, some antivaccination zealots may admit that a vaccine has been tested in human subjects, but then they claim that the vaccine was never compared to a placebo. That's a half-truth. Some studies do compare a new vaccine to a placebo. Still others compare a new vaccine to an injection that contains just the adjuvant. Still other studies compare a new vaccine to an old vaccine. The old vaccine is called an active control. Active controls are used because researchers are not allowed to expose research subjects to unnecessary risk.

The decision of what should be given to the control group in a study is not just a scientific question. It is also an ethical and legal question. It's not only immoral but illegal to ask research subjects to take unnecessary risks. This principle is clearly stated in the World Medical Association's Declaration of Helsinki, and it has been incorporated into law in many countries. So you can't ask someone to go without a tetanus shot just for the sake of some experiment.

Many people believe that the FDA turns a blind eye to the obvious dangers of vaccines. But in reality, the FDA oversees the research on all vaccines licensed in the United States and keeps careful track of all reports of bad things that reportedly happened to anyone who got any vaccine that is being used in the United States. As I'll explain in more detail below, the FDA sometimes takes action to prevent theoretical risks, even when there is no real evidence of an actual problem.

Vaccines are given to healthy people, especially to children, and are often required by law. For that reason, vaccines are held to a much higher standard of safety than many other medicinal products are. Fortunately, the risks of vaccination are amazingly low. Vaccines have been taken off the market in the United States because of extremely rare side effects. That's because the public health authorities have a much lower tolerance for side effects from vaccines than for side effects from other drugs.

We do have a serious problem with drug safety in the United States. An appallingly large number of people are dying from the effects of prescription drugs. Many of these deaths are due to deliberate misuse, such as drug abuse or even suicide attempts. Others are due to mistakes by consumers or healthcare professionals, such as dosing errors. Many problems result from drug interactions, especially when a patient is getting prescription medications from more than one doctor. Still other problems result from the fact that a patient is being given a drug treatment when conservative measures, such as diet and exercise, would have worked better. However, the decision of whether a potentially dangerous drug should be allowed to stay on the market is often hard to make. As always, the decision must be based on a balance of the benefits and risks.

The FDA also monitors the quality of all medicinal products, including vaccines, that are sold in the United States. The FDA can order defective batches of vaccine to be recalled. However, companies usually do their own recalls, without waiting for an order from the FDA. As anyone who has ever worked in the pharmaceutical industry can tell you, pharmaceutical executives will go to great lengths to avoid trouble with the FDA.

In the United States, we hear a lot of rhetoric about free speech and free markets. But the market for pharmaceuticals is tightly regulated, and so is pharmaceutical advertising. If you want to sell a drug or a vaccine in the United States, you must first get permission from the FDA. The FDA also puts extremely tight limits on what you can say in your advertising or other promotional materials for that product. The First Amendment of the U.S. Constitution protects free speech. However, the U.S. Supreme Court has consistently found that the federal government's broad powers to regulate commerce include the power to regulate advertising. In contrast, the antivaccination people can say whatever pops into their minds. They can get away with telling bald-faced lies.

Many people have told me that common vaccines are responsible for thousands of deaths and serious illnesses in the United States. But the results of the clinical trials tell a different story. When I review the reports of the studies of any of the vaccines that are on the market in the United States, I typically find that nearly all of the side effects are mild and last only a short time. Vaccines that obviously caused serious side effects in the clinical trials don't get approved. If the FDA finds out that a vaccine that is already on the market is causing a serious side effect, it will take that vaccine off the market. As computerization has made it easier to keep track of reports of adverse events, the FDA has been getting better and better at monitoring vaccine safety.

To understand what you read in a vaccine's prescribing information, you need to know something about how clinical trials are done. A clinical trial is any experiment that involves treatment of human subjects. In many clinical trials of vaccines, some subjects get the real vaccine while others get a placebo, which is a fake product that looks like the real thing. The purpose of a placebo-controlled clinical trial is to see whether using the product is better than doing nothing at all. Other clinical trials compare a new product to a similar product that has already been approved. The purpose of those active-controlled clinical trials is to see whether the new product is better than the standard treatment that is currently being used.

To make sure that the comparison is fair, the subjects are randomly assigned to receive either the new treatment or some sort of control: either a placebo or an active control. Neither the subject nor the person running the trial gets to pick who gets what treatment. This prevents investigators from rigging the experiment by putting the sicker people in the control group. Most vaccine trials are also double-blind, which means that neither the subject nor the person who is evaluating the results of the treatment knows who got which treatment. The purpose of this blinding is to keep people from making biased judgments about the effects of the different treatments.

It's theoretically possible for people who are running a clinical trial to provide false or inaccurate data. But doing so would be a federal crime. People who get caught committing fraud in a study of a drug or vaccine can be punished under the federal Pure Food and Drug Act. They could go to prison. At the very least, they go on the debarment list, which means that they will never be allowed to work for a pharmaceutical company in the United States ever again. The National Institutes of Health have a similar list of people who are not allowed to work on any NIH-funded project.

Clinical trial reports never talk about side effects. Instead, they talk about adverse events. There's a difference. An adverse event is any bad thing that happened *after* the person got at least one dose of some medicinal product. In contrast, a side effect is something that happened *because* the person took the medicinal product. Not all side effects are adverse events, and not all adverse events are side effects. Some side effects of drugs are desirable (which is why some people like to abuse prescription drugs), and some adverse events are completely unrelated to the medicinal product.

Double-blind placebo-controlled trials are the best way to figure out whether some adverse event is a side effect of a vaccine. If an adverse event is at least as common among the people who got a placebo as it is among the people who got the real vaccine, then the adverse event cannot be blamed on the vaccine. If there's no placebo group for comparison, it's hard to tell whether any kind of adverse event is likely to have been the result of the vaccine. That's why the reports of problems that have happened to vaccinated people should be interpreted with caution. Some of those problems had nothing to do with the vaccines that the person has received.

Some side effects are so rare that they might not show up in a clinical trial. Other side effects take so long to develop that they might not show up until after the clinical trial is over. To find out whether a vaccine is causing a small increase in the risk of some serious side effect, you may have to pool the results from several studies. To find evidence of a rare or delayed side effect, you need to look at population studies.

Some of the best population studies come from Denmark, which has an excellent health system and keeps careful records on everyone in the population. Danish researchers looked at the data from all of the 467,450 Danish children born from January 1990 to December 1996. They found that children who had received vaccines that contain the mercury-containing preservative thimerosal did **not** have a higher risk of autism or autism spectrum disorders. Nor did the total amount of thimerosal that the child had received make any difference.

In 1998, an article in the medical journal *The Lancet* suggested that autism could be linked to the MMR vaccine. (As I'll explain in chapter 18, this article was by Andrew Wakefield, who has since lost his medical license for ethical violations. The article itself was retracted.) Subsequently, Danish researchers studied the records for all of the 440,655 children born from January 1991 through December 1998. They compared the children who had received the measles-mumps-rubella (MMR) vaccine with the children who had not received it. (The MMR vaccine is a "live" vaccine and thus has never contained thimerosal.) The study found that the children who had received the MMR vaccine did not have a higher risk of autism or autism spectrum disorder. Nor did the timing of the vaccinations seem to make any difference in the risk of autism.

These two Danish studies are the largest and most persuasive, but numerous other studies done in other countries have come to the same conclusion. Autism is *not* more common among people who have been vaccinated with MMR or with vaccines that contain thimerosal. Thus, neither the MMR shot nor thimerosal can reasonably be blamed for causing autism.

Some antivaccination activists argue that combining the measles, mumps, and rubella vaccines into a single shot was responsible for causing autism. But data from Japan show otherwise. The MMR combined shot was withdrawn in Japan because of concern that the strain of mumps virus used in the combination product might be causing a few cases of aseptic meningitis, which is a common complication of natural mumps infections. (The Japanese vaccine makers used the Urabe strain of the mumps virus, whereas the Jeryl Lynn strain is used in the United States and Europe.) Yet the rate of autism diagnoses continued to rise in Japan, even after the combined MMR shot was replaced with separate shots.

In 1999, representatives from the CDC and the National Institutes of Health asked the Institute of Medicine to review the evidence on vaccines and autism. The Institute of Medicine is the health arm of the National Academy of Sciences. The National Academy of Sciences is an independent nonprofit organization. It works outside of government to provide unbiased, expert advice to government officials and the public. The Institute of Medicine has been doing reviews of the research on vaccine safety since the 1970s.

The Institute of Medicine's report, which was published in 2004, concluded that we should reject the idea that the MMR vaccines and/or thimerosal cause autism. The evidence simply does not support a cause-and-effect relationship. The authors of the report urged people to spend the dollars available for autism research on more promising areas of research.

All of these studies and the Institute of Medicine report eliminated any reasonable concern that vaccines are responsible for causing autism. In chapters 17 and 18, I'll explain why the controversy continued long after it should have ended.

Many antivaccination activists have made a huge fuss over the additives and contaminants in vaccines. Some people have even told me that evil people in government and in the pharmaceutical companies are putting poisons in the vaccines because they want to "thin the herd." Many antivaccination activists believe that Bill Gates is funding vaccine efforts because he wants to "depopulate" Africa, even though it is clear that the vaccinations he has been funding have been saving many children's lives.

In the United States, the FDA regulates what kinds of additives may be used in vaccines. The rules are spelled out Section 610.15 of Title 21 of the Code of Federal Regulations (21 CFR 610.15). There are several different kinds of additives, including diluents, preservatives, and adjuvants. These various additives serve important purposes.

A diluent is a diluting agent. It is a fluid that is used to dissolve solids and to make thick fluids thinner. Some vaccines are provided as a freeze-dried solid. These solids must be dissolved in a liquid before they can be injected. Thus, the vaccine maker provides the diluent that is used for that purpose.

The word *adjuvant* means helper. Vaccine adjuvants are irritating substances that create a mild inflammation at the injection site. This inflammation attracts white blood cells, which can then interact with the vaccine antigens. Adjuvants are used to make "killed" vaccines more effective, so that the patient develops a stronger and longer-lasting immune response.

According to 21 CFR 610.15, "An adjuvant shall not be introduced into a product unless there is satisfactory evidence that it does not affect adversely the safety or potency of the product." Aluminum salts are the most commonly used adjuvant. Mineral oil has also been used. Section 610.15 puts limits on how much aluminum any dose of vaccine can contain.

Vaccines are intended to keep healthy people healthy. But if a vaccine is contaminated by bacteria or fungi, it could make people sick. That's what happened in Bundaberg, Australia, in 1928. Twelve children died after catching a staph infection from their diphtheria vaccine (70 children died of diphtheria in Bundaberg that year). The vaccine had been packaged in a multidose vial. A bacterium called *Staphylococcus aureus* was accidentally introduced into the vial by the needle that was used to draw up one of the first doses of the vaccine from that vial. Then, the vial sat on a shelf for a while, giving the *Staphylococcus aureus* time to grow. Today, people are terrified of methicillin-resistant *Staphylococcus aureus* (MRSA). Back then, there were no antibiotics, so all strains of *Staphylococcus aureus* were as dangerous as MRSA is today.

As the Bundaberg disaster illustrates, changes in pharmaceutical regulations are usually reactive. Something bad happens, often unexpectedly. Then, the regulations are written or rewritten to keep that kind of thing from happening again. Few people outside of the pharmaceutical industry seem to understand this pattern. Most people who have never worked in the pharmaceutical industry know nothing about the regulations that pharmaceutical companies face. Of course, people naturally fill in the gaps of their knowledge with ideas that come from their political biases. For example, many liberals are aware of some disaster or scandal that occurred 10 or more years ago, but they are typically unaware of the reforms that were made in its wake. On the other hand, many conservatives are unaware that the disasters or scandals occurred. Thus, they may imagine that the pharmaceutical industry is over-regulated.

The FDA does not want anything like the Bundaberg vaccine disaster to happen in the United States. Thus, 21 CFR 610.15 specifies that most multidose vials of vaccine must contain a preservative and that the preservative must not be harmful to the patient or to the vaccine. The purpose of the preservative is to prevent dangerous bacteria and fungi from growing in the vaccine product. You can avoid the need for a preservative by packaging the vaccine in a single-dose vial, but that would be more expensive.

The Elixir Sulfanilamide disaster was another of the events that led to major advances in pharmaceutical regulations. In the 1930s, an antibacterial drug called sulfanilamide was a wonder drug. Many companies got in on the action of selling it. In 1937, one company decided to make a tasty sulfanilamide syrup for children. Their chemist found that sulfanilamide dissolved easily in diethylene glycol, so he used that to make the preparation. The product looked, smelled, and tasted good. There was only one problem. Diethylene glycol destroys your kidneys if you take it by mouth. More than 100 people, mostly children, died of kidney failure after taking the product.

Back in 1937, there was no federal law requiring drugs to be tested for safety before being sold to the public. Also, the FDA had no legal authority to remove unsafe drugs from the market. Fortunately, the drug had been mislabeled. Its label said it was an elixir, which is an alcohol solution, when the product was really a diethylene glycol solution. Because of this technicality, the FDA officials could legally seize the product, thus saving about 4,000 lives.

One bad thing and one good thing happened in the aftermath of the Elixir Sulfanilamide disaster. The bad thing was that the chemist whose mistake led to the poisonings committed suicide. The good thing was that Congress passed the 1938 Food, Drugs and Cosmetic Act, which empowered the FDA to require that drugs be tested for safety before they go on the market in the United States.

In 1960, a FDA employee named Frances Kelsey, MD, refused to approve a new tranquilizer called thalidomide. Dr. Kelsey felt that thalidomide had not been adequately tested for safety. She was particularly concerned about its use in pregnant women. Nobody could tell her whether the drug crossed the placenta. Dr. Kelsey held her ground, despite considerable pressure from the manufacturer. Thus, thalidomide was never approved in the United States. It was widely used in many other countries, until people realized that thalidomide causes severe birth defects if a woman takes it in early pregnancy. Many women had done so because thalidomide was being marketed as a remedy for morning sickness. In 1962, Congress granted the FDA even more power to regulate drugs, including the power to require that drugs be tested for effectiveness before they are approved for sale in the United States.

Most improvements in pharmaceutical regulations represent a response to some horrible tragedy. Once in a while, the FDA even acts proactively to prevent some theoretical harm to public health. The classic example is its decision to take the mercury out of practically all childhood vaccines.

Of all the preservatives that have been used in vaccines, thimerosal is the most controversial because it contains mercury. Thimerosal has been widely used as an antiseptic and as a preservative in vaccines since the 1930s. It has also been used as a preservative in contact lens solutions. Even a tiny amount of thimerosal is highly effective at preventing bacterial growth. Unlike many other preservatives that were available back in the 1930s, it did not interfere with the effectiveness of the vaccine.

Even though thimerosal contains mercury, the thimerosal in vaccines did not seem to cause health problems. Back in 1929, Indiana General Hospital tried using thimerosal as a drug to treat a terrible and then-untreatable disease called meningococcal meningitis (see chapter 35). The thimerosal had no effect on the meningitis. However, the doctors were amazed at how well the patients tolerated huge doses of thimerosal, doses that were far larger than the trace amounts that have been used in vaccines.

Antivaccine activists have told me that the FDA lets the pharmaceutical companies put thimerosal in childhood vaccines because the FDA employees don't care about children's health. The truth is that the FDA ordered pharmaceutical companies to start making practically all childhood vaccines thimerosal-free, even though there was no evidence that the thimerosal had caused any problems. Only after this decision was announced did the thimerosal become a hot-button issue for anti-vaccination and autism activists.

There has never been any evidence that the small amount of thimerosal in vaccines was causing any health problems. Back in the 1970s, only one childhood vaccine was likely to contain thimerosal: the diphtheria-tetanus-pertussis vaccine. In 1976, the FDA calculated the amount of thimerosal that people would be likely to get from vaccines over the course of a lifetime. It concluded that the amount was too small to worry about. But after that, there was a steady increase in the number of vaccines.

In 1997, Congressman Frank Pallone of New Jersey added a rider to the bill that provided FDA's funding. This rider required the FDA to look at the mercury content of all approved medicinal products. In response, the staff at the Center for Biologics Evaluation and Research (CBER), which is the part of the FDA that deals with vaccines, calculated how much thimerosal a baby was likely to get from vaccinations. It found that thimerosal exposure had gone up a lot since 1976.

Scientists at the CBER estimated that a baby could get as much as 187.5 micrograms of thimerosal from the recommended vaccinations. (A microgram is one millionth of a gram.) However, nobody knew whether this amount of thimerosal was enough to make someone sick. Since they had no guidelines for thimerosal, which is an ethylmercury, they decided to assume that thimerosal could be just as dangerous as methylmercury, which is the form of mercury commonly found in seafood.

The 187.5 micrograms of ethylmercury in thimerosal was higher than the accepted level of exposure for methylmercury. Of course, the difference between *ethyl* and *methyl* can be huge. If you get drunk on ethyl alcohol, you may have a hangover the following day. But if you got drunk on methyl alcohol, you would go blind and could die. Eventually, toxicologists realized that ethylmercury is less dangerous than methylmercury because ethylmercury is eliminated from the body much faster. That could help to explain why even the huge study from Denmark didn't show any adverse events from the thimerosal in vaccines.

In response to those findings, the CBER, the American Academy of Pediatrics, and the Centers for Disease Control and Prevention issued a joint statement on July 9, 1999. They noted that there was no evidence that the thimerosal did any harm. But just to be on the safe side, they agreed that thimerosal should be removed from practically all of the childhood vaccines as soon as possible. In other words, a group of scientists and government officials decided in 1999 that thimerosal should be taken out of childhood vaccines, even though there was no evidence that it was doing any harm.

The mercury in vaccines became a hot-button issue for antivaccination and autism activists only after the scientists at a government agency, in consultation with scientists and medical doctors, decided that thimerosal should be taken out of practically all childhood vaccines. Yet antivaccination activists have managed to use the specter of thimerosal to spread fear and distrust of not only vaccines but of the government, scientists, and doctors. Antivaccination zealots have used the fear of mercury poisoning to scare people away from having their children vaccinated, even though the mercury-containing thimerosal in the vaccines had never been shown to be a problem and had already been removed from the vaccines.

Some vaccines also contain trace amounts of contaminants, such as formaldehyde. Formaldehyde is used to turn the dangerous bacterial toxins that cause tetanus, diphtheria, and whooping cough into the harmless toxoids that are used in vaccines. Although the manufacturers try to remove as much of this formaldehyde as they can, trace amounts of it will remain.

Many people know that formaldehyde is a dangerous substance. Thus, they become upset if they hear that a vaccine contains even a trace amount of a substance that they think is dangerous. But they do not know that formaldehyde is also found naturally in the human body and in many wholesome foods. You would give a child 50 times more formaldehyde by feeding him a pear than he would get from a vaccination. A child would not get formaldehyde poisoning from eating a pear, and he certainly would not get formaldehyde poisoning from his vaccinations.

The people who try to frighten you by talking about the additives and contaminants in vaccines ignore one important point. Those additives and contaminants are already in the vaccine when the vaccine is used in clinical trials. If those additives and contaminants caused health problems, those problems would show up as adverse events that are more common in the vaccine group than in the placebo group. In population studies, those problems would be more common in vaccinated people than in unvaccinated people.

The fact that vaccinated people are not at greater risk for serious health problems such as autism should reassure us that "vaccine injuries" are actually rare. The common side effects of vaccines are not serious, and the serious side effects are not common. Injectable vaccines often cause some pain, swelling, and redness at the injection site. Some vaccines can cause a fever. However, these problems are usually mild and last only a few days. The severe and serious adverse events are remarkably rare. Not nonexistent, just rare. Nothing in this world is perfectly safe. That's why vaccines are still prescription medications. It's also why I would like to eradicate as many of the eradicable diseases as possible.

When people talk about the real or imagined side effects of a vaccine, they seldom put those side effects in context. They seldom compare those side effects to the effects of the disease that the vaccine is intended to prevent. Do you really think that a small dose of dead or weakened germs is more dangerous than an active infection with live, wild germs that are often deadly?

Some people fear that a baby's immune system would be overwhelmed by all the antigens from his or her vaccines. But as I explained in chapter 9, there are billions of bacteria swarming all over the baby's body, especially in the intestines. Babies also get exposed to lots of different viruses. In contrast, babies get exposed to surprisingly few antigens from vaccination, even if they get all of their recommended vaccines.

Of course, some vaccinations would be too risky for certain patients. For example, the "live" vaccines should not be given to pregnant women or to people with a suppressed immune system. Those vulnerable people must depend on the rest of us for protection. If everyone else is up to date with their vaccinations, then the vaccinated people will provide herd immunity to protect the people who cannot be vaccinated.

I imagine that we could deflate the antivaccination movement overnight if we allowed chiropractors and naturopaths and acupuncturists and maybe even yoga teachers to get paid to vaccinate people. Suddenly, a critical mass of the people who are currently spreading fear, uncertainty, and doubt about vaccinations in order to discredit the medical profession, which they view as their competition, could go into the business of selling vaccinations. Nevertheless, I believe that the state governments are right in concluding that vaccines should be provided only by people with certain kinds of medical or nursing training. The risks of vaccination are low, but they are not nonexistent.

A vaccine's prescribing information provides advice for avoiding serious and severe adverse events. This advice generally includes a list of contraindications. Patients who have one or more of the contraindications should not receive that vaccine. For example, "live" vaccines should not be given to pregnant women or to people with a suppressed immune system. Vaccines that were grown in eggs should not be given to people who are allergic to eggs.

The prescribing information will also include warnings and precautions, which are instructions for avoiding serious and severe adverse reactions. Vaccinations can occasionally cause a serious reaction, such as anaphylaxis, which is why they should be administered only by a licensed healthcare professional.

The purpose of a vaccine is to keep healthy people healthy. Thus, any vaccine that is likely to make a healthy person sick would not be approved. Vaccines have been taken off the market because they could cause a rare but serious side effect. For example, the first vaccine against rotavirus was taken off the market because it was linked to a serious intestinal problem in one out of 10,000 vaccinated babies. Sometimes, these decisions spark heated debates about whether the risk of a rare side effect in a vaccinated person outweighs the risk of the disease in an unvaccinated person.

In the United States, the pharmaceutical industry is heavily regulated. As I mentioned above, most of those regulations were written in response to some disaster that sickened or killed people. The regulations were designed to keep the same thing from happening again. One of the first of those bad things was a deadly epidemic of tetanus among children who had received diphtheria antitoxin in 1901.

At the turn of the 20th century, diphtheria was the 10th leading cause of death in the United States. The vaccine against diphtheria had not yet been invented, but diphtheria antitoxin could be used to save the lives of infected children. The antitoxin was made from the blood drawn from a horse that had been immunized against diphtheria. (I'll explain this in more detail in chapter 25). The antitoxins were generally produced by state and local boards of health, under no higher supervision. Unfortunately, a serum horse in St. Louis caught tetanus, probably from being jabbed with an unclean needle. Thirteen of the children who received antitoxin from that horse then died horribly of tetanus. In response, Congress passed the Biologics Control Act of 1902, which was signed into law by President Theodore Roosevelt.

The Biologics Control Act required federal licensing for anyone who wanted to manufacture and sell antitoxins, serum, or vaccines in the United States. These licenses had to be renewed annually. Since 1988, this licensing has been controlled by the FDA's Center for Biologics Evaluation and Research (CBER).

If you want to introduce a new vaccine in the United States, you must first get approval from the CBER. To get that approval, you must first go through the same process that is required for developing a new drug. Before you can give even the first dose of that vaccine to a human being, you must submit an Investigational New Drug application (IND) to the CBER. Your IND application will include lots of technical information on the vaccine, on how you plan to make the vaccine, and on how you plan to test it. You must also provide information on all of the preliminary studies, such as animal studies, that have been done on the vaccine. If you don't do a good job in putting together your IND, you won't get permission even to test the drug in human beings.

Once your IND has been approved, you can begin testing the

vaccine in human beings. The testing follows three phases. If you get good results in one phase, you may get permission to start the next phase. In Phase 1, the vaccine is given to only a small group of subjects. These subjects are carefully monitored to make sure that the vaccine produces the proper kind of antibody response without causing harmful side effects. In Phase 2, the vaccine is given to several hundred people, to help the researchers figure out the proper dosage. In Phase 3, the vaccine is given to thousands of people, to see whether it is effective enough and safe enough to be approved for the general public. The CBER can call for more studies or even put a halt to this process at any stage if the vaccine is ineffective or has harmful side effects.

Nearly all of the clinical trials are double-blind and controlled. The subjects who participate do not know whether they are getting the experimental vaccine or a comparator treatment, such as a placebo. Nor do the doctors who are evaluating the results of the treatment. Only after all the results are recorded does anyone find out who got what treatment. This blinding keeps the observations from being biased.

Some experimental vaccines, such as influenza vaccines, are compared to a placebo, which is generally an injection of plain salt water. However, placebo-controlled trials can be done only where the risk of receiving a placebo treatment, instead of the real vaccine, would be negligible. If using a placebo would be risky, an experimental vaccine would have to be compared to the best available vaccine.

If all goes well in Phase 1 through Phase 3, you may submit a Biologics Licensing Application. It includes all of your research results plus information on how you plan to manufacture the vaccine. At that point, the CBER will send inspectors to the factory where you plan to make the vaccine.

If the CBER approves your Biologics Licensing Application, the FDA's Advertising and Promotional Labeling Branch will tell you what you can and must say in the vaccine label. The CBER will also tell you what you can and cannot say in the advertisements and other promotional materials for your vaccine. If you make false or unfounded claims in your advertising or promotional materials, you can get into big trouble.

Once the CBER approves your Biologics Licensing Application, you can start selling the vaccine to doctors and pharmacies. Yet even then, the FDA is going to stay on your case. It will monitor your factory and your product to make sure that the quality is good. It will review your advertisements, to make sure that you are not making any false or unfounded claims. The CBER may even make you do some Phase 4 studies, to provide further evidence of effectiveness or safety. The FDA also maintains the Vaccine Adverse Event Reporting System (VAERS), which is also monitored by the CDC.

Many antivaccination activists claim that the VAERS data prove that vaccines are killing people or causing other serious illnesses. Yet the FDA stresses that VAERS data can do nothing of the sort. The VAERS data are not always complete and reliable, and the VAERS database does enable you to compare vaccinated people with unvaccinated people. So even if the reports in VAERS are true, they cannot show whether a particular kind of adverse event is more common in vaccinated people than in unvaccinated people, which is the first step toward proving that the vaccine causes the problem.

Some of the reports in VAERS might not even be true. Many of the VAERS reports were provided by ordinary people who know nothing about medicine. Some of the information may even have been provided by lawyers who are trying to win a lawsuit. Thus, the information that has been given to VAERS may be incomplete or even inaccurate. You can see this for yourself by reading the VAERS reports.

Anyone can go to the FDA Web site and download data and case reports from VAERS for any vaccine that is on the market. Yet before you can make sense of those data, you must understand one important principle. A vaccine is intended to prevent one particular disease. It is not a magic charm to ward off all evil. Thus, it is unreasonable to blame a vaccination for everything bad that happens to the patient from that point forward.

After I heard someone claim that many young women were being killed by the Gardasil vaccine, I downloaded the VAERS reports of deaths among patients who had allegedly received Gardasil. Most of these reports are so vague and incomplete that it is not clear that anything really happened to anybody. Here's one example:

> Information has been received via the internet concerning a 21 year old female who was vaccinated with GARDASIL. The patient died 4 days after vaccination. The cause of death was unknown. No further information is available.

If the cause of death is unknown, how can anyone honestly conclude that the death was due to Gardasil? Other reports provide strong evidence that the death was due to something other than Gardasil:

> None known -suicidal ideation denied at visit 4/26—known chronic depression she elected to stop her medications when she turned 18. Committed suicide 04/28/11. Hung herself.

The VAERS reports cannot prove that a vaccine is dangerous. But they could provide a warning about new, unusual, or rare side effects that did not show up in the clinical trials. Thus, the VAERS data could provide a signal that something bad might be happening. To see whether that signal represents a side effect of the vaccine, you have to do other kinds of studies. Two kinds of studies are particularly useful. One is the national population studies that are done in Denmark. The other is the studies of the health insurance claims databases from the United States. Some of these studies have looked for evidence of harm from Gardasil.

The Gardasil vaccine is intended to be given to girls and young women, a group who are also at risk for autoimmune diseases, such as lupus. One study looked at electronic medical records from a major insurance company to see whether girls who had received Gardasil were more likely to get a new diagnosis of an autoimmune disease than girls who had not received Gardasil. They weren't. Thus, it is unreasonable to claim that Gardasil is causing autoimmune disease.

The health insurance database studies can show whether any serious illnesses are more common in vaccinated than in unvaccinated patients. Unless a problem is more common among vaccinated patients than unvaccinated patients, it is probably not due to the vaccine. As healthcare databases improve, it will become easier to tell whether a particular adverse event really is likely to be due to a drug or vaccine.

Unless you have actually worked in the pharmaceutical industry, it's hard to appreciate how much better the FDA is getting at monitoring and interpreting adverse events in drug and vaccine trials. The www.clinicaltrials.gov Web site maintained by the National Institutes of Health is also making the reporting of clinical trials much more transparent. That Web site makes it easier for scientists and physicians and even consumers to find out the results of all of the clinical trials that have been done on a particular drug.

Like earlier reforms, these improvements in reporting and transparency were put in place because of problems that came to public attention. The purpose of these reforms was to make sure that the same kinds of bad things do not happen again. That's a principle that many critics of the FDA do not understand.

Some antivaccination activists have told me that the pharmaceutical companies can never be sued for damages that result from a vaccine. That's simply untrue. The real story is a bit complicated.

On April 19, 1982, the local NBC affiliate in Washington, DC, aired a documentary titled *DPT: Vaccine Roulette* (see chapter 18), which sparked fears about the safety of the diphtheria-tetanus-pertussis vaccine (see chapter 26). The documentary was long on pathos but short on logos. Like many antivaccination videos today, it pulled at the heartstrings by showing footage of seriously ill or disabled children. However, the statistics and quotations it provided were misleading. In reality, there was no scientific reason to believe that the disabled children had been disabled by their DTP shot. Nevertheless, the documentary led to a flood of lawsuits from parents who believed that their children had been injured by the vaccine. The pharmaceutical companies found it to be so costly to defend themselves against these lawsuits that most of them decided to stop making the vaccine. As a result, the cost of the vaccine rose and there were serious shortages of the vaccine.

When the last remaining manufacturer of the DTP shot threatened to quit making the vaccine, Congress passed the National Childhood Vaccine Injury Act of 1986. It set up a no-fault system for handling vaccine injury claims. The goal was to make sure that vaccine-injured children and their families were compensated quickly, generously, and fairly and without having to pay their own legal expenses. Its official title is the National Vaccine Injury Compensation Program, but it is often called the vaccine court. It is officially part of the Department of Health and Human Services, but several other federal departments, including the Treasury Department and the Justice Department, are involved in the program.

The Treasury Department collects an excise tax of $0.75 on each dose of each vaccine for a particular disease. The tax on a flu shot that covers three strains of influenza would be only $0.75, but the tax on a dose of the measles-mumps-rubella vaccine would be $2.25. The Treasury Department then puts the money into the Vaccine Injury Compensation Trust Fund. The money in this fund is used to pay claims. This money can go to the injured person, to the family of an injured child, or to the estate of someone who died.

To make it as easy as possible for these people to get compensation, the Department of Health and Human Services maintains a Vaccine Injury Table. The Vaccine Injury Table is a list of the injuries or conditions that are known to result from each of the vaccines recommended by the CDC. If you can show that you or your child got one of those recommended vaccines and then had a "Table injury" within the specified timeframe, and if the preponderance of the evidence does not show that the injury was not due to the vaccine, then you are entitled to compensation. For example, if someone got anaphylaxis within four hours of getting a tetanus shot, the anaphylaxis would be presumed to be the result of the tetanus shot, unless there were persuasive evidence that the anaphylaxis was due to some other cause, such as a bee sting in someone with a known allergy to bees. These simple rules make it easy to resolve most of the typical cases.

If a vaccinated person had a problem that is not listed in the Vaccine Injury Table, or if the problem did not occur within the specified length of time, that person or the person's family may still be able to collect. They just have to provide evidence to support their claim. This evidence may include their medical records as well as the testimony of expert witnesses. The family can be compensated even if the vaccine had been used in a way that goes against the instructions on the product label.

Once a claim is filed, a special master, who is a lawyer appointed by the judges of the vaccine court, decides whether the claim will be paid and how much will be paid. The petitioner can accept or reject the special master's decision. If either the petitioner or the Department of Health and Human Services doesn't like the special master's decision, they can make an appeal to a judge of the vaccine court, then to the U.S. Court of Appeals for the Federal Circuit, and finally to the U.S. Supreme Court.

Sometimes, antivaccination activists claim that a decision in the Vaccine Court "proves" that a vaccine causes a particular disease. It doesn't. The decisions of the vaccine court are based on the preponderance of the evidence. That is the standard used in civil lawsuits. Much higher standards of evidence are needed in science.

By 2002, thousands of families had petitioned the vaccine court, claiming that their children's autism was the result of vaccination. To deal with this huge caseload, the vaccine court established a special program called the Omnibus Autism Proceeding (OAP). The OAP combined many of the claims into two test cases. The decisions in those two cases maintained that there was simply no reliable evidence to support the idea that the measles-mumps-rubella vaccine or the thimerosal-containing vaccines, alone or in combination, are a causal factor in autism. Thus, autism spectrum disorders have not been added to the Vaccine Injury Table for any vaccine. Some of the petitioners have appealed this decision, but their appeals have not succeeded.

Nevertheless, some antivaccination activists claim that the decisions of the vaccine court actually prove that vaccines cause autism. They focus on two cases: that of Hannah Poling and that of Bailey Banks. Yet neither of those children really had autism.

When Hannah Poling was 19 months old, she received five shots in one day: tetanus-diphtheria-acellular pertussis, *Haemophilus influenzae* type b, measles-mumps-rubella, varicella, and inactivated polio. Two days later, she was irritable and running a fever. She broke out in a rash consistent with vaccine-induced varicella. A few months later, she was having problems with language, communication, and behavior. Her doctors found that she had an inherited defect in the mitochondria of her cells. This problem explained why she had a brain disorder. Although children with this problem often start showing signs of problems between their first and second birthdays, Hannah's parents felt that her brain disorder had been triggered by the vaccinations. They brought their case to the vaccine court and won.

The Poling case has confused many people, and some people disagree with the vaccine court's decision and fear that it will make people think that vaccinations might really cause autism after all. First of all, Hannah Poling did not have autism, although she did have some of the same kinds of language and communication problems that autistic children have. Second, there is no evidence that her vaccinations made her problem worse. In response to the vaccine court's decision in the Poling case, the United Mitochondrial Disease Foundation has released a statement saying, "There are no scientific studies documenting that childhood vaccinations cause mitochondrial diseases or worsen mitochondrial disease symptoms."

The vaccine-related varicella was not the only infection that Hannah Poling had had during that period. She had had so many fevers and ear infections that she eventually had a drainage tube placed in each ear. In fact, her frequent ear infections were the reason why she had fallen behind in her vaccinations, which was why she ended up getting so many shots on the same day.

The other case concerned Bailey Banks, who got a diagnosis of a brain disease called acute disseminated encephalomyelitis (ADEM) 16 days after his MMR shot when he was a toddler. This ADEM then led to a pervasive developmental delay. ADEM is similar to multiple sclerosis, in that both diseases result from the immune system attacking the myelin sheath that serves as insulation on nerve cells. Many different infectious diseases and several vaccines have been suspected as possible causes of ADEM. The only vaccine that is known for sure to increase the risk of ADEM is the Semple rabies vaccine, which the boy had not received. Nevertheless, the special master decided to rule in favor of the Banks family because the timing of Bailey's illness was suggestive.

Although Bailey Banks may have had some of the same symptoms as autistic children, he did not have autism. The ruling itself emphasized that Bailey Banks had a pervasive developmental delay but that he did not qualify for a diagnosis of "pervasive developmental disorder not otherwise specified" (PDD-NOS), which is part of the autism spectrum. Most children with autism have no signs of the kind of brain damage that Bailey Banks obviously had.

These two cases show that the vaccine court sometimes decides to rule in the plaintiff's favor when the cause of the plaintiff's health problems is unclear. Unfortunately, the antivaccine activists pretend that these decisions are evidence that the vaccines really cause health problems. Yet in reality, court decisions are legal decisions, not scientific decisions.

To help the vaccine court make fair decisions, the Health Resources and Services Administration, which administers the vaccine court, asked the Institute of Medicine to review the available research to see which adverse events are likely to be real side effects of eight of the 12 vaccines covered by the vaccine court. The Institute of Medicine's report, which was published in August of 2011, concluded, "Vaccines are not free from side effects, or 'adverse effects,' but most are very rare or very mild."

Among other findings, the Institute of Medicine concluded that several different vaccines could each be linked to anaphylaxis, which is a potentially life-threatening allergic reaction. It also found that injections of any kind could result in fainting or a problem with the shoulder joint. It listed some rare but serious side effects of the chickenpox and measles vaccines. But it also concluded that the MMR vaccine does *not* cause autism or type 1 diabetes, that the DTaP (tetanus) vaccine does *not* cause type 1 diabetes, and that the flu shot does *not* cause Bell's palsy or aggravate asthma.

In chapter 3, I explained the role of government in fighting infectious disease. I hope that from reading this chapter, you have begun to appreciate that the people at the FDA really do try to ensure that vaccines are safe. For example, they decided to err on the side of caution and demand that thimerosal be removed from practically all childhood vaccines. They came to that decision before Jenny McCarthy's son was even conceived. Yet several years after the mercury was removed from practically all of the recommended vaccines, McCarthy started campaigning for "mercury-free vaccines." Did she not get the memo?

There is a great deal of money at stake in questions about vaccines. The vaccine market may be small potatoes compared to the big blockbuster drugs, but it's still enough money for people to fight over. We do need activists to serve as watchdogs to make sure that FDA policies serve the public interest. Unfortunately, activists can do more harm than good if they misrepresent what goes on at the FDA.

17

The Recommended Vaccine Schedule

In the United States, the Food and Drug Administration (FDA) decides what vaccines you *can* get. The Centers for Disease Control and Prevention (CDC) suggest what vaccines that most people *should* get. State governments then decide what vaccines children *must* get. If you join the military, the Department of Defense decides what vaccines you *will* get. If you think that children get lots of vaccinations, just talk to anyone who has just been through basic training in the military!

People who join the military or who travel overseas get many vaccines that are not routinely recommended in the United States. Servicemen and -women and travelers get vaccines for diseases that are rarely if ever seen in the United States. Which diseases are people likely to get in the United States? What is the best strategy for preventing those diseases? These are hard questions. They are answered through a political process that involves people with several different kinds of expertise, including epidemiologists, immunologists, and economists. Most antivaccination activists believe that these decisions are based on the drug industry's business plans. Yet if you look at how any of these decisions are made, it's hard to support that idea.

The schedule of recommended vaccinations is produced by the Advisory Committee on Immunization Practices (ACIP). As an advisory committee, ACIP offers advice on how and when the vaccine products that are licensed in the United States should be used. The ACIP has no power to force anyone to follow its advice. However, the state governments may choose to base their vaccination laws on the ACIP's recommendations. Thus, the ACIP's recommendations may help to determine what vaccines a child must receive before the child may enter a public school.

ACIP consists of voting members, nonvoting ex officio members, and nonvoting liaisons. The voting members are experts on various aspects of immunology, preventive medicine, and so on who are appointed by the Secretary of Health and Human Services to serve a four-year term as a government employee. The ex officio members are people who are automatically included in the committee because they hold some other office (that's what *ex officio* means). For example, the Director of the CBER is an ex officio member of ACIP. Normally, the ex officio members of ACIP are not allowed to vote. However, they can be granted the permission to vote if too many of the voting members cannot vote, either because of absence or because of some conflict of interest.

The liaisons are people who represent various organizations, such as medical societies, the insurance industry, and the pharmaceutical industry. Although ex officio members can be allowed to vote in a pinch, when there aren't enough voting members because of absences or conflict of interest, the liaisons can never vote. So even though a pharmaceutical company can send a liaison to attend the ACIP meetings, their liaison is not allowed to vote.

ACIP establishes subcommittees and working groups who then do much of the background work of reviewing the science and drafting the recommendations. The working group meetings are not open to the public. The working groups draft some recommendations, which are then added to the agenda of the public meetings. For example, the working groups review the research on vaccines that have not yet been approved, so that the ACIP can make a recommendation as soon as the vaccine becomes available.

The ACIP holds three public meetings per year, which are announced well in advance. They are open to the public and are available online as a Webcast. The recommendations that are approved at those meetings are then sent to the CDC for approval. Then, they are published in the CDC's publication *Morbidity and Mortality Weekly Report*. The CDC does not have to approve the ACIP's recommendations, but it usually does.

If an ACIP member has some conflict of interest, such as owning stock in a company that makes the vaccine in question, he or she is not supposed to take part in any of the discussions about that vaccine. However, he or she can be granted a waiver, which would allow him or her to take part in the discussion but not to vote.

After the first rotavirus vaccine was taken off the market, the House of Representatives assigned a committee to study ACIP's decision-making process. The House committee concluded that the conflict of interest rules had to be tightened. It felt that too many waivers were being granted, and there was too much possibility for conflict of interest.

Conflicts of interest are a potentially serious problem because the ACIP is supposed to serve the public, not to serve the interests of private businesses. Even the appearance of a conflict of interest is a problem because it erodes the public's trust in the recommendations. Unfortunately, it's hard to find people who are knowledgeable enough about vaccines to render an expert opinion but have never been involved in research on any of the vaccines that are being considered. Often, some of the members must abstain from voting on recommendations related to the vaccines that they have studied.

The ACIP makes recommendations only for vaccines that have been licensed for use in the United States. Several considerations influence that decision. One consideration is the seriousness of the disease that the vaccine is intended to prevent. The ACIP recommends vaccines that are intended to prevent serious diseases that can cause hospitalization, long-term health problems, or death.

Another consideration is the likelihood that someone in the United States would get that disease. American children stopped getting smallpox vaccinations in the early 1970s because smallpox was no longer a threat to public health in the United States. Nor do we routinely vaccinate against yellow fever, typhoid fever, or cholera in the United States. Although those diseases are still circulating in some other countries, they are simply not a public health problem in the United States.

The ACIP could also recommend a vaccine for some people but not for everyone. For example, it does not recommend the routine use of the meningococcal vaccine for all infants. However, it does recommend the meningococcal vaccine for certain high-risk infants.

The ACIP also recommends a schedule for vaccination. The design of the schedule is a balancing act. On one hand, you want children to be protected against infectious disease as soon as possible. On the other hand, you would want children to get the extra protection they would receive from being vaccinated at the age at which the vaccine is most effective. The ACIP also considers the cost-effectiveness of the overall vaccination schedule.

Many parents and even some pediatricians want to deviate from the ACIP's recommended vaccination schedule. They argue that the body would be overwhelmed by having too many vaccinations too close together. Yet the schedule that the ACIP has recommended was based on studies of vaccine effectiveness and safety. None of the alternative schedules are supported by that kind of evidence.

In its 2011 evaluation of vaccine safety, the Institute of Medicine concluded that the ACIP's vaccination schedule is safe. The Institute of Medicine also warned that any alternative schedule that delayed vaccines is likely to be less safe because it leaves children at risk of catching vaccine-preventable diseases for a longer period.

18

The Antivaccination Movement

As long as immunization has been around, there have been people who have campaigned against it. To understand the antivaccination movement, you must understand why people get involved in it. How do they view the world, and what do they want to achieve? The debates about vaccination hinge on questions of authority. Whom should you trust? Should you trust your doctor about vaccinations? Or should you trust your minister or your chiropractor instead? Should you trust what government agencies and international health organizations say about vaccines? Or should you believe in the conspiracy theories you hear about over the radio and through the Internet?

I understand why many parents, especially mothers, are skeptical of the need for vaccines. Because of their previous experiences, many young women expect their doctor to give them a menu of choices. For example, women in the United States and many other countries can now choose from a broad array of contraceptives. When women decide to have a child, they can choose to have their baby delivered by a midwife or an obstetrician. Today, midwives and obstetricians often encourage their patients to fill out a detailed birth plan, detailing their choices with regard to where and how they want the baby to be delivered. (Of course, the birth does not always go according to the plan!) But once the baby is delivered, everything seems to change. Instead of asking the woman what she wants, doctors start telling her what must be done.

As soon as the baby is born, the doctor typically insists that the baby must have a vitamin K shot and a hepatitis vaccination. (These treatments are required by law in some states.) Later on, the pediatrician or family doctor insists that the baby should receive many more shots, all according to a standard schedule. Most of these shots are for diseases that the mother has never seen or even heard about. Sadly, doctors in the United States today are so pressed for time that they cannot take the time to explain the need for each vaccine. Thus, to many mothers, it may feel as if the doctor is jabbing the baby and making him or her cry for no reason. For these mothers, the antivaccine rhetoric just confirms their suspicions.

What do the leaders of the antivaccination movement want to achieve? Like anyone else, antivaccination activists get involved in political activism for any of three reasons: to serve the public, to serve God, or to serve themselves. It is hard to do all three at the same time.

I want to serve the public: I want to see measles and some other communicable diseases wiped off the face of the earth forever. After measles, mumps, and rubella are driven into extinction, there will be no more need for the MMR vaccine. The eradication of these diseases would be great for humanity, and especially great for children in poor countries. However, it would mean that the sales of the MMR vaccine will drop to zero as soon as those diseases are extinct. Thus, the pharmaceutical industry would lose a tiny percentage of its total sales.

Of course, many people support the antivaccination movement because they believe that the currently recommended vaccines are unsafe and/or unnecessary. Thus, they sincerely believe that their antivaccination activism is serving public health. But if the campaigns against smallpox vaccination had succeeded, human beings would still be dying horribly of smallpox. Unfortunately, the current antivaccination campaigns are leading to outbreaks of potentially deadly communicable diseases, such as measles, mumps, and whooping cough. Fears about polio vaccination have delayed the eradication of polio.

The movement to oppose immunization began in the 1720s, when news of variolation reached Britain and Massachusetts. Variolation was an early, risky approach to immunization. To variolate someone, you would take pus from someone with a case of actual smallpox and scratch it into someone else's arm. At first, many doctors in Britain and New England were against variolation because of cultural biases. Variolation was something that was done by black heathens in Africa and brown Muslims in Turkey. It had never been suggested by the ancient Greeks and Romans or by Western Christian theologians.

The variolation procedure was risky. Some people seemed to catch generalized smallpox from the variolation procedure. (Of course, a variolated patient could have caught smallpox naturally, since variolation could be performed only when someone with active smallpox was nearby.) Also, someone who had recently been variolated could spread smallpox to others. The variolation procedure could also spread other diseases, such as syphilis, which was called the great pox. Yet variolation usually produced only a relatively mild illness and scarring only on the arm, instead of all over the face and body.

When doctors counted the dead after a smallpox epidemic, they found that variolation reduced the risk of death by about 90%. More doctors started embracing variolation once they realized that the benefits clearly outweighed the risk, and once they realized that they could get paid for performing the procedure.

From the very beginning, some religious people were outraged by the very idea of variolation. On July 8, 1722, an Anglican minister named Edmund Massey preached that variolation was the work of the devil. He argued that as the Biblical character Job suffered from a plague of boils without complaint, Christians should accept smallpox without complaint.

In 1796, a British physician named Edward Jenner realized that pus from a person or animal with cowpox could be used to immunize people against smallpox. This procedure was called vaccination, after the Latin word for cow. Cowpox was a much milder disease than smallpox. Thus, vaccination was far safer and much better tolerated than variolation. It produced a much milder reaction at the inoculation site, and it could not spread genuine smallpox. Nevertheless, vaccination still involved some risk. It involved inoculating a healthy person with pus from a sick person or animal. Besides posing the risk of a generalized cowpox infection, Jenner's vaccination procedure could spread other kinds of infections.

Jenner's invention was rapidly adopted throughout the world. As a result, the rates of death from smallpox started dropping and life expectancy began to improve. In the late 19th century, smallpox outbreaks in the United States led to vaccination campaigns and ultimately to state laws requiring vaccination. In reaction, people who opposed vaccination got organized. The Anti Vaccination Society of America was founded in 1879, the New England Anti Compulsory Vaccination League in 1882, and the Anti-vaccination League of New York City in 1885.

In the 20th century, vaccines against many other diseases were developed. Vaccines also became much safer and more reliably effective. Scientists learned a lot more about microbiology and immunology, and the federal government got involved in regulating the vaccine business. Yet even as vaccine safety improved and the benefits of vaccination became increasingly obvious, the antivaccination movement persisted. With the rise of the Internet, it is growing.

Ironically, vaccination seems to be a victim of its own success. Most people in the United States today have never seen a case of whooping cough. Even most doctors in the United States today have never seen even one case of measles. Thus, most people have no idea how serious those diseases can be. As a result, many parents do not fear the vaccine-preventable diseases. Many of them fear the vaccines instead, mainly because of the lies being spread by antivaccination activists.

There have always been people who have religious reasons for opposing immunization. These people view disease either as a divine punishment or as some test of faith. Even today, many religious people feel that using any kind of medicine to prevent or relieve illness would be an insult to God. They recommend spiritual remedies, such as faith healing, instead. Although they view vaccination as a spiritual contamination, they may talk in terms of physical contamination. Thus, they may complain that vaccines contain poisons. As a result, some of their objections sound like scientific claims. Yet the complaints about the "toxins" in vaccines are not coming from toxicologists, who are the scientists who study poisons. Instead, these complaints are coming from people who know nothing whatsoever about toxicology.

The antivaccination zealots want you to trust them as authority figures. The religious ones want you to trust their spiritual authority. Yet many of them do not hesitate to bear false witness. The secular ones want you to respect them as scientific experts. But most of them have no scientific credentials, and none of them seem to have the credentials that really matter: advanced degrees in toxicology and epidemiology. The few who do have some sort of degree in science or medicine have published little if anything in the scientific literature, and nothing of value about vaccination. If they lack a publication record, they are not really medical researchers, regardless of what they say about their "research" and their "protocols." They have not done what it takes to build a good scientific reputation (see chapter 7). Nevertheless, their antivaccination activism puts them in the spotlight. They often become household names, unlike most real scientists.

Getting involved in the antivaccination movement is an easy way to get attention. Some people crave attention for its own sake. They love the limelight. They love to have a microphone in front of them. They love to be admired. Others seek attention because it's good for their business, whether it's a chiropractic or naturopathy practice, a retail business, a nonprofit organization that pays their salary, or their career in show business. Much of the antivaccination rhetoric on the radio and the Internet comes from people who are selling some alternative medicine product or service. Some of them are selling dietary supplements or herbal medicines. Others sell ad space to other alternative health businesses. For these businesspeople, antivaccination activism is an effective way for them to get free publicity, which helps them drum up business.

Many critics of vaccination realize that the pharmaceutical companies are for-profit businesses. Thus, it's understandable that these people would be suspicious of the pharmaceutical industry and its products. Yet critics of vaccination seem oddly unwilling to question the motives of the alternative medicine entrepreneurs. Alternative practitioners and the people who sell nutritional supplements by mail order are also in business to make money. Let the buyer beware.

People in the alternative health industry have political reasons as well as business reasons to speak ill of vaccination. The business reasons are clear enough. By attacking vaccination, they sow fear, uncertainty, and doubt about the medical profession, whom they view as their competition. It's a classic marketing strategy. By making people distrust mainstream medicine, the alternative medicine entrepreneurs also build their own political power base. Thus, they undermine the government's ability to regulate alternative medicine.

In the United States, the FDA can and does forbid people from selling ineffective or unsafe drugs. The FDA and the Federal Trade Commission can also forbid people from making false claims about the products that they sell. The state governments have the power to regulate the practice of professions such as medicine and dentistry by establishing each profession's scope of practice and by issuing and taking away licenses to practice those professions. But to exercise these powers, the executive branch of federal and state governments must have the support of their legislature. If the alternative medicine industry has enough support in Congress or the state legislatures, it can protect itself against government regulation. For example, the supplement industry in the United States is loosely regulated because that industry has been so effective in lobbying Congress.

People who resist vaccination become particularly angry when vaccination is mandatory. Some people simply resent being given orders or even advice from anyone. Others feel that public health and safety are not a legitimate aim of government. Antivaccination activists may frame their objection to vaccination in terms of freedom and human rights. Yet freedom entails protection from harm from other people. As the influential British philosopher John Stuart Mill wrote in his essay On Liberty, "The only purpose for which power can be rightfully exercised over any member of a civilized community, against his will, is to prevent harm to others. His own good, either physical or moral, is not a sufficient warrant."

Communicable disease is one of the situations where an individual's rights may be limited in the interest of public safety. Mary "Typhoid Mary" Mallon insisted on continuing to work as a cook. Unfortunately, typhoid fever kept breaking out in the households where she worked. Dozens of people fell ill, and at least three people died. When she refused to stop working as a cook, the state health authorities put her in quarantine for the rest of her life. Her right to come and go as she pleased and to work in the occupation she liked was less important than other people's right to be free of typhoid fever.

Although many antivaccination activists talk about the right to refuse vaccines, nearly all of the recommended vaccines are given to children, who are too young to make medical decisions for themselves. Thus, the real question is how much leeway parents should have in making medical decisions for their children.

Adults may refuse life-saving medical treatments that conflict with their religious beliefs. However, the Supreme Court has decided that parents do not have the right to martyr their children. In *Prince v. Massachusetts* (1944), the U.S. Supreme Court decided that "The right to practice religion freely does not include liberty to expose the community or the child ... to communicable disease or the latter to ill health or death." Parents who have withheld life-saving medical care from their children, even for religious reasons, can face criminal charges for child neglect. Theoretically, parents could be sued for negligence if their unvaccinated child passes a communicable disease on to other children. However, some states allow religious defenses in cases of child neglect and even the murder of children.

Many antivaccination activists feel that mandatory vaccination laws violate their Constitutional rights. Yet in *Jacobson v. Massachusetts* (1905), the U.S. Supreme Court upheld that states could impose quarantine or fines on people who refuse to cooperate with vaccination laws. The Court found that such laws are within the police power of the state, which is necessary to defend the public against communicable disease. In *Zucht v. King* (1922), the Supreme Court decided that a school system could refuse admission to unvaccinated children.

As I explained in chapter 16, the FDA goes to great lengths to ensure that the vaccines and other medicines sold in the United States are effective and reasonably safe. As I explained in chapter 17, the members of the CDC's Advisory Committee on Immunization Practices do try to make sound recommendations about how and when those vaccines should be used. Yet the federal government has no authority to force any civilians to be vaccinated. All it can do is give advice and support to the state and local governments. The state legislators then decide whether to take the CDC's advice when they write their state's vaccination laws.

All 50 states have laws that spell out which vaccines a child must have before the child may go to a public school or a public childcare facility. However, these laws have loopholes. All states allow exemptions for children who cannot receive a particular vaccine for medical reasons. All states except Mississippi and West Virginia allow exemptions for religious reasons. Some states also allow exemptions for "philosophical" reasons. Unfortunately, areas with higher rates of exemption do have higher rates of communicable diseases such as whooping cough.

In short, the federal government is not forcing vaccination on children. In theory, the state governments could force vaccination on children, but they seldom do so. All that they generally do is require either proof of vaccination or documentation of an exemption before a child may to go to daycare or a public school. As the antivaccination movement spreads its misinformation, more people seek exemptions. As more exemptions are granted, vaccination rates have been dropping and diseases like whooping cough have been spreading. As a result, more children have been getting sick and dying.

Many different individuals and organizations have been opposed to vaccination, for various reasons. As I mentioned above, many religious people oppose vaccination for religious reasons. The leaders of some small churches have been vocal opponents of vaccination. The leaders of some larger churches, such as such as the Church of Christ, Scientist (Christian Science), have taken a cautious stance in public.

Mary Baker Eddy, the founder of Christian Science, taught that illness is a mental error that can be healed by the Divine Mind. She taught that medicine was therefore incompatible with Christian Science. However, she allowed her followers to seek help from a doctor for setting broken bones, and she publically encouraged her followers to obey the state vaccination laws. Nevertheless, Christian Scientists have found loopholes in those laws. For example, they have lobbied for religious exemptions to vaccination or sent their children to church-run schools, as opposed to public schools. Vaccine-preventable diseases can spread rapidly among the unvaccinated students of those institutions. In 1972, eleven children at a Christian Science boarding school in Connecticut were paralyzed by polio. Between 1985 and 1994, there were four large-scale outbreaks of measles in Christian Science schools near St. Louis, Missouri.

From the time of its founding, the chiropractic profession led a vocal opposition to vaccination. After antibiotics became available, chiropractors spoke out against antibiotics, too. D. D. Palmer, the founder of chiropractic, did not believe in the germ theory of disease. He argued that all diseases resulted from misalignments of the joints, mainly the joints of the spinal column. He disapproved of the use of drugs of any kind, and he particularly opposed vaccination. He argued, "It is the very height of absurdity to strive to 'protect' any person from smallpox or any other malady by inoculating them with a filthy animal poison." Ironically, D. D. Palmer reportedly died of typhoid fever, a disease that is now preventable by vaccination and now survivable if the patient receives antibiotics and aggressive fluid therapy. The chiropractic profession's resistance to vaccinations and drug therapy probably peaked around 1940. This resistance softened somewhat after penicillin and later the polio vaccine proved their worth.

Nevertheless, many chiropractors are still active in spreading antivaccination messages. Many chiropractors feel that they have a financial incentive to oppose vaccination. Chiropractors cannot perform vaccinations. Thus, chiropractors cannot replace a family doctor or pediatrician as the family's primary care provider as long as the family has to keep taking their children to a regular medical clinic for vaccinations. Although the resistance to vaccination has probably been on the decline within the chiropractic profession, the Internet has made it possible for antivaccination chiropractors to reach a much larger audience with their message.

In the United States, the opposition to vaccination seems to be particularly strong in wealthy neighborhoods. Perhaps wealthy people feel that they should not have to follow the same rules as poor people. Wealthy people may believe that their children should receive custom-tailored, boutique medical care, rather than getting the same vaccines on the same schedule as everyone else's children. Yet the fact that rich people simply have more money to spend is important. Wealthy parents have more money to spend on alternative medicine: chiropractic and naturopathy and homeopathy and acupuncture and so on. Thus, they may be exposed to more antivaccination messages from alternative practitioners.

The modern antivaccination movement can be traced to a misleading television documentary that was aired in 1982. It was titled *DPT: Vaccine Roulette*. It showed footage of severely disabled children and then falsely claimed that the children's condition was the result of a reaction to the pertussis component of the diphtheria-tetanus-pertussis (DTP) vaccine. The movement grew even stronger in 1991, with the publication of a book titled *A Shot in the Dark*, which claimed that the whole-cell pertussis vaccine produced brain damage. As I explain in chapter 26, these claims were unfounded. Nevertheless, they caused many parents to fear vaccination and to lose faith in their doctors.

Just as the media started spreading these false rumors about vaccinations, family doctors and pediatricians were becoming less able to educate their patients' parents. Insurance companies in the United States have been paying less and less to primary care providers, such as pediatricians and family practice doctors. As a result, the family practice doctors and the pediatricians had to see more patients in less time, just to stay even. As a result, doctors had less time to devote to having long conversations about vaccines. Meanwhile, parents are being bombarded by antivaccination messages in many different media: radio, television, magazines, books, and the Internet.

The antivaccination movement gained even more momentum in Britain and the United States because of the fear that vaccines could cause autism. This story started with a minor safety problem with the mumps component of the measles-mumps-rubella vaccine. The MMR vaccine contains "live" viruses that are intended to produce a harmless infection that provokes a strong and long-lasting immune response. Several different strains of mumps virus have been used in mumps vaccines. The Urabe strain seemed to be somewhat more effective in producing immunity than the Jeryl Lynn strain that is used in the United States. It is also cheaper to produce. However, the Urabe strain was taken off the market in Canada and Britain in 1992 because it caused a few cases of aseptic meningitis: perhaps 1 case for every 4000 vaccinated children. (Note that the risk of aseptic meningitis is much higher with natural mumps infection than with the Urabe vaccine.) The children with aseptic meningitis from the mumps vaccine might have needed some supportive care in the hospital for a few days, but there were no deaths and all the affected children recovered with no lasting ill effects. (I'll talk more about mumps in chapter 23.)

To the surprise of industry insiders in Britain, this revelation of a problem with the mumps vaccine did not lead to a flood of lawsuits. Nevertheless, one attempt to build a class-action lawsuit against the vaccine manufacturers led indirectly led to a panic about the MMR vaccine. This panic was unleashed by a British surgeon named Andrew Wakefield.

Wakefield had just applied for a patent for a strange and completely unproven new form of measles vaccine. According to Wakefield's patent application, the co-inventor of the strange new vaccine was Hugh Fudenberg, who was an American medical doctor and clinical immunologist. Fudenberg had been claiming since the 1980s that the MMR vaccine caused autism. Fudenberg also claimed that he could cure autism by using a preparation that he made in his kitchen from his own bone marrow. In 1995, Fudenberg lost his license to practice medicine in South Carolina because of narcotics abuse and abuse of his prescribing privileges.

Even if Wakefield's alternative measles vaccine product had been effective, the patent for it would be worthless unless Wakefield could persuade doctors to stop using the combined MMR vaccine—which had an excellent track record for effectiveness and safety—and give separate shots for measles, mumps, and rubella.

In the patent application, which was dated June 6, 1997, Wakefield made some big claims. He claimed that the measles virus (either the wild virus or the strain used in the "live" measles vaccine) could lead to chronic inflammation of the intestines in some patients. He claimed that the introduction of the current measles vaccine in 1968 had caused an increase in inflammatory bowel disease in children. He claimed that the combination of the measles vaccine with the mumps and rubella vaccines in the MMR shot, which was introduced in 1988, had caused an epidemic of "regressive behavioural disorder" (autism). Wakefield claimed that he had studied 11 boys and a girl who had autism and inflammatory bowel disorders—all supposedly "associated with the presence of MMR viruses in the gut." He claimed that his new vaccine was not only safer than the conventional measles vaccine, it would serve as a curative treatment for inflammatory bowel disease and autism.

To provide support for his patent application, Wakefield wrote an article that was published in February 1998 in the medical journal *The Lancet.* (Eleven other people signed on as coauthors of the article.) However, there was an odd discrepancy between the patent application and the *Lancet* article. Both documents mentioned a group of 12 children who all supposedly had inflammatory bowel disorders and behavioral disorders. However, the patent application implied that measles, mumps, and rubella viruses had been found in inflamed intestinal tissue from the 12 children. In contrast, the *Lancet* article made no mention of any tests for the presence of these viruses in the tissue samples that had been taken from the children's intestines. Instead, the *Lancet* article merely claimed that the parents recalled that the symptoms started shortly after an MMR shot (for eight of the children) or after a natural case of measles (in one child).

In fact, the children's biopsy specimens had been tested for RNA from the measles, mumps, and rubella viruses. Nick Chadwick, who was a researcher who worked under Wakefield's supervision, had run the tests on samples from 22 patients, including the 12 patients described in Wakefield's *Lancet* article. The results for all 22 patients were negative—which may explain why Wakefield did not mention the tests in his *Lancet* article. Wakefield dismissed these negative test results and complained that Chadwick's test was not sensitive enough to find the viral RNA. Yet Wakefield could hardly quibble over the test that Chadwick had used; Wakefield was a coauthor of the article that described the validation of that test. The results for all 22 patients were reported in Chadwick's doctoral thesis, which was dated February 1998. However, this information was not published until November 18, 2004, when the British public television station Channel 4 ran a documentary titled *MMR: What They Didn't Tell You.*

The negative results of the viral tests were not the only important details that Wakefield left out of his *Lancet* article. In the *Lancet* article, Wakefield claimed that the 12 children were "consecutively referred to the department of paediatric gastroenterology." In reality, none of the 12 children had come to his clinic as a result of ordinary referrals by local doctors in London. Instead, Wakefield had sought these patients out. None of the children were from London. One had been flown in from the United States. Nearly all of the children had been recruited through an antivaccine group named Justice, Awareness, and Basic Support (JABS). Many of the children's parents were clients of a lawyer who was planning to bring a class-action lawsuit against the vaccine manufacturers. Wakefield had been paid £435,643 (roughly $780,000), plus expenses, to provide evidence that could be used in such a lawsuit.

In his *Lancet* article, Wakefield claimed that all 12 children had intestinal abnormalities, "ranging from lymphoid nodular hyperplasia to aphthoid ulceration." The medical records told a different story. A review of the children's actual medical records showed evidence of some sort of inflammatory bowel disorder for only three of the children. A review of the scoring sheets showed that the pathologist had rated the biopsy specimens for most of the children as normal.

To win a lawsuit against the vaccine makers, the children's parents would need to provide evidence that the children were healthy before they received the MMR vaccine but had become sick soon after vaccination. That was precisely the picture that Wakefield's *Lancet* article painted. The *Lancet* article claimed that all of the children had a history of "normal development followed by loss of acquired skills." The article claimed that all of the children had received an MMR vaccination before their behavioral symptoms started. The article claimed that in most cases, the behavioral symptoms started within 2 weeks of the MMR shot. However, the children's medical records suggested that some of the children had shown signs of developmental problems before they got their MMR shot. Of course, the plaintiffs would have to submit the children's actual medical records as evidence during the lawsuit.

Wakefield used his *Lancet* article as a springboard for launching a panic about the MMR vaccine. This panic would be a boon to a company that Wakefield had established to sell diagnostic test kits to the parents of autistic children.

This panic over the MMR vaccine came at a time when people were already worried about the mercury-containing preservative thimerosal (British people call it thiomersal). (The FDA had already decided to discontinue the use of thimerosal in practically all childhood vaccines, just as a precaution, even before the issue became controversial.)

When Wakefield's article appeared in *The Lancet*, Wakefield held a press conference and produced a video news release. He then went on a speaking tour in the United States. During that tour, he argued that the combined measles-mumps-rubella vaccine should not be used. He even appeared on the highly regarded CBS news program *60 Minutes*. The ensuing media frenzy created panic among parents, especially because the United States seemed to be having an epidemic of autism.

Unfortunately, it took several years for the truth to come to light. Brian Deer, who is a reporter for the *Sunday Times* of London, did an extensive investigation of this story. He reported his findings in articles in the *Sunday Times* and in documentaries on Channel 4, a public television station in Britain. He also provided extensive documentation on his Web site, www.briandeer.com.

On March 6, 2004, *The Lancet* published a letter in which 10 of Wakefield's 11 coauthors backed away from the suggestion that the MMR vaccine was causing autism (the other coauthor could not be contacted):

> We wish to make it clear that in this paper no causal link was established between MMR vaccine and autism as the data were insufficient. However, the possibility of such a link was raised and consequent events have had major implications for public health. In view of this, we consider now is the appropriate time that we should together formally retract the interpretation placed upon these findings in the paper, according to precedent.

On January 28, 2010, the General Medical Council struck Wakefield off the Medical Register, which meant that he could no longer practice medicine in Britain:

> The [Fitness to Practice] Panel made findings of transgressions in many aspects of Dr Wakefield's research. It made findings of dishonesty in regard to his writing of a scientific paper that had major implications for public health, and with regard to his subsequent representations to a scientific body and to colleagues. He was dishonest in respect of the [Legal Aid Board] funds secured for research as well as being misleading. Furthermore he was in breach of his duty to manage finances as well as to account for funds that he did not need to the donor of those funds. In causing blood samples to be taken from children at a birthday party, he callously disregarded the pain and distress young children might suffer and behaved in a way which brought the profession into disrepute.

After Wakefield was struck off the Medical Register, *The Lancet* formally retracted Wakefield's article. The editors gave this explanation:

> Following the judgment of the UK General Medical Council's Fitness to Practise Panel on Jan 28, 2010, it has become clear that several elements of the 1998 paper by Wakefield et al are incorrect, contrary to the findings of an earlier investigation. In particular, the claims in the original paper that children were "consecutively referred" and that investigations were "approved" by the local ethics committee have been proven to be false. Therefore we fully retract this paper from the published record.

Antivaccination zealots claim that the truth about the hazards of vaccines is being suppressed, and that Wakefield was being persecuted for telling the truth. However, the editors of *The Lancet* chose to publish Wakefield's article as an Early Report because they took even flimsy evidence of a safety problem with childhood vaccines seriously. The paper was retracted 12 years later only because a series of investigations showed that the "evidence" that Wakefield presented in his paper was not only flimsy but obviously false.

The fear-mongering about vaccinations raised such a ruckus because many parents had become alarmed by the rise in the incidence of diagnosed cases of autism. However, this rise was not due to a comparably large increase in the number of disabled children. It was at least partly due to a change in what was considered normal and how children were being labeled.

Autism is a developmental disorder that is diagnosed in early childhood. The word *autism* implies that the individual is abnormally self-absorbed, or lost in his or her own world. Some antivaccination activists point out that children were not receiving the diagnosis of autism in the 1930s. Of course they weren't. Back in the 1930s, the word *autism* was used to describe a symptom, not a diagnosis. The use of the word *autism* as a diagnosis started in 1943, when the syndrome called autism was described by a psychiatrist named Leo Kanner. Before that, there certainly were children who would have fit today's diagnostic criteria for autism. However, they would probably have been given a diagnosis of childhood schizophrenia or simply described as feeble-minded.

The number of cases of autism seemed to explode in the 1990s. However, this increase in the number of autism diagnoses was probably not due to a major increase in the number of autistic children. Instead, it was driven mainly by the publication of a book: the fourth edition of the American Psychiatric Association's *Diagnostic and Statistical Manual* (DSM-IV). Psychiatrist Allan Frances, who chaired the committee that compiled the *DSM-IV*, has explained that we have seen a 20-fold increase in autism *diagnoses*, but not a 20-fold increase in autism itself.

In his book *Saving Normal*, Dr. Frances explained that the autism "epidemic" has three causes. One is an improvement in case finding. In other words, more children who really have autism are getting a *correct diagnosis* of autism, instead of an *incorrect diagnosis* of childhood schizophrenia or mental retardation. Another cause was the addition of Asperger's syndrome to the *DSM-IV*. Asperger's syndrome is a broad category that could be extended to include a lot of children who would not previously have been considered to have a mental illness. In fact, some critics have suggested that the diagnosis of Asperger's syndrome is sometimes misused to label bright, intellectually engaged people as mentally ill. The third cause of the explosion in autism diagnoses was the need for parents to get some sort of psychiatric diagnosis for their child in order for the child to get special educational services. Dr. Frances warns that psychiatric diagnoses are often being used in an attempt to solve educational problems, as opposed to mental health problems.

Epidemiologists are still not sure of how much, if any, of the rise in the number of autism diagnoses represents a real increase in the number of children with autism. Epidemiologists are fairly certain that genetics, which stay stable in the population from one generation to the next, play a huge role in autism. Yet nobody knows what other risk factors may be important. Congenital rubella syndrome is one of the few things that are known to increase the risk of the symptoms of autism. Thus, if we stop vaccinating children against rubella before rubella is eradicated, we will end up seeing more cases of autism, not fewer.

Because the explosion of autism diagnoses occurred at the same time as the expansion in the vaccine schedule, many people feared that the vaccinations were responsible for causing autism. These fears were heightened by the fact that autism becomes noticeable at around the same time that children get their vaccination for measles, mumps, and rubella. Yet the signs and symptoms of autism simply tend to become obvious at that age, whether children were vaccinated or not.

We know from large population studies in Denmark and elsewhere that vaccinated children are not more likely than unvaccinated children to get a diagnosis of autism. Nor does the timing of the vaccinations or the total amount of the mercury-containing preservative thimerosal that a child got through vaccinations make any difference. Note that the autism diagnoses continued to rise long after the mercury was removed from practically all of the vaccines that children were receiving.

Although Wakefield has been exposed as a fraud, many antivaccination zealots still think of him as a hero. They turn a blind eye to his greed, his lies, and his other ethical lapses, such as ordering unnecessary medical procedures to be done on children. His supporters believe that vaccination is being promoted by an evil conspiracy that wants to poison children, perhaps to "thin the herd." They interpret any criticism of Wakefield as lies from this evil conspiracy.

The media have been providing undeserved support to the antivaccination movement through sensationalistic coverage of groundless vaccine scares, as well as by using a "false balance" approach to covering vaccine-related stories. For example, they have given publicity to Jenny McCarthy's campaign to "Green our vaccines!" But the fact that the commonly recommended vaccines are effective and remarkably safe isn't newsworthy. The media will give publicity to people who claim, without any evidence, that their child was injured by vaccination. Yet the media rarely show footage that would help people understand how horrible the vaccine-preventable diseases can be.

The antivaccination movement is strong because people want to be seduced by Ginger Grant, but their eyes glaze over when the Professor tries to explain things to them. Even reporters would much rather focus on celebrities than on scientists. Thus, we public health activists have a long, hard road ahead of us.

19

Disease Eradication Campaigns

Despite the best efforts of the antivaccination movement, mandatory vaccination eventually eliminated smallpox from the United States. The last case of smallpox in the United States occurred in 1949. In 1950, the Pan American Health Organization launched a campaign to eliminate smallpox from the Western Hemisphere. It succeeded in eliminating smallpox from all of the American countries except Argentina, Brazil, Colombia, and Ecuador.

In 1958, Viktor Zhdanov, the Deputy Minister of Health for the Soviet Union, presented a lengthy report on smallpox eradication to the World Health Assembly (the decision-making body of the World Health Organization). Professor Zhdanov argued that it would be feasible to drive smallpox into extinction within the following 10 years. Zhdanov had been inspired by the Soviet Union's success in stopping the transmission of smallpox in the 1930s, as well as the elimination of Guinea worm (dracunculiasis) from the Soviet Union's Central Asian republics. These successes made him think about what other diseases could be eradicated. Smallpox was a particular concern because cases kept being imported into the Soviet Union from Iran and Afghanistan. He thought that it would be cheaper as well as safer to eradicate smallpox than to keep vaccinating everyone against it. If smallpox could be driven into extinction worldwide, then nobody would have to be vaccinated against it ever again.

Zhdanov recommended compulsory vaccination in the countries where smallpox was endemic, along with identification and quarantine of potentially infected people. Nearly all of the delegates liked the idea, although some thought that the timeline was too optimistic. The Soviet Union and Cuba promptly donated smallpox vaccine to be used in the program. Today, many people take an antivaccine stance because they think of the vaccine industry as a way for capitalists to make money. In reality, the Communist countries warmly embraced vaccination and proposed the campaign to eradicate smallpox worldwide, thus freeing the children of the future from any need to be vaccinated against smallpox.

In the late 1950s, WHO was preoccupied with an ultimately unsuccessful attempt to eradicate malaria, which is also a deadly disease. It took seven more years before the WHA allocated the funds for the WHO to take on the smallpox eradication project. In the meantime, several countries had succeeded in eliminating smallpox within their borders. In 1966, an international team called the Smallpox Eradication Unit was created. It was led by an American, Donald A. Henderson, MD, MPH.

To eradicate smallpox, the Smallpox Eradication Unit of the WHO had to solve technical and political problems. The technical problems were relatively easy to solve. A stable, freeze-dried form of the vaccinia vaccine had just been developed. Also, a simple and effective two-pronged (bifurcated) vaccination needle had been developed. It took only 5 to 10 minutes to teach someone how to use the needle, which provided nearly 100% success in vaccine "take" with only a tiny dose of vaccine. (The vaccine against smallpox is scratched into the skin, not injected.) The political problems were far more difficult. The WHO had to work to support and coordinate the efforts of national and local health services, especially in areas stricken by civil war and famine.

Like the needle used for vaccination, the eradication campaign had two prongs. One was mass vaccination campaigns intended to immunize 80% of the population in countries where smallpox was endemic. The other was the attempt to find and contain local outbreaks. To find the cases, WHO created a network of consultants who helped countries set up their own surveillance and containment activities. Campaign workers showed people pictures of a patient with a smallpox rash and asked if anyone in the neighborhood had such a rash. When a case of smallpox was found, the patient was quarantined. Then, the campaign workers raced to vaccinate everyone nearby. That strategy was called ring vaccination.

It was hard to eradicate smallpox. Polio has been even harder to eradicate, and measles will be harder still. As I'll explain in more detail in chapter 20, smallpox is far less contagious than polio or measles. Since polio and measles are far more easily spread, a higher percentage of the population must be immunized to stop the spread of the disease. (For an explanation of the mathematics involved, see chapter 15).

Smallpox causes an obvious rash that leaves permanent scars. Even the vaccination leaves a permanent scar. Thus, it's easy to find and trace smallpox outbreaks. It's far harder to tell whether someone has been infected with poliovirus. Most cases of poliovirus infection cause no symptoms. Only a tiny percentage of cases lead to paralysis. Measles leaves no obvious scars. Nor does the vaccination against polio or measles leave a telltale mark on the arm. To tell whether someone is immune to polio or measles, you would have to run a laboratory test. Thus, it is far harder to track immunization and outbreaks of polio and measles.

The last naturally occurring case of the severe form of smallpox (variola major) occurred in 1975 in a two-year-old Bangladeshi girl named Rahima Banu. She survived. The last person to die of variola major was a British medical photographer named Janet Parker, who had been accidentally exposed to the virus from a medical laboratory in the floor beneath her darkroom. She died of the disease. Her mother caught it from her but survived. After Parker's diagnosis, the head of the microbiology laboratory from which the virus had escaped committed suicide. The last case of the milder form of smallpox, variola minor, occurred in 1977 in a Somali man named Ali Maow Maalin. Two years later, smallpox was declared officially extinct. Maalin survived and later worked as a vaccinator in Somalia's successful campaign to eliminate polio. Sadly, he died of malaria in 2013 while doing polio vaccinations after polio had been reimported to Somalia.

The smallpox virus is extinct in the wild. However, samples of the smallpox virus are still being maintained in laboratories in the United States and Russia. The World Health Organization has asked for them to be destroyed. Yet some experts are still asking for the destruction to be postponed because they feel that the virus can teach us so much about the human immune system.

Smallpox was a good candidate for eradication for several reasons. First, it occurs only in human beings. There is no wild reservoir of virus waiting to reinfect us. Second, the disease caused clear symptoms and left obvious scars. Thus, the diagnosis was easy to make, and it was easy to tell, from the scars, whether a person had had the disease in the past or had been vaccinated. Third, smallpox doesn't spread as easily or as quickly as polio or measles. Nevertheless, the eradication of smallpox was still a monumental achievement.

In 1988, the Global Polio Eradication Initiative was launched. It is a public-private partnership led by national governments and spearheaded by the WHO, Rotary International, the CDC, and the United Nations Children's Fund (UNICEF). Polio has proven to be much harder to eradicate than smallpox. It does occur only in humans, so there is no wild reservoir. Yet poliovirus can be spread by the fecal-oral route, so it could be spread by unclean water, as opposed to direct person-to-person contact. Also, people could have a case of poliovirus infection without becoming paralyzed, or even showing any obvious signs of illness. Thus, it is far harder to do surveillance and containment for polio. Yet the biggest hurdle in the polio eradication campaign has been distrust.

Some Muslim clerics in Nigeria were encouraging their followers to resist the vaccination program, out of fear that the vaccinations were really intended to sterilize Muslim girls. This fear was baseless. There is not yet an effective antifertility vaccine for use in human beings. The ones that are used for wildlife last for only about a year. Even if some madman had decided to give the animal vaccine to young girls, the vaccine's contraceptive effects would wear off before the girls went through puberty. Unfortunately, the resistance to the polio vaccination meant that polio persisted among people would then make a pilgrimage to Mecca (the Hajj), thus spreading polio to people who could then bring it back to many other countries.

As I write this, the Global Polio Eradication Initiative is in the final stages of eradication of polio. The first goal is to detect and interrupt all transmission of polio. Next will be the withdrawal of the oral polio vaccine. Then, the Initiative will certify that transmission has been interrupted. After that, they will work on redirecting their staff and other assets to work on other projects.

Meanwhile, another disease is on the verge of complete extinction: dracunculiasis, also known as Guinea worm. People catch it by drinking water contaminated by copepods (water fleas) that are infected with larvae of the guinea worm (*Dracunculus medinensis*). About a year later, the mature female worm forms a painful blister on the person's skin, usually on the leg or foot. Guinea worm is being eradicated by teaching people how to boil or filter their water and by keeping infected people from entering bodies of drinking water.

Yaws is another disease that is slated for eradication, even though there is no vaccine against it. Yaws is caused by a spirochete (spiral bacterium) that is related to the one that causes syphilis. Although yaws is seldom deadly, it can be disfiguring. From 1952 to 1964, the Global Control of Treponematoses program reduced the global prevalence of this disease by about 95%. The WHO projects that yaws can be completely eliminated by 2020.

The Measles and Rubella Initiative is a worldwide campaign of measles and rubella vaccination led by the American Red Cross, the United Nations Foundation, the CDC, UNICEF, and the WHO. The original goal of the M&RI was to reduce global measles mortality by 95% by 2015 and to eliminate measles and rubella in at least five of the six WHO regions by 2015. By 2013, it had reduced measles mortality by 75%, which is an important achievement. A worldwide vaccination campaign can ultimately drive measles, mumps, and rubella into extinction. Those diseases are caused by viruses that occur only in human beings and can easily be prevented by an effective vaccine.

Several other vaccine-preventable diseases also occur only in human beings and theoretically could be eradicated. The big exception is tetanus, which is caused by a bacterium that can live in the intestines of other animals and that is frequently found in soil. We will always need tetanus shots.

The antivaccination movement has done great harm to children. Yet many of the people who are involved in antivaccination advocacy really do care about children, especially their own. Yet if the antivaccination movement had been more successful, people would still be dying of smallpox in the United States. Thanks to the antivaccination scare tactics, babies are still dying of whooping cough in the United States. If this book achieves anything, I hope that it will persuade a few people to join in the effort to eradicate measles and other eradicable diseases. We no longer need to vaccinate children against smallpox. Once poliovirus is extinct, children will no longer need a polio vaccine. When measles, mumps, and rubella are extinct, then children will no longer need the MMR vaccine. Why try to scare people away from necessary vaccines when you could make those vaccines unnecessary by driving the diseases they prevent into extinction?

Part IV

Vaccines and Diseases

Some antivaccination activists claim that the vaccine-preventable diseases are harmless and are actually beneficial for the child in the long run. Thus, they ignore the deaths and the long-term disability that can result from these diseases: blindness, deafness, mental retardation, seizures, amputations, etc.

Some antivaccination activists claim that vaccines are unnecessary because the death rates from the disease were already going down before the vaccine came out. They gloss over the point that many children ended up in the intensive care unit of the hospital for an extended period, sometimes with a tracheotomy. Thus, they ignore children's suffering. They make a big deal out of the suffering of children who had supposedly been injured by vaccines, but typically without providing any evidence that vaccination had anything to do with the child's health problems.

Some antivaccination activists even claim that smallpox was never eradicated. But have you ever seen a person with a rash that looks like this (Figure 18)? In the days before vaccination, smallpox was common. It accounted for one out of every five deaths in Europe.

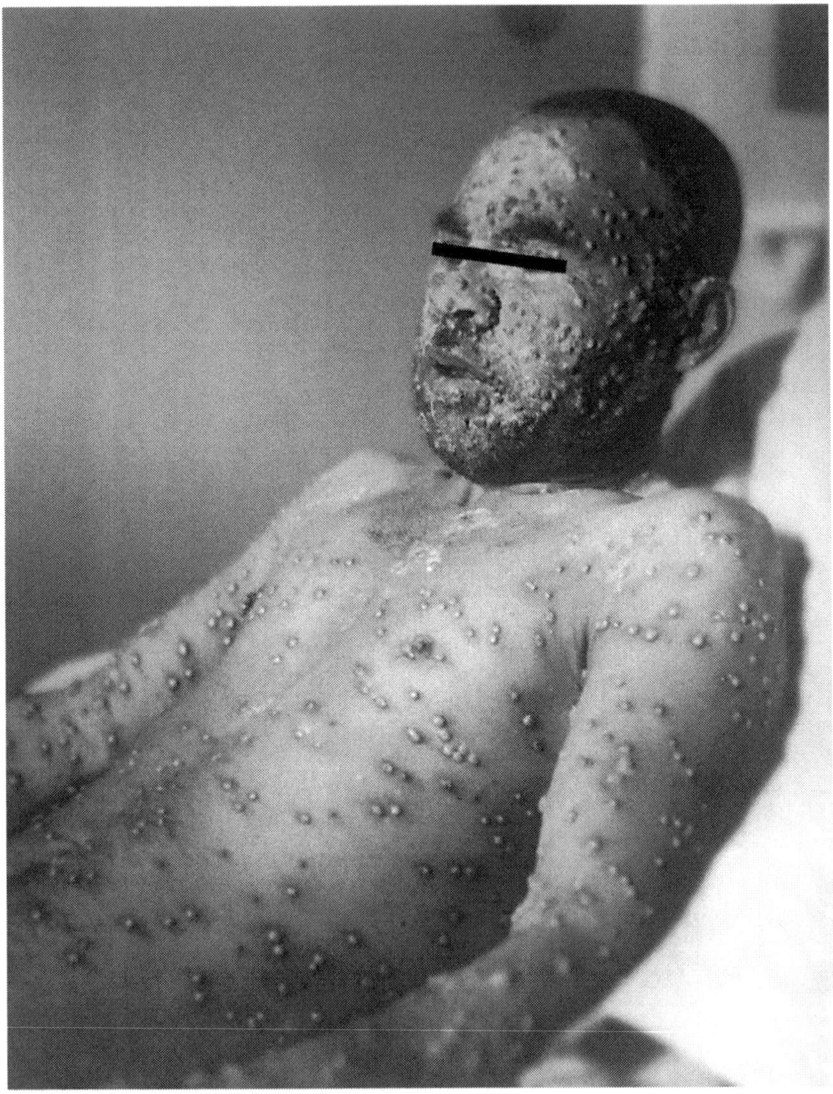

Figure 18. An Iranian man with smallpox in 1962. (Courtesy of Dr. Don Millar and the Centers for Disease Control and Prevention.)

In the following chapters, I will describe the diseases that the recommended vaccines are intended to prevent. I'll explain what causes them, what they do to the body, how they can be prevented, and whether they can be eradicated.

The only way to solve the conflicts over vaccination is to drive as many of the vaccine-preventable diseases as possible into extinction. A global campaign has already succeeded in eradicating smallpox. Polio is next. A parasitic disease called guinea worm is being eradicated through education. Next on the list for eradication should be measles, mumps, and rubella.

The recommended vaccines are remarkably safe, but they are not perfectly safe. We would all be better off if the disease that a vaccine is intended to prevent were driven into extinction. Then, there would be no need to vaccinate anyone against it.

20

Smallpox (Variola)

I was 7 years old when Neil Armstrong became the first human being to set foot on the moon. Like many people all over the world, I excitedly watched the event on live television. When Armstrong stepped off that ladder and onto the lunar surface, he said that it was a small step for a man, a giant leap for mankind. People all over the world took pride in the achievement, as if it had been achieved by humanity as a whole rather than by just the United States.

The moon landing was a landmark in history. It also gave rise to a cliché. Someone who was frustrated by the authorities' failure to achieve some simple goal might say, "If they can put a man on the moon, why can't they...?" Landing men on the moon and bringing them back safe and sound was a stunning achievement for the United States. However, it was far less important than something that all the nations of the world achieved cooperatively just a few years later. Together, the nations of the world drove smallpox into extinction.

Smallpox, which is also called variola, was a scourge of humanity for hundreds and possibly thousands of years. It often changed the course of history. Kings and queens died of it. The mummy of the Egyptian pharaoh Rameses IV, who died more than three thousand years ago, has lesions that look like smallpox blisters. Even as late as the 18th century, smallpox killed five reigning monarchs in Europe and rewrote many lines of succession. Large numbers of common people also died of it.

Smallpox was one of the main reasons why populations remained small even though birthrates were high. After the Spanish arrived in the Americas, smallpox epidemics devastated the indigenous peoples, including the Aztec and Incan empires. As a result, small forces of Spanish conquistadors were able to take control of what then became Latin America.

Smallpox also drew the northern boundary of the United States. A smallpox epidemic devastated the American forces in the Battle of Quebec during the Revolutionary War. The British soldiers, most of whom were already immune to smallpox, were therefore able to drive the Americans out of the Province of Quebec. As a result, the British retained control of Quebec, which is why Canada and the United States became separate countries.

People who became infected with smallpox virus would usually feel perfectly well until 10 to 12 days after infection. Then, they suddenly became ill with a high fever and aching pains that were so severe that the infected people usually became bedridden. Two or 3 days later, a rash would begin to develop on the skin, the mouth, and the tongue. At first, the pustules felt like tiny hard pellets under the skin. Later, they swelled and filled with thick, yellow pus. Each mature pustule had a small dimple, like a bellybutton (Figure 19). That was the hallmark of smallpox, as compared to other diseases that cause pustules.

The smallpox rash made the skin feel as if it were on fire. Some people had so many pustules that the pustules all ran together. Their skin slid off in sheets. Patients with that condition, which was called confluent smallpox, usually died. The pustules gave off a distinctive foul odor, as if the patient were already rotting while still alive. Experienced doctors could base the diagnosis on the odor alone. The rash was not only on the outer surface of the body but on the lining of the mouth and throat. Some smallpox victims died of thirst because swallowing had become unbearably painful.

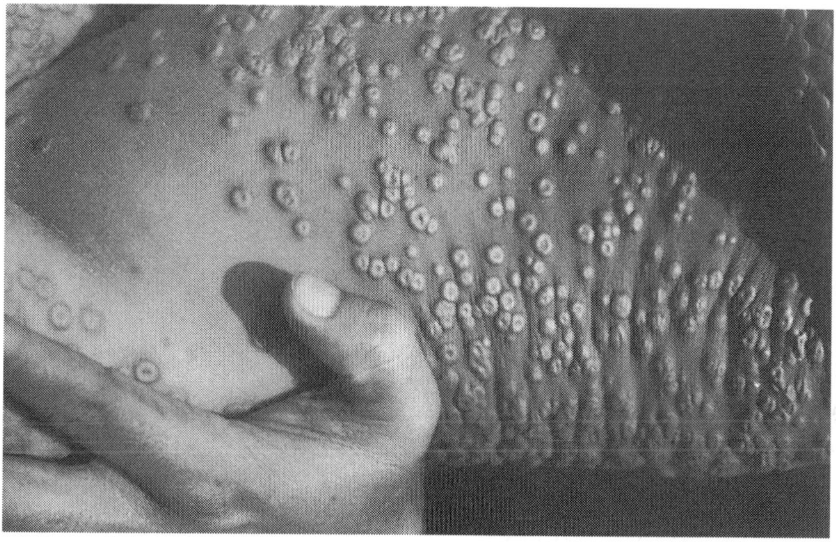

Figure 19. A smallpox (variola major) rash on a patient from Bangladesh in 1973. Note that each pustule has a dimple or indentation. This dimple was the hallmark of smallpox. (Courtesy of James Hicks and the Centers for Disease Control and Prevention.)

Overall, smallpox killed 10% or more of the people whom it infected. In some patients, smallpox took a hemorrhagic form. The skin turned black, and the patient bled from the eyes, nose, mouth, and every other bodily opening. Nearly everyone with the hemorrhagic form of smallpox died.

Smallpox had a high case-fatality rate, right up until it became extinct. Although the development of antibiotics decreased death rates from measles, it had no effect on smallpox deaths. Measles patients typically died of secondary bacterial infections, such as pneumonia. But smallpox patients died as a result of the damage that the smallpox virus itself did to their body. Even a dose of antibodies from someone who is immune to smallpox would provide only a limited benefit once the infection had taken hold. That's because antibodies have no effect on viruses that are already inside cells.

The death rates in "virgin soil" epidemics could be particularly high because so many adults would get sick at the same time. There would simply not be enough healthy people to tend to the sick. As a result, many sick people died of thirst and many babies and children eventually died of starvation.

If a smallpox patient survived, the pustules would become crusty and scabs would form. Most of the scabs would have fallen off by about three weeks after the rash appeared. When the scabs fell off, they revealed deep, permanent, pitted scars. Most of the people who survived a case of smallpox ended up horribly disfigured. Many were blinded.

Smallpox was spread by close, personal contact. Donald A. Henderson, MD, MPH, who led the World Health Organization's final push to eradicate smallpox, explained to me that smallpox patients did not become contagious until the rash appeared. Then, the lesions in the mouth started shedding virus. These viruses could then be expelled into the air when the patient coughed or spoke. Someone who was close to the patient—perhaps within 6 to 8 feet—could become infected by inhaling those infectious particles. Airborne spread over longer distances was extremely rare, unless the patient also had some illness that caused coughing. Smallpox by itself does not cause coughing.

Although the virus was also multiplying in the skin lesions, it would have been held in by the patient's skin, at least until the skin lesions started draining. Theoretically, smallpox could be spread by contact with the patient's contaminated clothing or bedding. However, this kind of spread seems to have been uncommon.

Dr. Henderson explained that in modern outbreaks of variola major (the severe form of smallpox), an infected person seldom infected more than 2 to 4 other people. Smallpox patients were generally too sick to get out of bed to wander around infecting other people. Also, smallpox generally didn't cause a cough. Coughing is an extremely efficient way to produce infectious airborne droplets.

For thousands of years, people sought divine help to deliver them from smallpox. Roman Catholics prayed to St. Nicasius (St. Nicaise), the patron saint of smallpox victims. Likewise, some polytheistic societies in Africa and Asia had gods that were specifically dedicated to smallpox. Yet no matter how hard people prayed, or how many sacrifices people made to their gods, smallpox still raged.

The one piece of good news was that you could get smallpox only once. If you survived one bout with smallpox, you would never catch smallpox again. So about a thousand years ago, people in India and China started trying to figure out ways to give someone a mild case of smallpox. Nearly everyone was eventually going to get smallpox anyway. So why not give them a mild case that wouldn't kill or blind them? These early methods of immunization were called variolation because they involved exposing someone to actual smallpox (variola).

By the 15th century, the Chinese started using a method that is now called insufflation, which means "blowing into" in Latin. They would take scabs from the mildest case of smallpox that they could find, grind the dried scabs into a powder, and then use a silver blowpipe to blow the powder up the patient's nose. The people who were infected with smallpox in this manner were then kept apart from everyone else until their rash had cleared.

By the 18th century, people in Africa and Western Asia had discovered that it was much safer to expose people to smallpox through a cut in the skin than through the respiratory tract. They would take fluid from a smallpox pustule and then rub it into a cut in the patient's skin, usually on the upper arm. This procedure, called inoculation, tended to produce a relatively small, localized smallpox infection. Since the patient was being exposed to genuine smallpox, this form of inoculation was called variolation. Ideally, the variolated patient would end up with one big scar on the arm, instead of scars all over the body. Yet this localized infection still provided lifelong immunity to smallpox.

Variolation was brought back to England from Turkey by Lady Mary Wortley Montagu, the aristocratic wife of the British Ambassador to the Ottoman Empire. Lady Mary was instrumental in introducing variolation to British high society. Her physician—Charles Maitland, who had served in Turkey in the diplomatic corps—eventually persuaded King

George I to let him variolate two of the king's grandchildren. Both children survived the variolation and never got smallpox.

At around the same time, the Puritan minister Cotton Mather in Massachusetts noticed that slaves who had been born in Africa seldom had smallpox scars on their faces. When Mather asked his African-born slave Onesimus about smallpox, Onesimus told Mather that he had "taken the smallpox" in childhood. Onesimus then showed Mather the scar on his arm.

When a smallpox epidemic struck Boston, Mather persuaded a local physician to variolate 248 people. Less than 3% of the variolated people died, as compared to 14% of those who caught smallpox naturally. Not only was Mather a prominent churchman, he was also a member of the Royal Society, a fellowship of the most prominent scientists in the British Empire. As a result, Mather played an important role in promoting variolation within religious and scientific circles.

At first, the medical profession largely opposed variolation. The procedure simply didn't make sense in terms of the medical theories that were being taught in the major universities back then. Germ theory hadn't yet been developed, and viruses had not yet been discovered. Back then, doctors were trained to think that disease resulted from an imbalance of the bodily humors, or perhaps from miasmata (bad odors), or occasionally from an unfortunate alignment of the planets. Furthermore, neither Hippocrates nor Galen had ever mentioned variolation. Thus, many prominent physicians dismissed the idea out of hand.

Of course, if you kept track of what was happening to actual patients, you would definitely choose variolation over a natural case of smallpox. People with a natural case of smallpox ran a much higher risk of dying. Even if they survived, they could be horribly scarred and perhaps blinded. On the other hand, if you were inoculated, your risk of dying of smallpox dropped by as much as 90%, unless your doctor killed you through "heroic" treatments such as bleeding or purging. The most likely result of variolation was that you'd end up with a nasty scar on your arm and lifelong immunity to smallpox.

Of course, variolation was still risky. It exposed people to active smallpox virus. Some people did die of generalized smallpox as a result. Also, the variolated patients had to be kept isolated from other people until their scabs fell off. Otherwise, they could pass smallpox on to others. Nevertheless, it was hard to judge the risks of variolation. That's because the variolation procedure could be done only during a smallpox outbreak. When patients who had just been variolated came down with generalized smallpox, it wasn't always clear whether they had gotten sick from the variolation or whether they had simply caught smallpox from someone else in the neighborhood.

Variolation was an unsanitary procedure that involved a break in the skin. As a result, it could result in an ordinary infection, which was often deadly in the days before antibiotics. Also, variolation exposed people to the bodily fluid of another human being. Thus, it could spread other infections, such as syphilis, from one person to another.

Wars have always produced epidemics of disease. Armies were a breeding ground for disease because so many young men were living in close quarters, often in unsanitary and stressful conditions. The movement of armies and refugees also tended to spread infectious diseases to populations that had not encountered them before. Thus, it should come as no surprise that the American Revolutionary War unleashed severe outbreaks of smallpox.

Smallpox wasn't unknown in Britain's North American colonies. However, it tended to occur in big epidemics every 10 to 20 years. Smallpox is like a wildfire. A wildfire quickly burns through all of the available fuel. Then it dies out on its own. For a few years after that, there's not enough fuel in the area to sustain a fire. Only after new trees have grown up is there enough fuel to have another wildfire. Smallpox epidemics act in a similar way. They burn through the population, striking a big proportion of the susceptible people. Once those people have either died or become immune, the virus can no longer find new people to infect. That's why epidemics fizzle out in small, isolated populations.

The population in the British colonies of North America wasn't large or dense enough to keep smallpox circulating for very long. As a result, smallpox epidemics in the colonies would quickly die out.

Then, the population would be free of smallpox for many years, until the population could sustain another major epidemic. In contrast, the population in Britain was so large and dense that smallpox was present all the time. In other words, smallpox was endemic in Britain. As a result, most British people caught it in childhood. Thus, most British soldiers had already had smallpox.

The British army offered variolation, on a voluntary basis, to those who had not yet had smallpox. Thus, most of the redcoats were immune to smallpox, while most of the American soldiers were not. For that reason, a smallpox outbreak was much more of a problem for the Americans than for the British. Some historians even suspect that the British spread smallpox deliberately during the Revolutionary War, as a means of biological warfare.

General George Washington was commander-in-chief of the Continental Army during the Revolutionary War. Washington had survived a bout of smallpox during a trip to Barbados in 1751, when he was 19 years old. John Adams, in contrast, had been variolated in Massachusetts in 1764; his wife Abigail and their children were variolated in July of 1776, while Adams was in Philadelphia signing the Declaration of Independence.

Two of the other signers of the Declaration were also strong advocates of variolation: Benjamin Franklin and Benjamin Rush. Their influence helped to persuade Washington to make what was probably the most important strategic decision that he made during the Revolutionary War. While camped at Morristown in 1777, Washington ordered immediate, compulsory variolation for everyone in the Continental Army who was not already immune to smallpox. The inoculations continued during the winter of 1778 at Valley Forge. The Continental Army also set up inoculation stations in Virginia to variolate recruits who came from the South. To keep the smallpox from spreading, the variolation was performed in inoculation hospitals, and the men were kept quarantined in inoculation huts until their scabs had dropped off.

The Continental Army was the first army to impose compulsory immunization for its recruits. At the time, the British army variolated its soldiers, but only on a voluntary basis. The British neglected to variolate an important group of people who could have helped them win the war: the black slaves who were offered their freedom in exchange for military service with the British forces. It may seem odd that the British did not bother to variolate these freedmen. However, Britain's goal in the war was to retain control over the North American colonies, not to undermine slavery. After all, the slave-based economy made the colonial enterprise in North America and especially the Caribbean profitable for the British Empire.

The biggest problem with variolation is that it exposed the patient to genuine smallpox virus that had not been weakened in any way. In contrast, most modern vaccines involve virus that has been inactivated or that has somehow been rendered less deadly. However, nobody in the 18th century knew anything about viruses, or even about the germ theory of disease.

In 1796, a British physician named Edward Jenner came up with a different means of immunization against smallpox. Jenner had heard the common folk wisdom that women who worked on dairy farms never got smallpox. The dairymaids themselves said that it was because they had caught a disease called cowpox from the cows. A case of cowpox looks like a very mild case of smallpox. However, it made the dairymaids immune to smallpox, as well as to repeated infections with cowpox.

Jenner inoculated a boy with pus from a cowpox pustule from the hand of a dairymaid. The inoculation produced a much milder reaction than you'd get from variolation. After the boy recovered from the inoculation, Jenner inoculated him with pus from a smallpox patient. The boy had no reaction to the variolation, which showed that the cowpox inoculation had made him immune to smallpox.

Inoculating someone with pus from a cowpox lesion was called vaccination, from the Latin word *vaccinus*, which means of or from cows. Since vaccination did not involve exposing the patient to genuine smallpox, there was no risk that vaccinated patients could transmit smallpox to anyone else. They could transmit cowpox for a short time after vaccination, but cowpox was a much milder disease.

Within only a few years, Jenner's report about vaccination was translated into many languages. Vaccination rapidly replaced variolation in many countries. The practice of vaccination was rapidly adopted in Europe and gradually spread throughout the world. It became much more widely accepted than variolation had ever been. By the 1830s, vaccination led to dramatic increases in life expectancy in France. Nevertheless, variolation continued to be practiced in some remote areas of Africa and Asia as late as the 1970s, when wild smallpox was finally driven into extinction.

The first vaccinations were done with pus from a cowpox pustule, often as an "arm-to-arm" inoculation from one human being to the next. This method of vaccination posed the risk of spreading other diseases, such as syphilis, from person to person. Although the vaccination material could be dried on threads or needles and transported for long distances, it sometimes lost its potency.

Much of the early resistance to vaccination programs was based on valid concerns about the safety and reliability of the early vaccination methods. As I explain in chapter 16, technical developments helped to make vaccines safer and more reliable.

When variolation was first invented, it was reserved for the wealthy people who could afford medical treatment. But in 1774, Benjamin Franklin raised money to provide free variolation for the poor. After the development of vaccination, many governments eventually required everyone to be vaccinated, whether they wanted to be vaccinated or not.

By the early 20th century, the rates of death from smallpox had gone down substantially in the United States. However, many people—especially poor whites and poor blacks in the South—continued to go unvaccinated. Thus, the decrease in death rates was only partly due to vaccination. Much of it was due to the spread of a milder form of smallpox, called variola minor. Variola minor killed only about 1% of its victims. It was also more easily spread because its victims were less disabled while they were contagious. Thus, they were able to come into contact with more people. Yet a case of variola minor would make you immune to variola major as well. Thus, variola minor was outcompeting regular smallpox (variola major).

The people who invented variolation and vaccination had no understanding of the germ theory of disease. They had no idea that viruses existed or what they were like. The first clue to the existence of the smallpox virus came in 1906, when an Italian microbiologist named Adelchi Negri showed that the infective agent from the vaccinia vaccine was small enough to pass through a porcelain filter. Thus, it was too small to be a bacterium.

Later research explained why a cowpox infection protects against smallpox infection. The viruses that cause variola major and variola minor are part of a family of closely related viruses called the orthopox viruses. Each orthopox virus tends to infect only a restricted range of possible hosts. For example, smallpox occurs only in human beings. However, the orthopox viruses closely resemble each other. They are brick-shaped, enveloped viruses that have their genes in a double strand of DNA.

For reasons I explained in chapter 12, double-stranded DNA viruses are far more genetically stable than single-stranded RNA viruses are. That could explain why antibodies against vaccinia virus would protect you against smallpox (variola major and minor), cowpox, and monkeypox, even though those viral lineages split a few thousand years ago. In contrast, the vaccine for last year's predominant strain of influenza virus (a single-stranded RNA virus) may be less effective this year. If a radically new version of the influenza virus starts circulating, a completely new version of the vaccine will be needed. (I'll talk about the effectiveness of influenza vaccines in chapter 29).

One puzzling discovery was that the vaccinia virus, which is currently being used for smallpox vaccination, is not really the cowpox virus. The vaccinia virus had been passed along from arm to arm and from laboratory to laboratory for so long that its pedigree was lost. However, it may have been descended from an otherwise extinct strain of horsepox.

During the 20th century, both variola major and variola minor were driven into extinction. First, they were eliminated from the industrialized countries. There has not been a case of smallpox in the United States since 1949. Then, an international effort organized by the World

Health Organization wiped them out of their last refuges by the late 1970s. The last natural case of smallpox occurred in 1977, and smallpox was declared extinct in 1980. Countries throughout the world stopped routine vaccinations by 1984.

Now that smallpox has been eradicated, the risks associated with the vaccinia vaccine itself would outweigh any possible benefits for the general population. That's why we no longer vaccinate children against smallpox. However, the vaccinia vaccine might still be useful for people who might be exposed to other orthopox viruses, such as monkeypox. However, those viruses are generally not a threat to public health in the United States.

After smallpox was declared extinct in the wild, the remaining samples of "live" smallpox virus were either destroyed or stored in one of two repositories: one in the United States and one in the former Soviet Union. Many people, including Dr. Henderson, have argued that these remaining samples of smallpox virus should be destroyed. The smallpox virus is not needed for making smallpox vaccine. Also, someone might decide to use smallpox virus as a biological weapon, or some madman might simply release the active virus, just as some madman sent anthrax spores through the U.S. mail in 2001. Several people died from the anthrax attacks, but anthrax does not spread from person to person. In contrast, a modern smallpox epidemic would be truly horrifying, considering that there is no treatment for smallpox and hardly anyone under the age of 40 in the United States has been vaccinated against smallpox.

The moon landings were impressive, but they had no lasting impact on most people's lives. In fact, many conspiracy theorists insist that the moon landings never really happened. In contrast, the eradication of smallpox was a tremendous achievement that has already saved millions of lives. (And of course, some antivaccination zealots insist that it never really happened.) Roughly 300 million people died of smallpox in the 20th century. Unless someone does something unimaginably stupid and evil, there will never again be even one case of smallpox anywhere in the world.

21

Polio (Poliomyelitis or Infantile Paralysis)

For thousands of years, people have known that children who got a fever while they were teething could end up permanently paralyzed. In the worst cases, the child simply stopped breathing and died. In milder cases, the child survived but lost the use of one or both legs, sometimes permanently. Paintings and carvings from ancient Egypt show children walking with canes, as well as adults with withered limbs—likely victims of infantile paralysis. Some historians suspect that the Roman emperor Claudius's limp was due to infantile paralysis. Usually, this disease occurred as isolated individual cases. However, the disease could also strike many people at once. For example, the Hippocratic writings include a description of an epidemic of a paralytic disease on the island of Thaos.

When pathologists in the 19th century started doing autopsies on people who had suffered from infantile paralysis, they found damage in the spinal cord. In particular, the gray matter of the anterior horn (part of the front of the spinal cord) had been damaged. Thus, they started calling the disease poliomyelitis: *polio-* comes from the Greek word for gray, *-myel-* comes from the Greek word meaning marrow and refers to the spinal cord, *-itis* means inflammation. In a particularly severe case of polio, the inflammation can extend upward into the brainstem or even the brain (polioencephalitis). Of course, we English-speaking people love short, simple words. So we started saying polio instead of poliomyelitis or infantile paralysis.

The paralysis caused by polio is often called acute flaccid paralysis. Acute means sudden. Flaccid means that there is a loss of muscle tone (i.e., the muscles go slack). This form of paralysis is typically due to a problem in the lower motor neurons, which are the nerve cells that start in the spinal cord and go to the muscles. Paralysis can also result from problems higher up in the nervous system (upper motor neuron disease). However, that kind of paralysis is usually associated with tight muscles (spastic paralysis).

The paralysis that results from a case of polio depends on what portions of the spinal cord have been damaged, and how bad the damage is. If only the lower part of the spinal cord is damaged, then only the legs are affected. In most cases of spinal polio, one or both legs are affected. In severe cases of spinal polio, the arms are weakened or paralyzed as well (quadriplegia).

The worst form of paralysis from polio is called bulbar polio. It results from damage to the brain stem. People with bulbar polio have trouble with swallowing, talking, and breathing. In the old days, people with bulbar polio simply died. But in the 20th century, the invention of a mechanical breathing device called an iron lung helped many people survive for years, or even decades, after they lost the ability to breathe on their own (Figure 20). In the aftermath of polio epidemics, hospital wards were filled with children in iron lungs.

As a case of polio develops, the legs tend to become paralyzed before the arms. This pattern is called ascending paralysis. In contrast, botulism produces a descending paralysis, which starts with the cranial nerves. In a case of botulism, the eye muscles are the first to become paralyzed. Then, the paralysis spreads to muscles lower in the body.

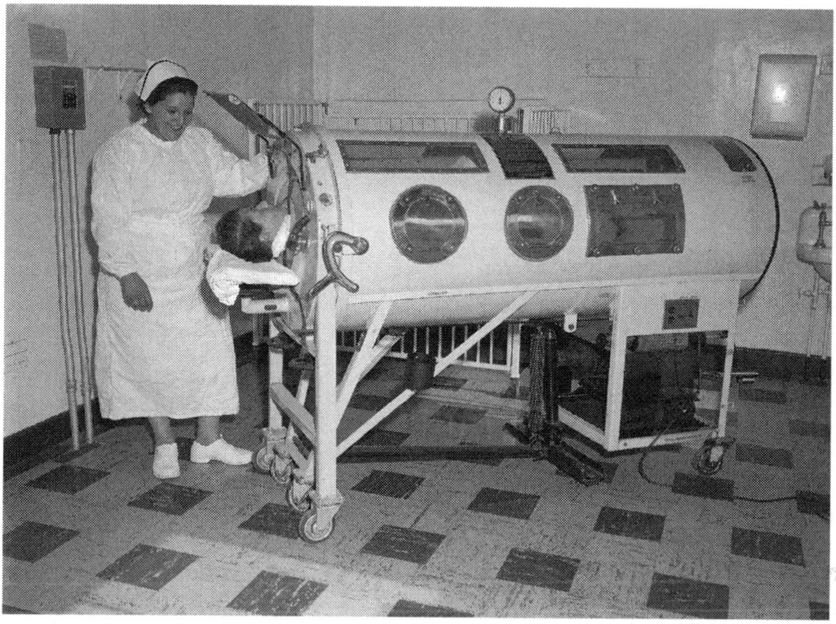

Figure 20. In this photograph from 1960, a nurse in Rhode Island cares for a patient inside an Emerson respirator. This so-called iron lung was needed to allow the patient to breathe. Note the mirror that lets the patient see something of his surroundings.

In 1909, the famous German doctor Karl Landsteiner and his assistant Erwin Popper proved that epidemic poliomyelitis is due to an infectious agent that is far smaller than a bacterium. In other words, it had to be due to a virus. They found that they could transmit the infection to monkeys, which then went on to suffer from paralysis. Landsteiner is also famous for discovering the ABO system of blood typing, which made blood transfusion much safer.

Poliovirus belongs to the genus *Enterovirus*. (Some other enteroviruses, such as EV-D68, can also occasionally cause acute flaccid paralysis.) The prefix *entero-* means intestines. As you might expect, the enteroviruses mainly infect the gut. Like other gut infections, they can be transmitted by water that has been contaminated with raw sewage. However, some enteroviruses, including poliovirus, can also infect the respiratory tract. As a result, they can be easily transmitted from person to person, just like the common cold. Poliovirus is highly infectious. If one person in a household catches poliovirus, the unimmunized children in that household have a nearly 100% chance of catching the infection. Unimmunized adults have about a 90% risk of catching the infection.

Until the late 19th century, most people first became exposed to poliovirus in infancy, while they were still being breast-fed and were thus being protected by their mother's antibodies. The mother's antibodies helped to protect the baby's nervous system from the effects of the virus as the baby's immune system was learning to make its own antibodies against the virus. As a result, there were relatively few cases of paralysis. Poliovirus is far more dangerous if a child's first exposure to the virus occurs after weaning, when the child is no longer protected by his or her mother's antibodies.

Before the late 19th century, polio was usually an endemic disease. In other words, an isolated case would occur every so often, usually in a young child. However, an epidemic of polio (a lot of cases at once) could occur if poliovirus started spreading among older people with no natural immunity, such as the isolated population on the island of Thaos.

Estimates of the risk of paralysis after poliovirus infection vary. They range from 1 in 3000 to 1 in 50 cases. The risk increases with age. The risk is also higher for malnourished and immunosuppressed people. Polio is particularly dangerous for pregnant women, although polio during pregnancy seems to have no effect on the fetus. Injury to the muscles during a poliovirus infection can increase the risk of paralysis. Thus, exercise or an intramuscular injection could trigger paralysis in someone infected with poliovirus.

Poliovirus normally infects the lining of the gastrointestinal tract. Like other gut infections, poliovirus can be spread by the fecal-oral route (e.g., by water contaminated by sewage). That's why poliovirus has been endemic in societies with poor sanitation. Fortunately, poliovirus can easily be inactivated by relatively low concentrations of chlorine. Because of the development of sanitary sewers and water treatment plants, fewer people became exposed to poliovirus. Unfortunately, the exposure tended to come at later age, when the risk of paralysis was higher. As a result, polio went from being an endemic disease (present all the time) to an epidemic disease (occurring from time to time in big clusters). Starting in 1881, Europe and then the United States started having epidemics of paralytic polio, usually in the summer. By that time, germ theory was well-accepted in scientific circles. Thus, scientists started to suspect that these epidemics of poliomyelitis were the result of an infection.

Although chlorination prevented polio from being spread through the water supply, poliovirus is resistant to soap and many conventional disinfectants. As a result, personal hygiene does little to stop the person-to-person spread. In temperate climates, polio epidemics tended to occur in the summer. Many people suspected that it was being spread in swimming pools. (Back then, some public pools were not chlorinated). In tropical climates, polio spreads all year round.

After the poliovirus begins to multiply in the cells of the intestines, it can invade the bloodstream. From there, it can make its way into the nervous system, where it spreads along nerve fibers. The poliovirus can destroy the lower motor neurons. Thus, poliovirus infection can cause acute flaccid paralysis. (However, it is not the only possible cause of acute flaccid paralysis.) After a while, the muscles shrink (atrophy) from lack of use.

If a nerve is merely inflamed, the patient can get some improvement as the inflammation subsides. Unfortunately, the dead nerve cells cannot be replaced. Thus, some degree of paralysis may be permanent. In the 1980s, physicians began to realize that many polio survivors go on to suffer from a post-polio syndrome many years after a case of polio. Their muscles progressively become smaller and weaker, and they suffer from joint problems and skeletal deformities, such as curvature of the spine.

It took a massive research effort to develop the vaccine that conquered polio. The person who should get the biggest share of the credit is Franklin Delano Roosevelt, who was President of the United States from March 4, 1933 to his death on April 12, 1945.

FDR came from a wealthy and prominent family. He was a distant cousin of President Theodore Roosevelt, who had been the uncle and guardian of Franklin's wife Eleanor. FDR's Delano ancestors had made a lot of money as international merchants, involved in the China trade.

From early on, FDR had political ambitions. In 1910, he was elected to the New York State Senate as an anti–Tammany Hall Democrat. During World War I, he served as Assistant Secretary of the Navy. In 1920, he ran for Vice President of the United States. Then, in August of 1921, when he was 39 years old, he was struck with an illness that left him permanently paralyzed from the waist down. In the 1920s, there were no laboratory tests to confirm the diagnosis of polio. Some medical historians have suggested that FDR's paralysis might have been due to Guillain-Barré syndrome, an autoimmune disease that can also cause an ascending acute flaccid paralysis. (Many cases of Guillain-Barré syndrome seem to be triggered by infection with a bacterium called *Campylobacter jejuni*.) Whether FDR had polio or Guillain-Barré syndrome does not really matter. What matters is that he did something about polio.

Roosevelt refused to accept that his paralysis was incurable, and he hoped that hydrotherapy would help him. In 1927, he bought a resort in Warm Springs, Georgia, where there was a natural spring whose water was always 88°F. At Warm Springs, he met many polio victims, many of them children. He eventually turned the resort into a nonprofit institute dedicated to the care of polio survivors.

FDR was elected to his first term as President in November 1932, during the depths of the Great Depression. Beginning in 1934, the annual Birthday Ball that was held in honor of the President's birthday was dedicated to raising money for polio research. In 1937, FDR issued a proclamation announcing the creation of the National Foundation for Infantile Paralysis, which would help polio survivors and work to develop a vaccine. FDR persuaded famous entertainers to get in on the act. In turn, they effectively reached out to the public.

In 1937, Vaudeville star Eddie Cantor suggested that all of the national radio programs originating in Hollywood should devote 30 seconds to an appeal for a million ordinary people to send a dime to the NFIP. The idea was that even in the depths of the Depression, nearly anyone could afford to donate a dime to help a child walk again. Cantor suggested, "We could call it the March of Dimes." (At the time, there was a popular radio show and newsreel series called The March of Time.) The radio appeal led to a deluge of dimes and dollars being sent to the White House. The National Foundation for Infantile Paralysis, which was later renamed the March of Dimes, eventually raised millions of dollars, which provided the funding that led to the development of the effective vaccines against polio.

The first effective vaccine against polio was the "killed" vaccine (i.e., made of viruses that can no longer infect a living cell) developed by Jonas Salk. His vaccine was tested in a nationwide field trial in 1.8 million schoolchildren. The trial's results, which were announced on April 12, 1955, the 10th anniversary of FDR's death, showed that the vaccine was not only safe, it dramatically reduced the risk of paralysis. This news was met with widespread rejoicing. Meanwhile, Albert Sabin was still working on an attenuated or "live" vaccine (made out of viruses that can infect living cells but without causing disease). This "live" vaccine would not only prevent paralysis, it would prevent a person from having a poliovirus infection of the intestine. Thus, it could stop the virus from spreading within the population.

Unfortunately, the Salk vaccine was only 90% effective in preventing paralysis from type 1 or type 2 poliovirus. It was only about 60% effective in preventing paralysis from infection with type 3. In the days before the introduction of the Salk vaccine, there were generally between 13,000 and 20,000 cases of paralytic polio per year in the United States. By 1960, the use of the Salk vaccine had caused that number to drop to 2525 cases. Fortunately, after the introduction of the Sabin's "live" polio vaccine in 1961, the number of cases dropped even further. In 1965, there were only 61 cases of paralytic polio in the United States. The use of the Sabin virus stopped the transmission of wild poliovirus in the United States. The last cases of endemic paralytic polio in the United States occurred among Amish people in the Midwest in 1979. They probably caught it from a relative who had become infected in the Netherlands. The last imported case of paralytic polio in the

United States occurred in 1993. Nevertheless, any disease that is circulating anywhere in the world is only a plane flight away.

The Sabin vaccine contains a "live" but weakened strain of poliovirus. It is intended to cause a mild infection that produces no symptoms and does no lasting damage. The virus in the "live" polio vaccine could also be spread to other people, just like wild poliovirus. Unvaccinated people might catch the vaccine strain from a vaccinated person. Thus, people could be immunized against polio even if they were not deliberately vaccinated. Unfortunately, the vaccine strain differs from the dangerous strains by only a few mutations. Because of their genetic instability, the "live" viruses used in the vaccine occasionally mutate back to a dangerous form. As a result, the "live" vaccine resulted in a few cases of paralytic polio in people who had been in contact with a recently vaccinated child. Thus, it caused about a dozen or so cases of paralysis per year. (Note that pregnant women and people with weakened immune systems should never receive a "live" vaccine and may need to avoid contact with people who have just received a "live" vaccine.)

After wild polio was eliminated from the Americas, the only people who were being paralyzed by polio were the handful of people every year whose paralysis resulted from the vaccine virus mutating back into a dangerous form. In 1988, a more effective "killed" polio vaccine became available. By 2000, the use of the "live" vaccine was discontinued in the United States. However, the "live" polio vaccine is still playing an important role in the efforts to eradicate polio in Africa and Asia.

There were two important safety problems with the early polio vaccines. One involved only the Salk vaccine. The other involved both the Salk and the Sabin vaccine. Some of the early batches of the Salk vaccine produced by Cutter Laboratories contained poliovirus that had not been completely inactivated. Despite warnings from Dr. Bernice Eddy, who had found that monkeys inoculated with the vaccine had become paralyzed, 120,000 doses of vaccine containing infectious poliovirus were produced. Among the children who received this vaccine, 40,000 developed polio infections that did not involve the central nervous system, 200 children ended up with some degree of paralysis, and 10 children died. The vaccinated children then spread the disease to other people; these secondary cases led to more cases of paralysis and more deaths. This tragedy, called the Cutter Incident, led to tighter federal regulation of vaccines, which in turn led to dramatic improvements in safety.

The other problem with the polio vaccine resulted from the fact that the vaccine had to be grown in monkey cells. The viruses for both the Salk and the Sabin vaccine were being produced in kidney cells from rhesus monkeys. Unfortunately, these cells were sometimes infected with a virus called SV40. The SV40 virus does not cause any health problems in the monkeys, unless they have immune suppression, such as from simian immunodeficiency virus (SIV). However, SV40 can cause tumors when injected into hamsters. After this problem was discovered, the vaccine makers stopped using rhesus monkey kidneys and started using African green monkey kidneys instead. The SV40 virus cannot infect African green monkey cells.

Because of this contamination of the early polio vaccine, millions of people worldwide were exposed to SV40 between 1955 and 1963. However, we have no evidence that this exposure led to any public health problem. Epidemiologists have found no evidence of a higher incidence of cancer or any other health problem in the people who were vaccinated between 1955 and 1963, as compared with those who were vaccinated later. Also, antibodies to SV40 have been found in serum samples that were stored before the polio vaccine was introduced. Thus, the SV40 virus, or something very similar to it, was already circulating in the U.S. population before the polio vaccine was introduced.

Many antivaccination activists have tried to stir up hysteria about the SV40 contamination. However, the SV40 contamination problem was recognized and solved more than 50 years ago, even though virology was far more primitive back then. The antivaccination activists also fail to point out the safeguards that have been put in place since then to prevent future contamination of vaccines by adventitious agents (i.e., by viruses that are not supposed to be in the vaccine). The antivaccine activists never discuss the precautions that vaccine makers must take to avoid contamination of the cell cultures used for making vaccines. Nor do the antivaccine activists explain the methods that are now used to test cultures for adventitious agents. The antivaccine activists also fail to point out that once a disease such as polio has been eradicated, everyone will stop vaccinating against that disease.

Some antivaccination activists have claimed that the AIDS epidemic in Africa was the result of polio vaccination. They claimed that chimpanzee kidneys were used to make the vaccine. These claims have been totally discredited. Even if you don't believe the scientists involved, the AIDS epidemic does not follow the pattern that you would expect if it had been spread by vaccination. From studying the genetic differences between different strains of the HIV virus, virologists now believe that HIV entered the human population around 1920 near Kinshasa, which is the capital of what is now the Democratic Republic of the Congo. It was able to spread rapidly from there because of strong railway connections and the sex trade. In other words, the AIDS epidemic broke out among sexually active adults, rather than within a cohort of vaccinated children.

The United States has been free of polio since 1979. Yet polio continued to circulate in some poorer countries throughout the world. In 1988, a Global Polio Eradication Initiative was launched. It is a public-private partnership led by national governments and supported by the WHO, Rotary International, the CDC, and UNICEF. Between 1988 and 2011, this global effort has decreased the worldwide incidence of polio by 99%. With any luck, polio will soon be a thing of the past.

Once polio has been eradicated, we can safely stop vaccinating children against polio. Yet the antivaccination zealots will not rejoice. Instead, they are already putting together their talking points. Some of them are claiming that the poliovirus infection did not cause acute flaccid paralysis. Some are even claiming that epidemics of acute flaccid paralysis are a bigger problem now than they were in the 1950s, and thus that the polio vaccine had no effect.

President Franklin Delano Roosevelt died in 1945. Shortly afterward, Congressman Ralph H. Daughton, a Democrat from Virginia, introduced legislation to put FDR's image on the dime, partly to commemorate his efforts in founding the March of Dimes. Lately, some conservatives have suggested that FDR's image should be replaced with Ronald Reagan's. Yet I would prefer the dime to stay as it is, to serve as a constant reminder of a time when we the people were united in a common cause that was true and pure and of lasting importance: the struggle to defeat infantile paralysis.

22

Measles (Rubeola)

Nearly everyone who was born before 1957 got measles in childhood. But thanks to an effective vaccine, along with laws requiring children to be vaccinated against measles, measles is no longer circulating in the Americas or Australia. As of 2005, measles was still responsible for 4% of all deaths of children under 5 years of age, worldwide. As I write this in 2015, measles is still circulating in Africa, Asia, and Europe. It is still killing large numbers of children in Africa. Because measles is still circulating overseas, it keeps being reimported to the United States and Australia, typically by unvaccinated travelers.

One nightmare scenario began in California in December 2014, when a measles outbreak centered on the Disneyland theme park. That kind of setting allows for many children, many of them unvaccinated, to be exposed to measles. The infected children could then carry the measles back to their home communities. More than 80% of the people who caught measles in this outbreak were unvaccinated, either because they were too young to be vaccinated or because their parents chose not to vaccinate them.

As I write this, the Measles and Rubella Initiative is working to drive measles into extinction. The M&RI is a worldwide campaign of measles vaccination led by the American Red Cross, the United Nations Foundation, the CDC, UNICEF, and the WHO. From 2000 to 2013, that vaccination campaign has decreased the worldwide annual death toll from measles by 75%—from 544,200 to 145,700. The ultimate goal is to decrease the number of measles cases, and therefore measles deaths, to zero. At that point, there will be no more measles, ever again. Once the measles virus is extinct, we can safely stop vaccinating children against it.

Measles can spread so fast because an early case of the measles looks and feels a lot like a common cold. The first sign of illness is usually a mild fever plus a cough, stuffy nose, and conjunctivitis (red, watery eyes). The infected person may feel achy and generally unwell. This relatively mild stage of the illness may last two or three days. At that point, tiny white dots (Koplik's spots) may appear inside the mouth. When those dots appear, the person can start shedding the measles virus. Because of coughing and sneezing, the infected person will produce clouds of airborne droplets that can efficiently spread the virus to other people.

Unfortunately, the measles virus spreads beyond the respiratory system. First, it makes its way to the lymph nodes. Normally, the cells in the lymph nodes are supposed to kill germs. But for some reason, they amplify the measles virus, which means that they make many new copies of it. These new copies of the measles virus then enter the bloodstream. Once this flood of measles virions enters the bloodstream, those virions can easily spread all over the body. At that point, the patient spikes a fever, often with a temperature of 104°F or higher. Then, the infected person breaks out in a rash. The rash consists of small red spots, some of which are slightly raised. The rash shows up first on the face and then spreads downward, over the arms, trunk, and legs. A few days later, the fever breaks and the rash starts to fade.

A case of measles can be deadly, for two reasons: the measles virus can spread to the brain, and the measles virus can suppress the immune system for several weeks. The brain infection is called encephalitis.

Measles encephalitis can lead to deafness, mental retardation, epilepsy, or even death. Measles can also cause blindness, especially in children with a vitamin A deficiency, which is a common problem among undernourished children in poor countries.

The measles virus can kill cells, especially the cells that line the respiratory tract. Just as a scratch in the skin leaves a person more prone to bacterial infections of the skin, damage to the respiratory tract leaves a person more prone to bacterial infections of the lung. These bacterial infections can be particularly severe because the measles virus was the first virus that was known to suppress the immune system. The measles virus interferes with the activities of white blood cells during the active measles infection and for several weeks afterward. The resulting immune suppression can linger for several years. This immune suppression can be particularly severe in people who are malnourished or have other causes of immune suppression, such as malaria or HIV infection.

Many people who die from a case of measles are actually killed by a secondary bacterial infection. That's why the case-fatality rate for measles started to go down after the development of antibiotics, even before the introduction of the measles vaccine. Antibiotics have no effect on the measles virus per se but can often cure the secondary bacterial infections that occur in someone whose immune system has been weakened by the measles infection.

Many antivaccination activists insist that the measles is no big deal. Some of the crazier ones even claim that a case of measles is actually good for the child. A few zealots even want to expose their children to wild measles virus by having their children attend a "measles party" with an infected child. But in reality, there is nothing good about having the measles. Even with modern medical care, one out of every 300 cases of measles leads to death. The death rate is far higher in Africa, where many children's immune systems are weakened by malnutrition (especially vitamin A deficiency), parasite infection (including malaria), and even HIV infection. In Africa, measles typically kills 5% to 10% of the children it infects. The case-fatality rate can be even higher (20% to 30% of infected children) during a famine or in refugee camps. It is roughly 30% among immunosuppressed people, such as AIDS patients. According to an African proverb, "Don't count your children until after the measles has passed."

To stop the horrible death toll among African children, the Bill and Melinda Gates Foundation has been funding UNICEF's measles vaccination campaign. The Gates Foundation has also been funding research for a measles vaccine that would protect babies younger than 9 months of age. Bill Gates has spent millions of dollars to save the lives of children in Africa. Yet some conspiracy theorists claim that Bill Gates's vaccine program is part of a program of genocide. They claim that the purpose of the vaccinations is to "thin the herd" and depopulate Africa. Of course, in reality, the vaccinations are saving lives. Scientists have estimated that 15.6 million more people throughout the world would have died of measles between 2000 and 2013 if the measles vaccine had not been invented.

No antiviral drug has been shown to be useful in treating the measles virus infection. However, doctors have gotten much better at managing the bacterial infections that occur in patients whose immune system has been weakened by a case of measles. Antibiotics can be used to treat bacterial pneumonia. Intravenous fluids can be life-saving in cases of severe diarrhea. That's why the number of deaths due to measles in the United States started to fall even before the measles vaccine became available in the 1960s.

Before the measles vaccine was developed, there was no effective way to avoid catching the measles. Even quarantine measures did little good because infected people could start spreading the virus a day or two before it became clear that they had measles. The virus can remain infectious for up to two hours after leaving an infected person. Thus, you could catch measles just from being in a room where an infected person had been up to two hours before. That's why nearly everyone who was born before 1957 has had the measles.

Failure to vaccinate even a few children against measles can lead to serious outbreaks of measles. In 2011, an intentionally unvaccinated child from New Zealand brought the measles back from a family vacation in England. The child then passed the infection to several other unvaccinated children at school. These children became ill and then passed the infection along to still others. All told, there were 489 confirmed cases of measles in that outbreak. Of those patients, 82 needed to be hospitalized.

Fortunately, the "live" measles vaccine that has been used for many years remains highly effective and provides long-lasting protection. Nearly 99% of the people who have received two doses of the "live" measles vaccine that is currently being used become immune to measles. That's why most, but not all, of the measles cases in a measles outbreak occur in unvaccinated people. The immunity produced by the live measles virus may even be life-long. In contrast, the effects of the "killed" measles vaccine that was introduced in the 1960s tended to wear off after a few years. The patients could then be at risk for a severe reaction called atypical measles if they became infected with wild measles virus. (See chapter 12 for a discussion of "live" and "killed" viruses.)

The "live" vaccine itself produces some suppression of the immune system. However, this immune suppression is much milder than the immune suppression produced by the wild measles virus, and it does not last as long. Like other "live" viruses, the measles virus should not be given to pregnant women or people with a suppressed immune system. Those vulnerable people need to be protected by the herd immunity produced by vaccinating practically everyone else.

Thanks to measles vaccination, the measles virus is no longer circulating in the Americas. Unfortunately, it keeps being reimported, often by unvaccinated people who belong to communities where many of the young people are unvaccinated. In 2013, an intentionally unvaccinated teenager from an orthodox Jewish community in Brooklyn, New York, brought back measles from a trip to London. As a result, 58 other unvaccinated people, mainly children, caught the measles. One of the infected children ended up with pneumonia. Two pregnant women had to be hospitalized because of the measles, and one of them miscarried. In 2014, an unvaccinated Amish humanitarian aid worker brought back a case of measles from the Philippines. As a result, more than 380 people caught the measles.

An outbreak of measles is a public health emergency. Measles can kill. Also, it spreads very fast among communities with a low vaccination rate. When a measles outbreak occurs in the United States, the federal, state, and local public health authorities go to great lengths and considerable expense to contain it. First, they must identify everyone with a known or suspected case of measles. Then, they must find everyone who has come into contact with a possibly infected person. During the outbreak in Brooklyn, the public health authorities identified 3500 people who had been exposed to the infected people.

Public health authorities can do two things to keep a measles outbreak from spreading: isolate the sick people and vaccinate the susceptible people. In many cases, isolation is simple. Patients simply stay home, to be cared for by people who are already immune to the infection. If a person with measles needs hospital care, the hospital must take special precautions to keep that patient from infecting other people. If you have a suspected case of measles, state governments have the legal authority to detain you and hold you in isolation until you no longer pose a threat to other people.

The measles-mumps-rubella (MMR) shot may be offered to unvaccinated people who have been exposed to measles up to 3 days earlier. Since the MMR vaccine is a "live" vaccine, it must not be given to pregnant women or to people with a suppressed immune system. However, those patients and newborn babies may be given a shot of immune globulin if they have been exposed to someone with a suspected case of measles within the past 72 hours or at most the past six days. The immune globulin contains antibodies from people who are already immune to measles.

The measles virus belongs to the genus Morbillivirus, which in turn belongs to the family Paramyxoviridae. The genes in this family of viruses are in the form of negative-sense single-stranded RNA. Nevertheless, the measles virus is surprisingly stable genetically, which suggests that most of the mutants are weeded out by natural selection.

The genes of the measles virus are contained in a protein capsid that is surrounded by a fatty envelope. As I explain in chapter 12, a virus's envelope can make it easier for the virus to enter a host cell.

However, the envelope can be damaged by drying, heat, or detergents. As a result, enveloped viruses generally don't last long outside their host, which is why they are usually spread by fairly close person-to-person contact.

Enveloped viruses can sometimes cause persistent infections. In rare cases, the measles virus can cause a persistent infection called subacute sclerosing panencephalitis (SSPE). This condition occurs in people who had a natural case of measles, usually before the age of 2 years. Often, these cases arise in people who caught measles when they were still too young to be vaccinated. People with SSPE seem healthy for several years after their bout with the measles. But then they go on to suffer from problems with thinking and coordination. Then, these cases always get worse, leading to coma and death. There is no effective treatment. The number of reported cases of SSPE has been declining sharply since the introduction of the measles vaccine. After the measles virus has been extinct for a few years, there will be no new cases of SSPE.

The measles virus is closely related to the virus that caused rinderpest, a now-extinct disease of cattle. Other morbilliviruses include the virus that causes distemper in dogs. Another morbillivirus was responsible for massive die-offs of marine mammals. Other members of the family Paramyxoviridae include the mumps virus and the respiratory syncytial virus. All of these viruses infect the upper respiratory tract. All of them are rapidly spread by airborne droplets. As I explained in chapter 3, vaccination is the only effective way to prevent the transmission of diseases that spread by airborne droplets.

DNA studies suggest that the split between measles and rinderpest occurred only about a thousand years ago. Rinderpest had probably been killing domestic cattle for thousands of years before that. Ancient Roman writings describe a disease that was probably rinderpest. Rinderpest was deadly to cattle, Asian water buffalo, and yaks. Some of the severe strains of rinderpest could kill 95% of a herd. Fortunately, however, veterinarians were able to develop an effective rapid diagnostic test, as well as a vaccine that remained stable for months without refrigeration. As a result, an international campaign led by the United Nations' Food and Agriculture Organization was able to drive rinderpest into extinction. The last recorded case of rinderpest was observed in 2001. The disease was declared officially extinct in 2011.

So far, vaccination campaigns have driven two infectious diseases into extinction: smallpox and rinderpest. Polio will be next. There are several reasons to believe that measles could also be driven into extinction. First, measles occurs only in human beings. Thus, there is no wild reservoir of measles virus to reinfect the human population. Second, measles can easily be prevented by a cheap and highly effective vaccine that provides lifelong protection. In contrast, people need booster shots against diphtheria and tetanus every 10 years or so. Third, the measles virus is genetically stable, which is why people get the measles only once, and why the same measles vaccine continues to be effective year after year.

Yet at the same time, there are several reasons why it will be hard to eradicate measles. Measles is far more contagious than smallpox. Both are spread by airborne droplets, but smallpox generally doesn't make people cough. Also, smallpox is such a devastating illness that most patients are bedridden by the time they become contagious. Measles does cause coughing and sneezing, which means that the infected person will produce lots of infectious droplets. Also, the infected person's symptoms are mild enough at first that they can go about their normal routine, exposing everyone they meet to the virus. That's why measles outbreaks spread so fast in unvaccinated populations.

Another problem is that measles doesn't leave telltale signs behind. Smallpox left people scarred for life. Even the vaccination left a scar on the arm. An actual case of smallpox left obvious scars all over the face and body. Because of these scars, public health workers could tell, just from looking at you, whether you were immune to smallpox. In contrast, neither the measles nor the measles vaccination leaves an obvious mark on the outside of the body. People who were born before 1957 are presumed to be immune to measles. To tell whether a younger person is immune to measles, you have to test their blood for measles antibodies.

Measles is so contagious that you have to vaccinate nearly everyone in order to drive it into extinction. In contrast, smallpox did not spread nearly as quickly as measles. Thus, public health workers could use a ring vaccination strategy in the last stage of the smallpox eradication campaign. Instead of trying to vaccinate everyone on the planet, they concentrated on vaccinating people who lived near known cases of smallpox.

Smallpox was the first disease to be driven into extinction by a vaccination campaign. Rinderpest was second. Polio is likely to be the third. Measles should be next on the list, along with mumps and rubella. Once those diseases are extinct, there will never be any need to vaccinate anyone against them.

23

Mumps

Mumps was once a common childhood disease. It has probably been around for thousands of years. The Hippocratic writings from around 400 BC describe a disease that involved swelling of the testicles, as well as a swelling near the ear, on one or both sides. In the 1930s, the famous American pathologist Ernest William Goodpasture and his coworker Claude D. Johnson proved that mumps was caused by a virus, as opposed to a bacterium. They were even able to find the virus itself and make a vaccine against it.

The mumps virus belongs to the genus Rubulavirus in the family Paramyxovirus. Thus, it is distantly related to the measles virus. The mumps virus is a tiny ball, about 200 nm in diameter, surrounded by a fatty envelope. The fatty envelope helps to make it easy for the virus to infect the host cells. However, the envelope means that the virus does not stay infectious for long outside of the body. As a result, the disease is usually spread by fairly close personal contact. Like many other respiratory infections, the mumps is generally spread by airborne droplets. These droplets are produced when an infected person talks, sneezes, or coughs. As I explained in chapter 3, vaccination is the only effective way to prevent diseases that are spread by airborne droplets.

The genes of the mumps virus are in a linear single strand of negative-sense RNA that is 15,384 nucleotides long. Twelve different genotypes of the mumps virus have been identified. However, all of these genotypes look the same to the human immune system. In other words, all 12 genotypes belong to the same serotype. Five different genotypes of the mumps virus have been used for making a mumps vaccine. There were concerns that one of these strains, the Urabe strain, could cause aseptic meningitis. Viral or aseptic meningitis is usually a benign condition. Someone with the condition may need to be hospitalized for a few days of supportive care, but there are almost never any long-term effects.

The Urabe strain was derived from a mumps virus that had been isolated in Japan. However, the vaccine used in the United States and Britain is based on the Jeryl Lynn strain of the mumps virus. It was derived from the mumps virus that Dr. Maurice Hilleman at Merck isolated from his daughter Jeryl Lynn. Had the Jeryl Lynn strain been unavailable, we would be using the Urabe strain in the United States. Even though the Urabe strain produces a few cases of aseptic meningitis, even a case of vaccine-associated aseptic meningitis is still far less serious than a natural case of mumps. In fact, patients are less likely to get aseptic meningitis from the Urabe vaccine than from a natural case of mumps. The Urabe vaccine is also more effective than the Jeryl Lynn strain and cheaper to produce. For that reason, it is still preferred in some poor countries where natural mumps infection is still a serious public health problem.

The mumps virus infects the upper respiratory tract. Some cases look just like an ordinary cold. However, many cases progress to full-blown mumps, which means severe swelling in the glands that produce saliva (spit). These glands may swell up so much that the whole jaw looks swollen. The word *mump* originally meant grimace. The classic test for mumps was to give the patient a sour pickle to eat. If a patient can eat the pickle without pain, he or she probably doesn't have the mumps.

Some antivaccination activists claim that mumps is no big deal. But a friend of mine nearly died of mumps when he was eight years old. It left him deaf in one ear. Being deaf in one ear is a nuisance because it means that he cannot figure out which direction a sound is coming from. It also meant that he could never serve in the military. However, my friend was lucky. If he had been a few years older when he caught the mumps, it could have left him unable to father children. After puberty, mumps attacks the testes in males and the breasts and ovaries in girls. Adults are far more likely than children to suffer from complications from the mumps.

Up until the invention of the mumps vaccine, the mumps was a major problem for the military. Because so many young men were in close quarters, the mumps would spread like wildfire among the troops. The men who had grown up on farms were particularly hard hit. Most of the city boys had already had mumps in childhood. During World War I, mumps ranked third in terms of the diseases that caused men to lose time from duty. Not only was mumps common, but about 30 percent of the men who got mumps were temporarily disabled by painful swelling of the testes.

Before the introduction of the mumps vaccine, nearly everyone eventually caught the mumps virus. But thanks to the mumps vaccine, there are now only about 300 cases of mumps per year in the United States. In bad years, there are outbreaks that affect several thousand people. Many of the cases occur in people who had been vaccinated. The mumps component of the MMR vaccine is only about 88% effective in protecting someone from the mumps. Thus, we must vaccinate practically everyone in the population to keep the mumps from circulating.

Mumps occurs only in human beings. There is no wild reservoir. Thus, we could drive mumps into extinction through vaccination. After that, nobody will have to be vaccinated against mumps ever again. The hard part will be surveillance. Many mild cases of mumps virus infection look just like a common cold.

24

Rubella (German Measles)

In most children and adults, rubella is no big deal. It generally produces a mild illness that looks like the common cold, but with a red rash that fades after three days. Some rubella infections produce no obvious symptoms at all. But in a pregnant woman, rubella can lead to disaster. Rubella during pregnancy can lead to miscarriage or still-birth. Even if the baby is born alive, it could be born prematurely and/or with serious birth defects, including mental retardation, blindness, and deafness as well as problems with the liver and bone marrow. This collection of problems is called congenital rubella syndrome.

Fortunately, rubella and thus congenital rubella syndrome can easily be prevented by vaccination. In fact, the virus that causes rubella can be driven into extinction through an international vaccination campaign. After the rubella virus becomes extinct, there will no longer be any need to vaccinate anyone against rubella. Currently, an international partnership called the Measles and Rubella Initiative is working to eradicate both measles and rubella.

Many parents are afraid to have their children vaccinated with the measles-mumps-rubella (MMR) vaccine. They have been told that the MMR vaccination causes autism. It doesn't. In reality, the rubella vaccine has probably prevented many cases of autism. Congenital rubella infection is one of the few known causes of autism-like symptoms. If we stopped using the rubella virus vaccine, we'd end up with more cases of autism-like conditions, not fewer.

Rubella is one of the six classical exanthems. These were childhood diseases that caused the body to break out in a red skin rash, or exanthem. The first of these diseases to be recognized was measles, which is also called rubeola. Thus, measles was called first disease. By 1627, it became clear that measles and scarlet fever are two separate diseases. Thus, scarlet fever was called second disease. Rubella was called third disease.

The first known description of what is now called rubella (which means "little red" in Latin) was written in 1740 by a German physician named Friedrich Hoffmann. He thought that it was just a mild form of regular measles. But in 1814, another German doctor, George de Maton, suggested that the disease that was being called Rötheln (which means little red in German) or three-day measles was not just a mild case of regular measles. He believed that it was an entirely separate disease. English-speaking people called it German measles because so much of the literature about it came from Germany.

Until the 1940s, doctors thought that rubella was only a minor disease of childhood. Then, there was a major epidemic of rubella among Australian men in army camps. The epidemic then spread among civilians. In 1941, an Australian eye doctor named Norman McAlister Gregg noticed a huge increase in the number of babies born with cataracts, along with other birth defects. He overheard some of the afflicted babies' mothers saying that they had had rubella during their pregnancy. Gregg knew of 13 cases of babies with congenital cataracts among his own patients. By asking his colleagues, he was able to find a total of 78 cases. In 68 of those cases, the mothers reported that they had had rubella while pregnant with the afflicted child. After he published his findings in an Australian medical journal, he was contacted by women who had given birth to deaf children after having rubella during pregnancy. Gregg's theory that rubella could cause birth defects was later confirmed by other researchers in Australia, the United States, and Sweden.

After World War II, scientists made great progress in growing various kinds of cells from animal tissue in cell culture. These advances made it possible for other scientists to identify the rubella virus, and to grow a weakened version of the virus to use as a vaccine. The rubella virus is the only member of the genus Rubivirus, which is a member of the togavirus family. The other togaviruses are alphaviruses that are carried by mosquitoes.

Before the development of the rubella vaccine, a minor epidemic would break out in the United States once every 9 years or so. There would be a major epidemic of rubella once every 30 years. The last major epidemic of rubella in the United States occurred in 1963 through 1965. There were about 12.5 million rubella cases. These cases led to about 2,000 cases of encephalitis, more than 11,000 lost pregnancies, 2,000 deaths among newborns, and 20,000 cases of congenital rubella syndrome. Dr. Stanley Plotkin recalled,

> Those of us who were practicing pediatrics or obstetrics during those years remember with poignancy the many tragedies we witnessed as families struggled with decisions about therapeutic abortions and severely damaged infants. In Philadelphia, I calculated that at the height of the epidemic 1% of all births were affected.

Thanks to the rubella vaccine, which was introduced in 1969, rubella has been eliminated from the Americas. Today, the rubella virus is incorporated into the measles-mumps-rubella combined vaccine. However, rubella still continues to circulate in some other countries, including Japan.

Japan had introduced rubella vaccination in 1972, but the vaccine was given only to girls in junior high school. The boys were not vaccinated against rubella because they could never become pregnant. The

MMR vaccine was introduced in 1989, targeting boys and girls between the ages of 2 and 6. As a result, large numbers of Japanese men are still susceptible to rubella, which is why rubella is still circulating in Japan. Most of the cases are occurring in adult men, but a few cases have occurred in pregnant women.

Between October 2012 and June 2013, ten cases of congenital rubella syndrome were reported in Japan. Six of the babies were born to women who had never been vaccinated. The other four were born to women whose vaccination history was unknown. If rubella had not been circulating amongst the unvaccinated men, these women would never have become infected.

To prevent congenital rubella syndrome, we need to keep pregnant women from catching rubella. The problem is that you cannot vaccinate pregnant women against rubella. The rubella vaccine, like other "live" vaccines, must not be given to a pregnant woman or to anyone with a suppressed immune system.

Unfortunately, many parents in the United States and some other countries are refusing to allow their children to receive the MMR vaccine. Many of them have become convinced that mercury in the MMR shot causes autism. Yet the MMR shot contains "live" vaccines. The mercury-containing preservative thimerosal has been used only in "killed" vaccines. Thus, the MMR shot has never contained thimerosal. Nor have any vaccines ever been shown to increase the risk of autism.

The MMR vaccine does not cause autism. In reality, it might actually prevent a few cases of autism-like syndrome. An autism-like syndrome is one of the things that can result from congenital rubella syndrome. Epidemiologists from Emory University's Rollins School of Public Health estimated that by preventing congenital rubella syndrome, the MMR vaccine has prevented hundreds or even thousands of cases of autism, besides preventing deaths and cases of blindness and deafness and other problems.

25

Diphtheria

Diphtheria is a potentially deadly infection caused by a bacterium (*Corynebacterium diphtheriae*) that is in turn infected with a virus called beta phage. These infected bacteria produce a toxin that kills cells in the infected person's throat. These dead cells can then build up to form a tough gray film, called a pseudomembrane, that can block the person's airway. As a result, the person may suffocate. But even if a doctor puts a tube down a patient's throat to allow the patient to breathe, the patient could still die. That's because the toxin from the bacteria can travel through the bloodstream and can damage the heart and brain.

Like other respiratory infections, diphtheria can be easily spread from person to person by the clouds of airborne droplets that are produced when a person coughs or sneezes. Like many other dangerous respiratory infections, a case of diphtheria starts off looking and feeling like a common cold. As a result, the correct diagnosis may not be made in time to save the patient's life. That's why the vaccine to prevent diphtheria is so important.

Back in 1910, diphtheria was one of the 10 leading causes of death in the United States. Fortunately, the death rate started dropping in the early 20th century because of the development of diphtheria antitoxin to treat the disease. The death rate dropped even further after the development of a reasonably effective and remarkably safe vaccine to prevent the disease. Although a *Corynebacterium diphtheriae* infection can be treated with antibiotics, such as penicillin, the antibiotic does not destroy the toxin that the bacteria have already released. Even the antitoxin does not affect the toxin that has already become bound to the person's tissue. As a result, diphtheria remains a deadly disease. Even with the best of modern medical care, about 5% to 10% of the people with respiratory diphtheria die of the disease. The death rate is even higher (roughly 20%) among patients under 5 years of age and older than 40 years of age.

The diphtheria vaccine prevents people from dying of diphtheria, and it helps to prevent people from spreading the disease to other people. Since the bacterium that causes diphtheria is found only in human beings, we could eradicate diphtheria if we managed to stop it from being spread from person to person.

Tragically, diphtheria is still circulating in countries with poor vaccination coverage. As a result, epidemiologists do not think that diphtheria will be eradicated anytime soon. Unfortunately, it takes repeated doses (booster shots) of the vaccine to maintain immunity. Also, it can be hard to track a diphtheria outbreak. Mild cases of respiratory diphtheria can be mistaken for a common cold. Diphtheria can also produce a nasty skin infection, particularly among poor and homeless people. This skin infection is particularly common in the tropics, which is probably why many people in tropical countries develop natural immunity to diphtheria.

Diphtheria is a Greek word, but there's no evidence that the ancient Greeks knew about this disease. The oldest recorded epidemic of what was probably diphtheria occurred in Spain in 1613, which was called el Año de los Garotillos (the year of strangulations). By the mid 17th century, French physicians realized that diphtheria was contagious. French doctors coined the name *diphtheria* (from the Greek for "pair of leather scrolls") to refer to the pseudomembrane that can strangle the patient.

In the 1880s, diphtheria was linked to infection with a particular bacterium, a gram-positive club-shaped rod called *Corynebacterium diphtheriae*. This bacterium can be found inside samples of pseudomembrane taken from human beings with diphtheria. The *Corynebacterium diphtheriae* from human diphtheria patients caused a diphtheria-like condition when given to other animals, such as guinea pigs and pigeons. Yet *Corynebacterium diphtheriae* could often be found in the respiratory tract of some perfectly healthy people. Eventually, microbiologists realized that some strains of *Corynebacterium diphtheriae* cause diphtheria while others are harmless.

Although a case of diphtheria can cause serious damage in the heart and brain, the *Corynebacterium diphtheriae* organisms are aerobic (oxygen-loving) bacteria that are found only in the upper respiratory tract or in skin lesions. How can bacteria in the throat or in the skin cause problems in the heart and brain? Microbiologists began to suspect that the dangerous strains of *Corynebacterium diphtheriae* release a toxin that kills cells in the lining of the throat, thus causing the pseudomembrane. If this toxin entered the bloodstream, it could damage the heart and brain. Starting in 1949, microbiologists could use a laboratory test (Elek's test) to tell whether a strain of *Corynebacterium diphtheriae* can produce toxin.

The recipe for the diphtheria toxin is in a gene carried by a virus called beta phage. Only the strains of *Corynebacterium diphtheriae* that have been infected by this virus can produce the diphtheria toxin. Without that viral gene, *Corynebacterium diphtheriae* cannot make the diphtheria toxin and thus cannot cause diphtheria. Diphtheria was the first disease to be linked to a bacterial toxin. Later on, microbiologists found that bacterial toxins play an important role in other diseases, including tetanus, botulism, and cholera.

At first, a case of diphtheria looks and feels like a common cold. But after a few days, the symptoms worsen. The lymph nodes in the neck may become so swollen that the patient may seem to have the mumps. A pseudomembrane may start to cover the tissues at the back of the throat. If the disease is left untreated, the pseudomembrane may choke the patient to death. Meanwhile, the toxins from the bacteria attack the heart and nervous system.

The clinical diagnosis of diphtheria is based on an upper respiratory illness with low-grade fever and a gray membrane that is stuck to the tissue in the back of the throat. The diagnosis can be confirmed by laboratory tests, such as a throat culture. However, any patient who is suspected to have diphtheria should be isolated and should start receiving treatment with antibiotics and antitoxin right away. Any delay, even to wait for confirmation of the diagnosis, could be deadly.

Anyone who has been exposed to someone with diphtheria should also be treated with antibiotics, even if they have no signs or symptoms of infection. The apparently healthy people who have been in contact with the patient may be in the early stages of the infection or may be carriers of the disease. Antibiotic treatment can prevent these people from becoming sick or from spreading the infection to other people.

Because the diphtheria toxin is a protein, the human immune system can make antibodies against it. Unfortunately, it takes time for the body to learn to make those antibodies. The purpose of an antitoxin treatment is to give the patient a dose of someone else's antibodies (actually, antibodies from a horse), to fight the infection right away. In contrast, the purpose of the diphtheria vaccine is to prepare patients to make their own antibodies, in case they become exposed to diphtheria later on.

Diphtheria antitoxin was the first effective treatment for diphtheria. It was originally developed in 1890 by a German physiologist named Emil von Behring. Diphtheria antitoxin was made by injecting a horse with a tiny dose of diphtheria toxin. A few of the horses died as a result. The horses that recovered then went on to a long career as blood donors. Every so often, a few pints of blood were drawn from each horse. The blood was allowed to clot. Then, the antibody-rich liquid portion, or serum, was separated and used to make the antitoxin. In 1901, the New York State Department of Health set up a laboratory to manufacture antitoxin for diphtheria and anthrax. The antitoxin was provided free of charge to state institutions and the poor. The New York State

Department of Health also developed methods for establishing the purity and potency of the product.

In the early 20th century, diphtheria antitoxin was a wonder drug. It cut the death rate from diphtheria significantly. In 1896, a randomized study of hospitalized diphtheria patients found that only 3.3% of the patients who got antitoxin died, as opposed to 12.2% of the untreated patients. People throughout the United States became aware of the importance of diphtheria antitoxin because of an outbreak in Nome, Alaska in 1925.

The native people in the area surrounding Nome had no natural resistance to European diseases. Roughly half of the population of Nome had died in the Great Pandemic of influenza a few years earlier. Now, the survivors were being threatened by an outbreak of diphtheria, which was likely to kill a high percentage of the people who caught it. Unfortunately, the diphtheria antitoxin that the local doctor had on hand had expired and was probably no longer effective. The new shipment that he had ordered had failed to arrive before the port became icebound for the winter.

When the diphtheria epidemic broke out in January of 1925, the local doctor sent a radio telegram to the US Public Health Service, begging for antitoxin. However, temperatures in Alaska had dropped to 20-year lows. At Fairbanks, the temperature was -50°F (-46°C). The available airplanes could not be flown in such cold weather because they had open cockpits and water-cooled engines. Thus, the Public Health Service decided to ship the antitoxin by a relay of dogsleds. The Governor of Alaska Territory asked the US Postal Service Inspector to arrange a relay of dogsleds to deliver the antitoxin.

Together, the dogsled teams carried the antitoxin 674 miles (1,085 km) in 127½ hours, which was considered a world record, incredibly done in extreme subzero temperatures, made worse by near-blizzard conditions and hurricane-force winds. A number of dogs died during the trip. One of the heroes of the run was a dog named Togo, who led his team across the open ice of Norton Sound. Togo managed to find the roadhouse at Isaac's Point despite a blinding blizzard, thus saving his entire team from certain death.

The Great Race of Mercy made headlines in newspapers all over the United States. The mushers and their dogs were portrayed as heroes by an exciting new medium: radio. Today, Balto, the lead dog from the team that ran the final stretch into Nome, is immortalized by a statue in New York City's Central Park. Every year, the 1925 serum run to Nome is commemorated by the Iditarod Trail Sled Dog Race.

Although diphtheria antitoxin did save many lives, it has some serious drawbacks. It does a good job of neutralizing the diphtheria toxin that is floating free in the bloodstream. However, antitoxin has no effect on diphtheria toxin that has already become bound to tissue. Thus, the antitoxin is most effective if it is given early in the course of the disease. Another problem is that the antitoxin product contains many other foreign proteins. Thus, it can cause an allergic reaction called serum sickness. The signs and symptoms include swelling, fever, rash, and joint pains. Yet another problem is that since diphtheria antitoxin comes from an animal, it could be contaminated with other infectious agents.

In 1901, there was an epidemic of tetanus in St. Louis, Missouri. Fourteen children died horribly. All of the children had received diphtheria antitoxin that had been made by the city's health department. An investigation revealed that the antitoxin had come from a serum horse that the city had been using for several years. Unfortunately, the horse got tetanus, probably from an unsanitary needle-stick injury, and had to be put down. The contaminated antitoxin reached the children because the city had failed to follow proper safety precautions, including proper labeling and bacteriologic tests. At around the same time, nine children in Camden, New Jersey died of tetanus after receiving a smallpox vaccine produced by the Camden Board of Health.

In response to these disasters, the US Congress passed the Biologics Control Act of 1902. It was the first federal law to address the quality of medicinal products. The act required licensing of manufacturers and products. It also required uniform labeling of the products, including identification of the item, the manufacturer's name and address, and the expiration date and license number. Eventually, the responsibility for regulating biological medicinal products, which are medicinal products made from a living organism or its products, fell under the Center for Biologics Evaluation and Research, which is part of the FDA.

In 1907, von Behring showed that giving someone a dose of diphtheria toxin combined with antitoxin produced safe and long-lasting immunity to diphtheria. The trick was to provide enough toxin to stimulate the immune system and just enough antitoxin to prevent the toxin from making the patient sick. (In the early days, some people got sick and a few people died because of toxin-antitoxin preparations that contained too much free toxin.)

In 1914, William H. Park, MD, from the New York City Board of Health launched a massive campaign of diphtheria vaccination. Children were first given a skin test called the Schick test to see if they were already immune to diphtheria. Those who were not immune were then inoculated with the toxin-antitoxin mixture.

In 1923, two researchers—Gaston Ramon at the Pasteur Institute in France and Alexander Thomas Glenny at Wellcome Research Laboratories in London—independently found that they could denature the diphtheria toxin by treating it with formaldehyde. The denatured toxin, called a toxoid, couldn't cause diphtheria. However, the toxoid did stimulate the immune system to make antibodies that prevented diphtheria toxin from attacking cells.

Formaldehyde is commonly used to turn bacterial toxins into harmless toxoids for use in vaccines. The toxoid is then refined to remove as much of the formaldehyde as possible. The FDA has set strict limits on the amount of formaldehyde that a vaccine product can contain. The antivaccination activists try to scare people away from vaccinations by pointing out that some vaccines contain formaldehyde. However, they hide the fact that vaccines contain only trace amounts of formaldehyde, and that small amounts of formaldehyde are produced naturally in your own body during normal metabolism. In fact, formaldehyde plays an essential role in the process by which our cells switch their genes on and off. As a result, a newborn baby's body already contains 50 to 70 times as much formaldehyde as the baby would get from his or her vaccines. Thus, there's no reason to expect that the trace amount of formaldehyde in vaccines is any cause for alarm.

Unfortunately, the immunity produced by an injection of toxoid is not permanent. Glenny eventually realized that the toxoid did a better job of eliciting immunity if there was slight inflammation at the injection site. To provoke a mild inflammatory response that would lead to a stronger immune response, Glenny started to add aluminum salts to the vaccine. The substances that are used for this purpose are called adjuvants, from the Latin word *adjuvare*, which means to help. According to US federal law (21 CFR 610.15), "An adjuvant shall not be introduced into a product unless there is satisfactory evidence that it does not affect adversely the safety or potency of the product."

Antivaccination activists tell you to be afraid—be very afraid—of the aluminum salts in vaccines. They tell all sorts of horror stories about the supposed dangers of the tiny dose of aluminum salts in a vaccine. Yet they never point out that aluminum is the third most common element in the earth's crust. Nor do they petition the FDA to ban aluminum foil or aluminum beverage cans or the products such as antacids or baking powder that contain aluminum salts. Antivaccination activists have no problem with aluminum, per se. They simply hate vaccines.

In 1928, twelve children in Bundaberg, Queensland, Australia, died after receiving injections of diphtheria toxin-antitoxin from a multidose vial. The Commission that investigated these deaths concluded that the vial had become contaminated with bacteria. The bacteria were carried into the vial by the needles used to draw up one of the first few doses. The bacteria then multiplied while the vial sat on a shelf between doses. Unfortunately, the vial did not contain a preservative to kill bacteria or at least suppress their growth. To prevent similar tragedies from happening in the future, the regulatory agencies in various countries, including the US FDA, require that some sort of preservative be added to multidose vials.

US federal law (again, 21 CFR 610.15) requires most multidose vials of vaccine to contain preservative. The preservative has to be effective against the bacteria and fungi that could contaminate the vaccine. Yet the preservative cannot interfere with the effectiveness of the vaccine. The preservative must also be "sufficiently nontoxic" that the dose that you get through vaccination is not harmful.

The antivaccination activists want you to be terrified of the preservatives in vaccines, especially the mercury compound thimerosal, which had been used in vaccines for more than 70 years but has been phased out of nearly all childhood vaccines. They want to use the specter of mercury poisoning to scare parents away from vaccinating their children. Yet the antivaccination activists don't seem to be worried about mercury in general, only the mercury in vaccines. Antivaccination activists never seem to speak out against the dangers of eating tuna or other fish. As I explained in more detail in chapter 16, vaccine products are tested with the adjuvants and preservatives already in them. If these additives really do pose a threat to health, then health problems would show up as adverse events in the clinical trials and in postmarketing surveillance.

Antivaccination activists want you to be terrified of the "toxins" in vaccines. Yet they are strangely silent about the diphtheria toxin that a dangerous strain of *Corynebacterium diphtheriae* would release into the human body. My grandfather was born in Pittsburgh, Pennsylvania, in 1899. While he was growing up, some children from his neighborhood died of diphtheria. Not one person in my neighborhood got diphtheria while I was growing up. Nor was anyone killed by a vaccination. So from my perspective, diphtheria vaccination seems to have been a good deal. Today, the diphtheria vaccination is given in a combination vaccine against diphtheria, tetanus, and whooping cough.

Diphtheria is still a deadly disease, and epidemics can break out if people stop vaccinating children and if adults don't get their boosters. In the disruptions that ensued after the collapse of the Soviet Union, there was a major resurgence of diphtheria in the Russian Federation. It was the worst outbreak in a developed country since the 1960s. Tens of thousands of people got sick. During the early stages of the outbreak, more than 20% of the cases in some countries were fatal, owing to the lack of antitoxin and antibiotics. In areas where the antitoxin was consistently available, only about 3% of the cases were fatal. The epidemic was eventually brought under control by a massive vaccination campaign.

After diphtheria is eradicated, we can stop vaccinating people against diphtheria. But it would be madness to stop before then.

26

Whooping Cough (Pertussis)

A friend of mine from Texas begged me to write this book on vaccination. He was angry because a midwife—yes, a licensed healthcare provider—had told him and his wife that they should *not* vaccinate their children. That midwife was actually breaking the law. According to state law (Texas Health and Safety Code 161.501), she was supposed to be promoting vaccination. Specifically, she was supposed to give prospective parents a brochure that explained how important it is for children to be vaccinated against pertussis (whooping cough) and for the parents of newborns to get a booster shot against pertussis.

My friend knew that many people in his town were refusing to have their children vaccinated against pertussis and refusing to get their own booster shots. That meant that there would be gaps in the herd immunity that is supposed to protect his baby. Newborn babies are the people who are most likely to die from pertussis, but they are too young to be vaccinated against it. The best way to protect babies against pertussis is to make sure that all children are vaccinated against pertussis and that all adults, especially those who have contact with infants, get their booster shots. That way, the newborns will be surrounded by a cocoon of immunized people. The pertussis vaccine is usually in the same shot as the tetanus and diphtheria booster.

Pertussis is a severe respiratory syndrome that is caused by infection with a bacterium called *Bordetella pertussis*. The word *pertussis* also refers to the coughing. The prefix *per-* means "thoroughly" in Latin. *Tussis* means cough. A person with pertussis is therefore "coughing thoroughly." Pertussis is called whooping cough because it can cause coughing fits that are so severe that the person ends up gasping desperately for air afterward. This gasp makes a "whoop" sound. It's called an inspiratory whoop (inspiratory means related to inhalation). The coughing fits can be so bad that they make the person vomit.

A *Bordetella pertussis* infection starts off with an incubation phase that lasts for a week to 10 days. During that time, the person shows no symptoms. The next phase is called a catarrhal phase because it looks and feels like the common cold. During the catarrhal phase, which usually lasts 1 to 3 weeks, the person typically has a runny nose, a mild cough, and a low-grade fever. The symptoms are generally so mild that most people don't bother to seek medical help for themselves or for an afflicted child. Unfortunately, the catarrhal phase can be followed by a paroxysmal phase, in which the person has severe coughing fits. This paroxysmal phase can be severe and can last for 6 to 10 weeks. If the person survives that, the coughing fits gradually subside during a convalescent phase that can last several weeks.

The coughing fits can be so bad that the person cannot breathe. As a result, the person may turn blue. Although the person may look fine between coughing fits, the coughing fits make it impossible for the person to eat or sleep or to keep food down. Thus, the coughing fits from pertussis can take a heavy toll on a person, especially on a newborn.

Some babies with pertussis don't have coughing spells with the classic whooping noise. Instead, they simply stop breathing. Often, babies with pertussis have repeated episodes where they turn blue and their heart slows down. Sometimes, they simply die without warning.

If you think that this sounds a lot like sudden infant death syndrome (SIDS), which is often called cot death, you are right. A German autopsy study published in the July 1 2004 issue of *Pediatrics* showed that about 5% of babies who were thought to have died of SIDS had actually died of an unrecognized case of pertussis.

Some antivaccination activists try to scare parents away from vaccination by claiming that vaccination causes SIDS. But that's an outright lie. In reality, vaccination *decreases* a baby's risk of sudden death. However, it's hard to say by how much the vaccination decreases the risk of death. Unvaccinated babies are also at risk for other forms of medical neglect. People who refuse to vaccinate their children often refuse to provide other kinds of medical care, as well.

Bordetella pertussis was discovered in 1900 by two Belgian microbiologists: Jules Bordet and Octave Genou. They took some phlegm from Bordet's son Paul, who had whooping cough, and did a Gram staining procedure on it. When they looked at the stained phlegm through the microscope, they saw tiny pink ovals. They suspected right away that these gram-negative coccobacilli were the cause of whooping cough. However, it took them six years to figure out how to grow those bacteria in the laboratory so that they could fulfill Koch's postulates. To grow these bacteria, they had to create a special growth medium that included blood and potato starch. The blood provided nutrients that those bacteria cannot live without. The potato starch absorbed some fatty acids that would otherwise suppress the growth of the bacteria. The bacteria were eventually named *Bordetella pertussis*, in honor of Bordet.

In the 1930s, two women who worked for the Michigan Department of Health Laboratory—Pearl Kendrick and Grace Eldering—developed a practical diagnostic test for pertussis and the first useful pertussis vaccine. Back in those days, public health laboratories often hired female scientists because the women could be paid less than male scientists. Kendrick and Eldering's boss allowed them to do their pertussis research in their spare time, after they had finished all of their routine work of testing water and milk samples. Kendrick and Eldering reached out to local doctors, local public health departments, and even

First Lady Eleanor Roosevelt for support for their pertussis research. Not only did Kendrick and Eldering succeed in developing a safe and effective vaccine, they conducted well-designed field trials to show how effective and safe their vaccine was. The Michigan Department of Health began mass-producing the pertussis vaccine in 1938.

By 1940, pertussis vaccine was available nationwide. As a result, the number of cases and the number of deaths from pertussis fell sharply. It reached a historic low in 1976. Sadly, we are now seeing increasing outbreaks of pertussis because of parents' refusal to vaccinate their children.

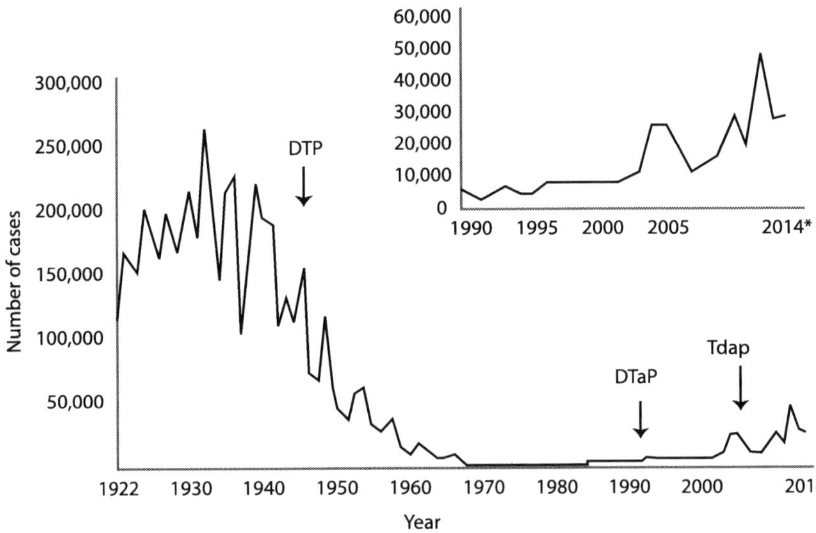

Figure 21. Pertussis cases in the United States, 1922 to 2014. Source: Centers for Disease Control and Prevention.

Bordetella pertussis and a related species, *Bordetella parapertussis*, both seem to be descended from *Bordetella bronchiseptica*, the bacterium that causes kennel cough in dogs. Both *Bordetella bronchiseptica* and *Bordetella parapertussis* can cause respiratory infections in humans. *Bordetella parapertussis* can even produce an illness that looks like a mild version of pertussis. However, *B pertussis* is far more dangerous than the other two *Bordetella* species: it's the only species that produces pertussis toxins.

Bordetella pertussis bacteria secrete two dangerous toxins, which are small proteins: pertussis toxin and adenylate cyclase toxin. Both toxins do things that are good for the *Bordetella pertussis* bacteria but bad for their human host. The pertussis toxin paralyzes the cilia, which are the hair-like projections on the cells that line the airways. The cilia normally act like tiny brooms that sweep mucus and trapped particles, including bacteria and viruses, up and out of the respiratory tract. Normally, this mucociliary escalator does a good job of carrying dirt and germs up and out of the lungs. Unfortunately, the pertussis toxin binds to the cilia so that they can no longer sweep. As a result, mucus and other crud can build up in the lungs. When the mucociliary escalator stops working, then coughing is the only way to clear the crud out of the lungs. Of course, with every cough, the patient spews out a cloud of tiny airborne droplets, teeming with *Bordetella pertussis* bacteria. All that coughing is an effective way to spread the disease to other people.

As if the buildup of crud in the lungs weren't bad enough, pertussis toxin and the adenylate cyclase toxin also suppress the immune system. As you may remember from reading chapter 14, the white blood cells are an important part of the immune system. White blood cells are supposed to swallow the germs and other bad things that they find in the body. But when a white blood cell swallows pertussis toxins, those toxins jam the white blood cell's internal signaling system. Thus, the pertussis toxin makes it hard for the white blood cell to fight infections. This suppression of the immune system helps the *Bordetella pertussis* survive longer in the host. As a result, the host may remain contagious for a longer period and pass the disease on to a larger number of people. However, the immune suppression also leaves the host open to other kinds of bacterial and viral infections of the lung.

Besides having crud in their lungs and suppressed immunity, people with whooping cough are also at risk for aspiration pneumonia. Because of all the coughing, vomiting, and gasping, they sometimes end up inhaling their own vomit. This means that they inhale a dangerous mixture of food, bacteria, and caustic stomach acid.

Pertussis can cause other serious complications, besides pneumonia. Some infants end up with brain damage, possibly because of oxygen deprivation and possibly because of the effects of the pertussis toxin, which can pass from the bloodstream into the brain. The severe coughing can cause broken ribs, hernias, rectal prolapse, and bleeding into the brain. The violent wrenching of the head due to the severe coughing can also cause bleeding within the eyes, sometimes leading to blindness. The coughing fits can also lead to pneumothorax, a dangerous condition in which air leaks from the lung into the chest cavity, potentially suffocating the person. More than half of the babies who get pertussis must be hospitalized.

At the beginning of the 20th century, pertussis was a major cause of death, mainly in infants and young children. Most of them didn't die of the pertussis itself. They died of complications, mainly pneumonia. Thus, the death rate from whooping cough started to decrease as doctors got better at treating pneumonia, even before the pertussis vaccine became available. One important advance was the development of antibiotics.

The macrolide antibiotics, such as azithromycin, are effective at clearing *Bordetella pertussis* from the respiratory tract. If the appropriate antibiotic is given early enough in the course of the infection, the patient will have a milder illness and will be less likely to spread the infection to others. Nowadays, people who have come in contact with someone with a suspected case of pertussis are given a macrolide antibiotic to prevent the *Bordetella pertussis* infection from taking hold. Other antibiotics can be useful in treating the secondary bacterial infections that cause pneumonia in pertussis patients.

Pertussis patients may also need hospitalization for other forms of supportive care, such as intravenous fluids to fight dehydration. Nurses and respiratory therapists also use many techniques, such as postural drainage and suction, to clear the patient's lungs. Pertussis patients may also need supplemental oxygen, sometimes in an oxygen tent or through a ventilator. If those methods don't provide enough oxygen, a form of heart-lung machine may be used. It's called extracorporeal membrane oxygenation (ECMO). It takes the patient's blood out of the body and runs it through an artificial lung that lets oxygen into the blood and lets carbon dioxide out.

Although these treatments have dramatically improved survival, pertussis still kills people, mainly newborns. Unfortunately, we are seeing outbreaks of pertussis in the United States and other industrialized countries. In 2012, there were 41,880 reported cases of whooping cough in the United States. There were 18 recorded deaths, including 13 babies under 3 months of age. These were just the reported cases. It's possible that many relatively mild cases of *Bordetella pertussis* infection went undiagnosed. It's also possible that some cases that were classified as SIDS were really pertussis in disguise. Although the disease surveillance system probably does miss many cases of pertussis, it nevertheless gives us disturbing evidence that pertussis is becoming more common. Although a pertussis outbreak can occur even where vaccine coverage is high, antivaccination movements are having the effect of making pertussis more common.

Antivaccination activists want you to believe that vaccination played no role in decreasing the death rate from pertussis. They also want you to think that pertussis is nothing to worry about. Sometimes, they do and say appalling things to further their case.

In 2009, a healthy newborn baby in Australia came down with pertussis; she then died at 4 weeks of age. After her death, her grieving parents spoke out, wanting to know why they hadn't been warned about the pertussis outbreak in their community. At that point, a prominent local antivaccination activist contacted the Director of Public Health. She disputed that the baby had died of pertussis and demanded that the child's medical records be made public. Her antivaccination group then harassed the grieving parents, accusing them of lying about the cause of their baby's death.

Antivaccination activists and some proponents of alternative medicine don't want you to realize that pertussis is a serious disease that causes great suffering and can lead to serious complications, including death. The advice they give about how to manage pertussis shows how ignorant they are. If you do an Internet search for whooping cough and alternative medicine, you'll see plenty of advice about using honey or garlic or some sort of herbal tea to treat whooping cough. Such advice seems to be coming from people who are clueless because they have never seen a real case of whooping cough, or any other serious illness for that matter. If that kind of old-fashioned, homemade remedy really worked, whooping cough would never have been a major cause of death. The death rates from whooping cough started to come down only after the development of modern medicine.

Since most babies with pertussis need to be hospitalized, and since many families in the United States have no health insurance or are underinsured, they cannot afford hospital care for their child. Nor can they afford to take a month or two off from work to care for a sick child. Thus, a case of pertussis can drive a family into bankruptcy, even if the child is lucky enough to survive with no serious lasting effects. In other words, people who refuse to vaccinate their children and who fail to get their own booster shots are exposing themselves and other people to serious risks.

Because *Bordetella pertussis* lives only in human beings, we could theoretically eradicate it through an effective vaccination program. Once pertussis is extinct, nobody will need to be vaccinated against it. Unfortunately, it will be technically difficult to eradicate pertussis, for two reasons. One results from problems in diagnosis, the other from limitations of the currently available vaccines. However, the main problem is political, not technical. It results from political resistance that stems from irrational fear of the vaccine.

The first technical problem is diagnosis. Many *Bordetella pertussis* infections go undiagnosed. That's because the classic cases of whooping cough generally happen only in people who have never been exposed to *Bordetella pertussis* in the past. That's why whooping cough was once a disease of childhood. A child's first case of *Bordetella pertussis* infection would cause whooping cough. Children who survived that first infection developed protective immunity for a while. As their immunity faded, they could become infected with *Bordetella pertussis* again, but they might have only a mild illness that could be mistaken for a cold, if they had any symptoms at all. Yet even if they had mild symptoms or no symptoms, they could still pass the infection on to other people. The same thing happens as the effects of pertussis vaccination wear off. Adolescents and adults can catch a *Bordetella pertussis* infection and pass it on to others, without having the classic signs of whooping cough.

In other words, a *Bordetella pertussis* outbreak can "fly under the radar" until the bacteria find their way into a highly susceptible person, who gets an obvious case of whooping cough or simply dies of something that looks like SIDS. We see the same problem with polio. Many of the people who catch and pass on a wild poliovirus infection show no signs of illness or seem to have only a "gut bug." Thus, an outbreak can go unnoticed until someone ends up paralyzed. We didn't have that problem with smallpox. The signs of smallpox are so clear and obvious that tracing the outbreaks was like tracking a large herd of elephants.

To confirm a diagnosis of *Bordetella pertussis* infection, you have to do laboratory testing. This testing is important because other kinds of illness can cause a severe chronic cough with an inspiratory whoop. A few years ago, another friend of mine e-mailed me to tell me that he'd just been given a diagnosis of pertussis. He'd been coughing for 2 months. He also had a severe case of hives (urticaria). Yet something about his story made no sense. He didn't have young children. Nor did he work around children. Nor was he the sort of person to neglect his booster shots. Besides, a nagging cough or hoarseness is one of the seven warning signs of cancer. So I did an Internet search for "cough inspiratory whoop urticaria." To my alarm, that search brought up a bunch of hits for lymphoma, which is a form of cancer. I e-mailed him back, asking him if any laboratory test had been done to confirm the pertussis diagnosis. None had. As it turns out, he did have lymphoma—the same rare form of lymphoma that had killed his brother at precisely the same age. Fortunately, despite the inexcusable delay in diagnosis, my friend survived.

We will not be able to eradicate pertussis until scientists develop a better vaccine. There were some legitimate concerns about the safety of the original pertussis vaccine. Also, some of the people who receive the pertussis vaccine don't develop protective antibodies as a result. That problem is called primary vaccine failure. But even if the vaccine does work, its effects are not permanent. Sometimes, the effects wear off faster than expected. That problem is called secondary vaccine failure. Even though there are occasional cases of primary and secondary vaccine failure, we theoretically could drive *Bordetella pertussis* into extinction through vaccination. It's simply a matter of maintaining high vaccine coverage and responding appropriately to outbreaks.

It would be nice to have a longer-lasting pertussis vaccine. However, the biggest roadblock to the eradication of pertussis is not technical. It's political. It stems from irrational fear of the vaccine. People are far more frightened of the theoretical problems that they imagine that the vaccine *might* cause than they are of the real problems that pertussis *does* cause. This irrational fear of vaccination has always been a problem. However, it has become even more serious as people forget what the vaccine-preventable diseases are really like. As the vaccine-preventable diseases disappeared, people stopped fearing them. All they had left to fear was the vaccines.

The original whole-cell pertussis vaccine occasionally caused a side effect that caused no lasting damage to the children but scared the living daylights out of their parents. This led to fears, which turned out to be groundless, that the vaccine could cause significant, permanent brain damage.

The vaccines that are made of whole, dead cells of *Bordetella pertussis* contain an endotoxin. An endotoxin is a toxin that is usually inside the bacterial cell but can be released after the cell dies. In some children, the *Bordetella pertussis* endotoxin caused a minor but alarming fever. Some children had a febrile seizure as a result. A febrile seizure is a convulsion that is triggered by a fever. Febrile seizures are common. They often occur in many otherwise healthy children between 9 months and 5 years of age. They can be triggered by any fever, such as the fever that results from a common cold or an ear infection. I had several febrile seizures (not vaccine-related) when I was a toddler. They terrified my parents. I had one of the febrile seizures in the doctor's office, and it startled him, too. Fortunately, there is no evidence that simple febrile seizures cause any serious problems. Most children outgrow the problem by the time they are 5 years old.

There was no evidence that the febrile seizures were doing any lasting damage. Nevertheless, some people started to worry that the pertussis vaccine could lead to chronic seizure disorders and brain damage. As a result, people started talking about "vaccine-related encephalopathy," even though they had no evidence that any cases of encephalopathy were truly vaccine-related. The fact that a child got a diagnosis of a seizure disorder after vaccination does not mean that the seizure disorder was necessarily due to the vaccination.

To see whether pertussis vaccination was linked to vaccinations, the British government undertook an enormous study called the National Childhood Encephalopathy Study (NCES). In that study, children with neurological problems were followed up and compared with matched controls. The results were released in 1991.

The NCES wasn't a perfect study. From a scientific standpoint, it tended to overstate the risk of vaccine-related injury. For example, the study didn't exclude children whose brain disease was due to some other obvious cause. Also, there were problems with bias in the data. For example, people had to think back to remember when the child's problem became obvious, relative to the timing of the vaccination. That introduces a problem called recall bias. Even so, the study showed that the risk of vaccine-related injury, if it existed at all, was very low.

The authors of the NCES estimated that there might be 1 case of neurologic disease for every 330,000 vaccinations. Yet when those presumed cases were reviewed in more detail, not a single one could honestly be blamed on the pertussis vaccination. Some of the children turned out not to have a brain disease after all. In other cases, an autopsy study or a viral culture showed that the problem was due to some unrelated problem. A similar study in the United States showed no evidence of a relationship between pertussis vaccination and neurologic disease.

In 1994, the US Institute of Medicine reviewed the evidence on pertussis vaccination and brain disease and concluded that the DPT vaccination probably did cause a few cases of brain damage, but only a very few cases. However, later studies cast doubt on even that conclusion. A study of children from Australia, New Zealand, Canada, and Scotland found that many of the children whose seizures had originally been blamed on the pertussis vaccine actually had genetic forms of epilepsy. In short, there's no clear evidence that the pertussis vaccination had caused brain disease in anyone. In contrast, there's plenty of evidence that a natural case of pertussis can cause brain damage or even death. No vaccine is risk-free, but a pertussis vaccine is much safer than an actual case of pertussis.

Vaccination, like any medical treatment, poses some risk of side effects. Fortunately, the clinical trials and the postmarketing surveillance have shown that nearly all of the side effects of the pertussis vaccine are mild and temporary. The potentially serious side effects are extremely rare. We have no evidence that the pertussis vaccine has caused any cases of encephalopathy. But even if there really were a 1 in 330,000 risk of getting encephalopathy from the vaccine, the risk from vaccination would still be far lower than the risk of encephalopathy or death from getting a natural case of pertussis. If you think that getting a dose of dead germs in a vaccine is dangerous, what do you think would happen if the child had an overwhelming infection with live germs?

Ideally, we would have vaccines and other medicines that have no bad side effects. But in reality, we have to choose from the options that actually exist. Rather than waiting for science to develop a vaccine that poses no risks whatsoever, we have to weigh the risks of using an existing vaccine versus letting children run the risk of getting a deadly disease. Clearly, the best course of action is to use the vaccine, unless it is contraindicated for medical reasons, such as if a child has a suppressed immune system because of cancer or chemotherapy. Our current vaccines are not completely risk-free, but they are remarkably safe. If we make full use of our existing vaccines, we can prevent children from suffering and dying from whooping cough. Perhaps with a more effective vaccine, we might be able to drive *Bordetella pertussis* into extinction. After that, nobody would need the pertussis vaccine.

The disputes over vaccination go on largely because most people don't know how to use evidence to draw reasonable conclusions. Few people understand the difference between the absence of evidence and the evidence of absence. Before the NCES and other large studies were undertaken, we had an *absence of evidence* that pertussis vaccination was causing brain disease. After those studies were done, we had *evidence of absence*—a large body of evidence that suggested that the pertussis vaccine is *not* responsible for causing brain disease. As a result, it is no longer reasonable to blame cases of childhood epilepsy or other brain diseases on the pertussis vaccine. Nevertheless, many people remained convinced that the pertussis vaccine harms children. These ideas were spread by books and documentaries and by parent advocacy groups.

Of course, the antivaccination activists are also trying to frighten people about the other ingredients and contaminants in the pertussis vaccine. (Note that the pertussis vaccine is usually included in the same shot as the diphtheria and tetanus vaccines.) In particular, they try to frighten people about the aluminum that is used as an adjuvant in the pertussis vaccine or the trace amount of formaldehyde that remains in the vaccine. They have also made a big deal about the mercury-containing preservative thimerosal. Yet thimerosal has been removed from the routine childhood vaccines, including the pertussis vaccines.

The hysteria over the nonexistent problem of vaccine-related encephalopathy scared many people away from vaccinating their children. Thus, it led to pertussis outbreaks that led to real suffering and death. The hysteria also led to changes in vaccine policy that increased the cost of the vaccination, while undermining its effectiveness. Because of the concern over febrile seizures and the fear of the nonexistent problem of vaccine-related encephalopathy, there has been a shift from the whole-cell to the acellular pertussis vaccine.

The acellular pertussis vaccine doesn't contain the bacterial endotoxin. As a result, it is less likely to cause fever and febrile seizure. However, the acellular vaccines are not only more expensive, they seem to be less effective. The lower cost-effectiveness of the acellular vaccines could represent a real problem in poor countries. These questions of effectiveness and cost-effectiveness are going to become important as we try to achieve worldwide eradication of pertussis.

Bordetella pertussis is found only in human beings. We have an effective vaccine to prevent clinical cases of whooping cough. Perhaps with a better, longer-lasting vaccine, we could drive *Bordetella pertussis* into extinction. After that, there would be no more need to vaccinate anyone against pertussis and we could stop worrying about even the theoretical risks of pertussis vaccination.

27

Human Papillomavirus (HPV)

For more than a hundred years, doctors had suspected that cervical cancer was the result of a sexually transmitted infection (venereal disease). Then, in the 1980s, a German scientist named Harald Zur Hausen finally showed that practically all cervical cancers are due to infection with some type of human papillomavirus (HPV), which can be sexually transmitted. This discovery led to a Nobel Prize for Zur Hausen and to the development of some remarkably safe and effective vaccines for preventing not only most cases of cervical cancer but also most cases of genital warts. These vaccines might also protect men as well as women from some cancers of the mouth, anus, and lung.

Antivaccination zealots are against the use of all vaccines. Thus, they are against the HPV vaccine as a matter of principle. However, many critics of the HPV vaccine are not against vaccines, per se. They simply dislike the idea of vaccinating 11-year-olds against a sexually transmitted disease. They complain that 11-year-olds are too young to be having sex. But that's beside the point. The best time to give a vaccine is when the vaccine is most effective. Giving two doses when a child is 9 to 13 years old is as effective as giving three doses to patients aged 15 to 26. So it's better and cheaper to vaccinate early. Note also that the HPV vaccine is most effective if it is given before the patient is exposed to HPV. So the best time to immunize people against HPV is while they are still too young for sex.

Many parents worry that the HPV vaccine might make young girls feel that it is okay for them to have sex. Fortunately, several studies have shown that getting the HPV vaccine does not alter a girl's feelings about sex. A vaccine against warts is not an aphrodisiac. Vaccinating your 11-year-old daughter against HPV will not turn her into a nymphomaniac. But it could help keep her from dying of cervical cancer in her 30s. Cervical cancer can kill. It can also leave a young woman unable to have children.

When the HPV vaccine first came out, a friend of mine asked why her daughter, who is not sexually active, should be vaccinated against HPV. My friend was worried about what she should say to her daughter about the vaccine. I pointed out that she might not have to say anything at all. The girl had never asked any questions about any other shot. If she asked questions about this one, I would just tell her the truth: that it's against human papillomavirus, which can cause cancer.

Most parents have a hard enough time accepting that their children are growing up, and especially that their daughters may eventually choose to have sex. Many parents want their children to have only one monogamous sexual relationship in their lifetime. Yet even if those children take that path in life, there is no guarantee that their spouses will stay faithful. (In fact, it is highly unlikely that they will.) So the HPV vaccine is a reasonable precaution.

The first clue to the existence of papillomaviruses was discovered in the 1920s, when scientists realized that warts are contagious. They found that warts can spread from person to person. The germ that causes warts is so small that it passes right through a filter made out of porcelain. Thus, the germ was too small to be a bacterium. It had to be a virus. The proper medical name for a wart is a papilloma, which literally means "tiny, nipple-like growth." For that reason, the viruses that cause warts are called papillomaviruses. Later work showed that the papillomaviruses are non-enveloped viruses whose genes are in a double strand of DNA.

Since then, hundreds of types of papillomaviruses have been found. Each is specifically adapted to a particular body surface in a particular species of animal. The human papillomaviruses (HPVs) are found only in humans. HPV type 1 causes warts on the soles of the feet (plantar warts). HPV type 2 causes warts on the palms of the hands. Several types of HPV cause genital warts, which are warts on the sex organs. Roughly 90% of genital warts are due to HPV type 6 or type 11. Other types of HPV lead to cancer of the cervix, which is the neck of the womb. (HPV type 6 and type 11 rarely if ever cause cancer.)

Doctors had long suspected that cervical cancer, which was a common cause of cancer death in women, was somehow the result of sexual activity. In 1842, an Italian surgeon named Rigoni-Stern reported that cervical cancer was rare among nuns. In 1950, a gynecologist from Quebec found the same thing. He reviewed the causes of death for 13,000 nuns. Not one of the nuns had died of cervical cancer, although several of them had died of other reproductive system cancers. The women who were most likely to get cervical cancer were prostitutes and the wives of men who often visited prostitutes.

It was easy to tell that cervical cancer is caused by some sexually transmitted infection. The hard part was figuring out which sexually transmitted infection was the culprit. The original suspect was herpes simplex 2, the virus that causes genital herpes. It was a reasonable guess. Herpes simplex 2 is sexually transmitted, and it is a herpesvirus. The first virus that was shown to cause cancer in humans was another herpesvirus, the Epstein-Barr virus. But in the 1970s and 1980s, Harald Zur Hausen and his team isolated and cloned four types of HPV: types 6, 11, 16, and 18. They found that type 16 was present in roughly 50% of all cervical tumors, and type 18 was present in another 17% to 20% of cervical tumors. They found types 6 and 11 in genital warts but not in cervical tumors. Eventually, other researchers found more types of HPV in genital warts and cervical tumors. Later work by other researchers showed that more than 99% of cervical cancers are infected with some strain of HPV.

The first available HPV vaccines (Gardasil and Cervarix) protect against HPV-16 and HPV-18, which are the most important causes of cervical cancer. Together, HPV-16 and HPV-18 account for about 70% of cervical tumors, including the most aggressive cervical tumors. Gardasil also protects against HPV-6 and HPV-11, which together account for about 90% of all cases of benign genital warts but almost never lead to cancer. In January 2015, the FDA approved Gardasil 9, which provides coverage against nine types of HPV, including the four types included in the original Gardasil vaccine. Gardasil 9 provides protection against the HPV strains that have been responsible for about 90% of cervical cancers. However, even Gardasil 9 cannot provide 100% protection. There are still some rare cancer-causing strains of HPV that are not yet included in the vaccine. Also, the vaccine cannot cure the HPV infections that the patient caught before vaccination. Thus, even women who have been vaccinated against HPV will still need regular screening for cervical cancer. Nevertheless, the HPV vaccine represents an opportunity to drive the most dangerous strains of HPV to extinction through vaccination.

As Zur Hausen explained in his Nobel lecture, it's hard to show the links between infections and cancer. The main reason is that no human cancers show up right after the infection. Often, the cancer doesn't show up until many years afterward. Also, the infections that cause cancer are extremely common, but only a few infected people get the cancer. By the time the cancer is diagnosed, the evidence of the infection may have vanished.

To understand how HPV causes warts, you need to know something about the normal growth and development of the outer layer of the skin (the epidermis). If you look at a cross section of a bit of epidermis through a microscope, you can see that it is made up of several different layers. The bottom layer of the epidermis is the basal layer. It consists of living cells that are actively dividing. As these cells divide, they push some of their daughter cells outward. As those cells pass into the outer layers of the epidermis, they transform themselves. They produce lots of keratin, which is the hard, tough protein in your hair and fingernails. By the time they reach the surface, those skin cells have become toughened, dried-out husks of their former selves. That's why the surface of the skin provides a tough and dry protective surface.

The outer surface of the skin is continually flaking off. As the outer cells are shed, they are replaced by maturing cells from underneath. Human beings are continually shedding tiny flakes of dead skin. These tiny flakes build up as dust in our homes. Wherever we go, we leave a trail of tiny flakes of dead skin, just as Hansel and Gretel left a trail of breadcrumbs. Dogs can smell these skin flakes. That's why bloodhounds find it so easy to track us down.

HPV takes advantage of this normal life cycle of skin cells. It generally enters through a small break in the skin. It then infects the cells of the basal layer of the epidermis or of the mucous membranes. Like all viruses, HPV can be copied only by living cells. Unlike many other viruses, however, HPV does not kill or rupture its host cell. Instead, the HPV-infected cells go on living and dividing. By keeping a low profile, HPV avoids attracting the attention of the immune system. HPV generally makes its host cell divide a bit faster, which is why HPV infection gives rise to a small benign tumor, or wart. HPV also suppresses the local immune defenses, which is why the infection can persist for a long time. Eventually, infected cells make their way to the surface and are shed. Then the virus can be passed on to someone else, or to a fresh area of skin or mucous membrane on that same person, and the cycle repeats.

The tiny flakes that people are constantly shedding from their skin can carry HPV that can infect other people. You can catch HPV-1 if your bare feet come into contact with HPV-1 virus from someone else's feet. The strains of HPV that affect the hands and feet are easy to catch because people often run around in bare feet and touch things with their bare hands. The strains of HPV that affect the insides or the outsides of the private parts are much harder to catch, for the obvious reason.

Many types of HPV cause no obvious symptoms. The worst thing that most strains of HPV do is cause warts. As long as the HPV infection doesn't cause inflammation or spread too far, it can avoid triggering an immune response. Eventually, however, the immune system may notice the HPV infection and effectively clear it. Wart infections seldom cause major problems unless the immune system is suppressed, such as in someone with HIV infection. Then, the warts can grow out of control.

One severe case of HPV infection occurred in an Indonesian man named Dede Koswara, who became famous as the Tree Man because his entire body, especially his hands and feet, was covered with warts that grew so thick that they looked like bark. His problem was eventually found to be a rare hereditary defect of the immune system. It allowed warts caused by an ordinarily harmless type of HPV to grow out of control.

In contrast, some women are genetically resistant to cervical cancer. Doctors had known for many years that Jewish women rarely get cervical cancer. At first, epidemiologists suspected that the Jewish women were being protected by some lifestyle factor, such as their husband's circumcision. Later research showed that a gene mutation that helps to protect women against cervical cancer just happens to be more common in Jewish women than in the general population. This phenomenon is a result of the founder effect. A large percentage of Jewish women just happened to be descended from a woman who carried that mutation.

It's easy to understand how HPV can get transmitted from person to person. What's harder to understand is why some strains of HPV only cause warts, while others cause cancer, and why even the cancer-causing types cause cancer in only a small percentage of cases. The explanation has to do with both the HPV virus itself and with the infected person. Most warts are benign, and most people's immune systems can eventually clear the infection. Unfortunately, if the immune system fails to clear the infection, some strains of HPV can cause the warts to become malignant.

The dangerous strains of HPV produce proteins that interfere with two natural tumor-suppressing proteins in human cells: p53 and pRb. This interference is good for the virus but bad for the host. In a healthy cell, pRB controls the rate at which the cell makes copies of DNA. By suppressing pRB, the HPV virus can cause the cell to make more copies of the viral DNA, as well as the cell's own DNA. The result would be more viruses and more infected cells. For this process to work, the virus must also suppress p53. Besides helping to repair damaged DNA, p53 helps to slow down the rate at which DNA is copied. If the damaged DNA cannot be repaired or if the cell keeps copying DNA too fast, p53 can tell the cell to kill itself. If both p53 and pRB are inactivated, a damaged cell can keep reproducing itself without being repaired. Thus, the dangerous strains of HPV can allow a cell to collect enough gene mutations to become malignant.

It was hard to develop a vaccine against HPV, but for a simple reason. Most of the common antiviral vaccines are against viruses that cause acute infections, such as influenza or measles. An influenza virus or a measles virus is in a desperate race against time. It must reproduce itself in large numbers very quickly if it is to have any chance of being transmitted to another host before the current host's adaptive immune system destroys it. When you try to amplify an influenza virus or a measles virus in a cell culture, you can produce many virions (infectious virus particles) very quickly. In contrast, the HPV virus causes a chronic infection. The HPV infection will last for a long time. Therefore, its best strategy would be to multiply slowly, to avoid killing its host cell and to avoid attracting the attention of the immune system. This strategy would enable the infected tissue to shed small amounts of virus over an extended period, as the skin cells are shed. For that reason, it was simply impractical to develop a "killed" vaccine for HPV. The cell cultures simply didn't produce enough virions to yield a useful vaccine.

The other standard kind of vaccine, an attenuated ("modified live") vaccine, was completely out of the question. It would be unthinkable to give healthy people a dose of a "live" virus that causes a chronic infection that could lead to cancer years later.

Recombinant DNA technology made it possible to create an effective HPV vaccine. To make a recombinant vaccine, you must first find the gene for an important protein, typically a protein from some outer structure of a bacterium or from the protein coat of a virus. The key is to pick a protein that is harmless to a human being but that would enable the human immune system to learn to recognize and fight the germ. Once you find that gene, you put it into some cell that you can grow in large numbers, such as yeast cells. Those transgenic yeast cells can then produce large amounts of that protein, which can then be purified and used in making a vaccine.

Through recombinant DNA technology, you can easily make a protein that has exactly the right sequence of amino acids. The tricky part is to get that protein to fold itself into exactly the right shape. Some proteins don't always fold into exactly the right shape, especially if they were made in a foreign cell. And in immunology, the exact shape matters a great deal.

Some proteins are complexes that are made up of two or more kinds of subunit, each kind coded for by a different gene. Fortunately, the protein coat of an HPV virus is made up of repeating units of just one protein, which is called L1. When a human cell is infected by HPV, it makes many copies of L1. Those L1 subunits then stick together in groups of five. Then, 72 of those groups of five assemble themselves into a spherical shell that forms the protein coat of the virus.

Geneticists found a way to get yeasts to make the L1 protein. Then, chemists found a way to get those L1 subunits to assemble themselves into an empty shell that looks just like the protein coat of a natural HPV virus (Figure 22). Those empty shells are called virus-like particles. To the immune system, they look like the natural virus. As a result, these virus-like particles can be used to immunize a patient against the natural virus. Unlike the natural virus, however, the virus-like particles do not contain the genes that cause infected cells to give rise to warts or malignant tumors. The HPV vaccines are mixtures of VLPs made out of the L1 proteins from the various strains of HPV.

The pivotal clinical trial of Gardasil involved 12,000 women age 16 to 26 from 13 countries. Each group received a series of 3 injections over the course of 6 months. One group received Gardasil. The other received a dummy injection that contained only the adjuvant of the vaccine. An adjuvant is a substance that creates mild inflammation, to boost the immune system's response to the vaccine. The Gardasil vaccine was so effective at preventing precancerous lesions that the trial was stopped early, so that the women in the placebo group could get the vaccine. The clinical trials of Gardasil have shown it to be practically 100% effective at preventing disease from the four targeted strains of HPV in girls and women who have never been exposed to those viruses before. It was less effective in women who had already been infected with one of those viruses. As a result, the CDC recommended that the Gardasil vaccine be given to 11- to 12-year-olds. Gardasil is currently indicated for females and males between the ages of 9 and 26.

Figure 22. A virus-like particle is made by giving a yeast cell the gene for a protein called L1, which makes up the virus's protein coat. The yeast cell then makes many copies of the L1 protein, which naturally fit together into groups of five, which then combine in groups of 72 to make an empty shell called a virus-like particle. A virus-like particle looks like a real virus, but it does not contain the viral genome. As a result, it can be used to immunize a patient but does not cause a viral infection.

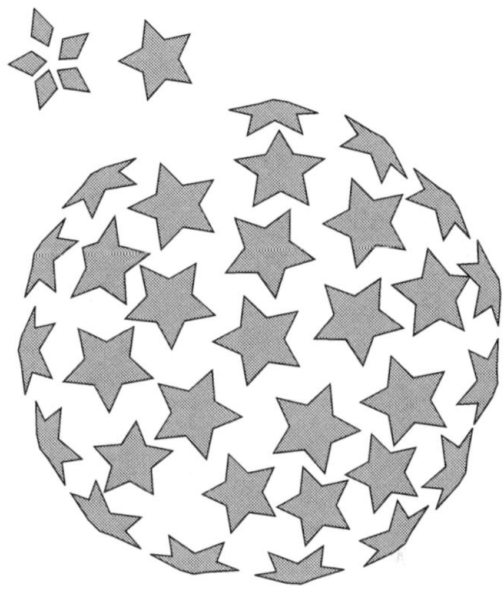

In Australia, which has made the HPV vaccine available for free to girls and women since 2007, the incidence of genital warts among women under age 26 decreased by 93% by 2011. There has also been a striking decrease in precancerous lesions of the cervix. The incidence of genital warts in men has also decreased. It takes several years for HPV-infected cells to give rise to a malignant tumor. We will have to wait a few years to see a significant decrease in cervical cancers in Australian women. Because of the widespread use of the HPV vaccines, the dangerous strains of HPV are becoming less prevalent. As a result, we will probably see an overall decrease in cervical cancers, in unvaccinated as well as vaccinated women.

I've seen a lot of anti-Gardasil rhetoric over the Internet. I'm shocked by how misleading it can be. For starters, I see the standard lies that the germ in question doesn't really cause a serious disease. Some people point out that only a small proportion of the people with an HPV infection actually die of cancer. Yet they use this fact to imply that the infection doesn't really cause the cancer, when in fact the infection must be present for cervical cancer to occur. Not everybody who buys a lottery ticket wins the lottery. But you have to play to win. Likewise, you probably have to get an HPV infection in order to get cervical cancer. As Harald Zur Hausen told an interviewer from *Cancer World*, "I frequently ask colleagues to provide us with tumour samples which are in their opinion negative and we have never got any."

Other antivaccine activists point out that the death rates from cervical cancer started to fall before the vaccine was invented. That's true. But that is because the detection and treatment of cervical cancer improved. In 1927, a Greek doctor named Georgios Papanicolaou developed a screening test—the Pap test—that can help detect cervical cancer in the earliest, most treatable stage. A comprehensive program of testing and treatment can reduce the death rate from cervical cancer by 80%. When my father was in the army in the 1950s, he was assigned to work for a military pathologist. My father says that the pathologist insisted on reviewing all of the Pap test slides himself, for fear that a case of cervical cancer might otherwise be missed.

Despite an effective program of early detection, women still die of cervical cancer. In the United States, there are roughly 12,000 new diagnoses of cervical cancer and roughly 4,000 deaths from cervical cancer per year. Also, the burden of disease from cervical cancer remains high. Often, the treatment involves major surgery. Sometimes, this surgery can leave a young woman unable to bear children.

I've also seen many transparent lies about the Gardasil studies. For example, many people complain that in the studies, Gardasil was compared to a control that contained the vaccine adjuvant, rather than just plain saline solution (salty water). Yet if people simply look at the prescribing information, they could see that one of the Gardasil studies did use a saline control. Critics of the vaccine also make a big fuss over the number of adverse event reports in the studies. Yet as with most vaccines, most of the adverse events were mild and temporary. The important ones weren't significantly more common with Gardasil than with the saline injection. Severe and serious adverse events were rare and were unlikely to be related to the vaccine.

There are two ways to figure out whether a problem is being caused by a vaccine. One is to look at the comparison of vaccinated versus unvaccinated subjects in the clinical trials. The other way is to look at the studies of health insurance databases. If the vaccine really does cause a problem, then that problem would be more common in the vaccinated patients than in unvaccinated patients. Both kinds of studies have strengths and weaknesses. The clinical trials randomly assign some subjects to a control group, but the size of the studies may be too small for a rare side effect to show up. The health insurance database studies are larger, but the treatments were not randomly assigned. As a result, you have to worry about the effects of confounding variables.

If a problem is just as common among unvaccinated people as among vaccinated people, and the study is large enough for the results to be meaningful, then we can rule out the vaccine as a cause of the problem. The clinical trials of the HPV vaccines showed no evidence of common problems. So far, the database studies have shown no evidence of rare problems. Thus, we have plenty of evidence that the HPV vaccines are remarkably safe.

We already have good reasons to believe that HPV vaccination will dramatically reduce a woman's risk of genital warts and precancerous lesions of the cervix. We are also seeing evidence that Gardasil could help to prevent some other cancers, including some cancers in men.

I've seen antivaccination activists quibble that the clinical trials of Gardasil used precancerous lesions rather than cervical cancer as an endpoint. Normally, I'm cautious about accepting surrogate endpoints in clinical trials. However, we shouldn't expect to see any cancers among the girls and women in the clinical trials. Those research subjects are being very closely monitored. Any precancerous lesions are noticed early and surgically removed. It would be a violation of research ethics to allow a precancerous lesion to go untreated, just to see if it becomes malignant. Note also that cervical cancer takes several years to develop. Thus, evidence of the effect of HPV in preventing cervical cancer will not come from the clinical trials. It will come from other kinds of studies, such as population studies and studies of health insurance companies' databases.

I've also seen a lot of misleading commentary about the postmarketing surveillance of HPV vaccines. As I explained in chapter 16, the Vaccine Adverse Event Reporting System (VAERS) includes reports of bad things that may or may not have actually happened, and that may or may not have been due to the vaccine. Some antivaccination zealots assume that anything bad that happens to a vaccinated person must have been due to the vaccination. So far, more than 100 million doses of HPV vaccine have been administered. Within that enormous population of vaccinated people, there have inevitably been some deaths. However, we have no evidence that the HPV vaccination *caused* any of those deaths. Gardasil may do a good job of preventing HPV infection, but it cannot ward off all evil. A wart vaccine cannot cure type 1 diabetes, cardiomyopathy, or seizure disorders. Thus, it will not prevent the patient from dying from those other problems.

Not every adverse event reported to VAERS was the result of the vaccine in question. As I explained in detail in chapter 16, the VAERS reports aren't useful for proving cause-and-effect relationships. However, they are useful for alerting the regulatory authorities to the possibility of serious problems that are rare or that take a long time to develop. That possibility must then be addressed in other kinds of studies. For example, researchers from Kaiser Permanente analyzed the electronic health records of 189,629 young women who had been vaccinated with Gardasil. These patients' records were compared with those from a group of matched, unvaccinated controls to see if the risk of any of 16 autoimmune diseases went up during the 180 days after vaccination. Not only was this study large, it involved reliable, unbiased data on the diagnosis and timing of illnesses, relative to the timing of the vaccinations. The analysis showed no sign that Gardasil increased the risk of any autoimmune disease. Instead of having no evidence that

Gardasil causes autoimmune disease, we now have good evidence that it does not. A similar study showed that Gardasil does not increase the risk of blood clots. Of course, the antivaccination zealots are never persuaded by evidence of any kind.

The anti-Gardasil rhetoric often includes a sad story about some unfortunate girl who became ill or even died of some mysterious disease after being vaccinated with Gardasil. The antivaccination activists assume that since the mystery illness happened after the vaccine, it must have been caused by the vaccine. Thus, they are committing an error in reasoning called the *post hoc ergo propter hoc* (after it therefore because of it) fallacy. All causes happen before their effects. Yet not everything that happens after some event is the result of that event.

As any medical historian can tell you, human beings have been suffering and dying from mysterious illnesses since prehistoric times. However, we have not seen a sudden increase in any important health problem now that huge numbers of girls and now boys have received Gardasil. Nor have any studies shown that any important health problem is more common in vaccinated patients than in unvaccinated patients.

Why do the antivaccination activists imagine that two or three doses of noninfectious virus-like particles would be far more dangerous than a chronic infection with an active, potentially cancer-causing virus? The antivaccination zealots want me to think that the proteins from the viral coat of HPV are dangerous, unless they come from a chronic active infection with the actual virus—in which case they want me to think that the proteins are harmless. The whole thing makes no sense.

Some antivaccination activists complain that the Gardasil vaccine contains traces of "recombinant DNA" from the virus. Yet they never explain that this "recombinant DNA" would be just the DNA for the L1 protein, which itself seems to be harmless. The vaccine does not contain the genes that cause a cell to give rise to warts and tumors. Those genes were never transferred to the yeast that is used to make the vaccine! The antivaccination activists never point out that a natural infection with wild HPV would cause extended exposure to the gene for the L1 protein, along with the truly dangerous genes from HPV. The antivaccination activists want me to think that being exposed to a trace amount of the DNA for a harmless protein would be dangerous, while being chronically exposed to the entire genome of a wild, cancer-causing virus would be somehow less harmful.

If you vaccinate your daughters and sons against HPV, you are helping to protect them (and your future sons- and daughters-in-law) against some nasty and aggressive cancers. Vaccinating your children against a common cause of cancer does not give them "permission" to have sex. Nor will withholding the HPV vaccination persuade them and their future spouses to remain virgins until their wedding night, and to remain faithful to each other forever after. If the fear of contracting HIV or genital herpes in the short run does not scare teenagers away from having sex, then the risk of dying of cancer when they are "old" (i.e., in their 30s) would probably not sway them. Yet if we vaccinate our children against HPV before they become sexually active, we can reduce their risk of dying of cancer. The choice really is that simple.

28

Tetanus

Tetanus is unusual among the vaccine-preventable diseases. Tetanus is infectious but not contagious. In other words, it is caused by a germ, but not by one that is passed from person to person. You can't catch tetanus from another tetanus patient, not even indirectly, such as by being bitten by the same mosquito. Instead, you catch tetanus from the environment, through an open wound.

Tetanus has been around for thousands of years. The ancient Egyptians and later the ancient Greeks knew that patients with open wounds, even minor ones, were at risk for deadly muscle spasms. Those ancient writings provide detailed descriptions of cases that a modern doctor would clearly recognize as tetanus.

The early symptoms of tetanus are irritability, muscle cramps, soreness or weakness of the muscles, and difficulty in swallowing. The later symptoms are the result of the severe muscle spasms. The muscles that are served by the shortest nerves are affected first. That means the muscles of the face. When the facial muscles go into spasm, the patient can no longer open his or her mouth. That sign is called lockjaw.

Another result is a peculiar facial expression called a sardonic smile (risus sardonicus). Eventually, the disease affects the muscles of the neck and back. The result can be a severe arching of the back (opisthotonos). The muscle spasms can be severe enough to break bones and dislocate joints. If the muscles controlling the vocal cords and the diaphragm are affected, the patient will be unable to breathe without help from a ventilator. Tetanus can also cause high blood pressure and abnormal heart rhythm.

Up until the 20th century, tetanus was nearly always a death sentence. It was also a horrible death. During World War II, a US Army surgeon named Col. Glenn wrote, "In my clinical experience I have never seen such a terrifying disease as tetanus." However, practically none of the tetanus cases during World War II occurred in U.S. servicemen or –women. Practically everyone in the US Army was vaccinated against tetanus. As a result, there were only 12 tetanus cases, 5 of them fatal, in the entire US Army during World War II. Six of those 12 tetanus cases occurred in soldiers who had not been vaccinated. Another two cases were in soldiers who had not received all of their vaccinations.

Thanks to vaccination, tetanus has gone from horribly common to practically nonexistent. In the late 19th century, there were roughly 200 tetanus cases per 100,000 persons per year in the United States. Nearly all of those cases were fatal. By 1947, the number had dropped to only 0.4 cases per 100,000 per year. Nowadays, there are roughly 50 tetanus cases per year in the entire United States. Thanks to antibiotics and tetanus antitoxin, as well as improved supportive care, only about five of those cases are fatal. Most tetanus cases nowadays are among elderly people whose immune systems are weak. There are also a few cases among newborns whose mothers were not immune to tetanus.

The ancients knew that tetanus was typically the result of an open wound. But before the development of germ theory, nobody knew why an open wound could lead to tetanus. That mystery was unraveled in 1884, when two Italian scientists were able to induce tetanus in laboratory animals by injecting them with pus from a human being with tetanus. That result suggested that tetanus was caused by an infection. That same year, a German physician named Arthur Nicolaier induced tetanus in animals by injecting soil into them. Nicolaier identified a soil bacterium (*Clostridium tetani*) that he believed was the likely cause of tetanus. However, he was unable to grow a pure culture of the bacterium. Five years later, a researcher at Robert Koch's laboratory in Berlin succeeded in culturing *Clostridium tetani*. He then proved that tetanus was due to a toxin that was released by the bacterium.

Once the cause of tetanus was understood, scientists could develop an effective treatment. They used the same method that had been used for making diphtheria antitoxin. First, horses were immunized against tetanus. Then, blood was drawn from those horses. The horses' blood serum, which is the liquid left after the blood clots, is then used to make the antitoxin product. During World War I, tetanus antitoxin was used to prevent and treat tetanus in wounded soldiers. In the 1920s, scientists found that they could denature the tetanus toxin with formaldehyde. The denatured toxin is called a toxoid. The toxoid has been damaged just enough that it cannot cause tetanus. However, it can still provoke the body to produce protective antibodies against tetanus toxin.

It was a bit surprising that the tetanus vaccine worked. The few people who survived an untreated case of tetanus did not become immune to tetanus. The tetanus toxin is so powerful that even a lethal dose is too small to provoke an immune response. However, people can tolerate a big enough dose of tetanus toxoid to develop antibodies to protect against a natural case of tetanus.

The *Clostridium tetani* bacteria live in the intestines of human beings and animals. *Clostridium tetani* bacteria are also commonly found in soil. When microbiologists started studying *C tetani* in the laboratory, they learned some basic facts that explain a lot about tetanus. The first is that *C tetani* is anaerobic. In other words, it needs an environment with little or no oxygen in order to grow. Because it thrives inside the intestines, it is commonly found in manure. The fact that *C tetani* is anaerobic also explains why it thrives inside deep wounds, such as puncture wounds.

When I was growing up, I heard people say that you catch tetanus from stepping on a rusty nail. That kind of injury would produce a deep puncture wound, which is exactly the sort of environment where *Clostridium tetani* can thrive. However, tetanus is caused by bacteria, not by rust. If you stepped on a nail in a barnyard, where the soil is teeming with *C tetani* from manure, you were particularly likely to get tetanus.

Another significant clue about *Clostridium tetani* comes from its peculiar shape. *C tetani* is classified as a bacillus, which means a rod-shaped bacterium. However, the *C tetani* bacteria are sometimes shaped more like a club or a tennis racket. Those oddly shaped bacteria are in the process of turning into spores. If oxygen levels are too high, a *C tetani* bacterium can convert itself into a spore. It makes a tough, hard coat for itself and goes into a state of suspended animation. *C tetani* spores can survive in soil or elsewhere in the environment for many years. When conditions improve, the spore can germinate, which means going back to its vegetative form.

Clostridium tetani produces two different toxins: tetanospasmin and tetanolysin. Both are small proteins. Tetanospasmin causes the symptoms of tetanus. Tetanospasmin causes tetanus by preventing nerve cells from releasing GABA (gamma-aminobutyric acid). GABA is an inhibitory neurotransmitter. GABA normally acts as a brake on nerve activity. It prevents nerve cells from firing. When tetanospasmin prevents the release of this inhibitor, it's like cutting the brake lines in a car. The nerve cells become overactive. The result is uncontrolled contraction of the muscles. Tetanospasmin has to travel the length of a nerve fiber before it has this effect. That's why the muscles that are served by the shortest nerves are affected first.

Tetanospasmin is the second most deadly toxin known to medical science. The only known toxin that is more deadly is botulinum toxin D, which is produced by a related bacterium, *Clostridium botulinum*. Botulinum toxin D is the cause of botulism, which also affects the function of the nerves. Ironically, botulinum toxin (Botox) is useful as a drug.

Many people have tiny doses of Botox injected into their face to paralyze some of their facial muscles, so they won't end up with frown lines. Jenny McCarthy, who has done so much to frighten people away from vaccinating their children, freely admits that she gets Botox injections in her face. If no toxin should ever be injected into the human body, why does she allow the deadliest toxin known to science to be injected into hers?

Clostridium tetani also produces a toxin called tetanolysin, which causes tissue destruction. Thus, it may help *C tetani* survive in a wound. Several other clostridia produce dangerous toxins. One example is *Clostridium perfringens*, the cause of gas gangrene. I have no idea why the clostridia produce so many dangerous toxins.

Since tetanus is not spread from person to person, you can't get any benefit from herd immunity. In other words, you can still get tetanus even if every other human being on the planet is immune to tetanus. Since tetanus is caused by a bacterium that can be found in other animals and in soil, tetanus will never be eradicated. Thus, there will always be a need for tetanus shots.

The tetanus toxoid vaccine has been spectacularly successful in reducing the number of people who get tetanus. Unfortunately, toxoid vaccines do not provide permanent protection. The CDC recommends that people get booster shots for tetanus every 10 years. Today, the tetanus toxoid vaccine is combined with a diphtheria toxoid vaccine and a vaccine against whooping cough.

To boost their effectiveness, the toxoid vaccines contain an adjuvant, usually an aluminum salt. As I explained in the diphtheria chapter, the antivaccination activists make a huge fuss over the tiny dose of aluminum salts in the vaccines, but they do not complain about the huge dose of aluminum salts in baking powder and antacids. They also complain about the preservatives that are used in the multidose vials of these vaccines. Yet many of them also tell horror stories about the problems with contamination that occurred before the vaccine manufacturers started putting preservative in the multidose vials. The antivaccination activists want to eat their cake and have it, too.

The side effects of tetanus vaccination are usually mild and temporary. There may be soreness, redness, or swelling at the injection site. There may also be fever, headache or body aches, and fatigue. A severe allergic reaction to the vaccine is very rare (less than one case per million doses) and usually occurs within minutes of the injection.

People who have had a severe allergy to the tetanus vaccine or to any component of the tetanus vaccine should not get the vaccine.

On a sad note, I have to point out that Arthur Nicolaier, the discoverer of *Clostridium tetani*, did not die of natural causes. Nicolaier had been a professor of medicine at the Charité, a prestigious medical school in Berlin, Germany. However, he was removed from office in 1933, when the Nazis took power and passed laws that made it illegal for Jews to be civil servants. Nicolaier committed suicide in August 1942, at age 80, when he learned that he was about to be sent to a concentration camp. It was a tragic end for a man whose work saved so many people from such a horrible death as tetanus.

29

Influenza (the Flu)

I get a flu shot every year. In a good year, my flu shot will decrease my risk of catching the flu by about 60%. In a bad year, it decreases my risk of catching the flu by only about 20%. But even that seems like a good deal to me. The cost is covered by my health insurance, and I'd gladly get a jab in the arm for even a 20% decrease in the risk of a week or more of misery.

The flu shot might not give me complete protection against the flu, but it gives me some protection. I will be less likely to catch the flu; and if I do catch the flu anyway, I will be less likely to have a severe case. I will also be less likely to spread the flu to other people, especially to sick or elderly people and to babies who are too young to be vaccinated. Getting the flu shot may be an act of hope, not faith—but it is also an act of charity.

I hear more nonsense about the flu vaccine than I hear about the childhood vaccines. Many people claim that they once caught the flu from the flu shot (which is simply impossible because their vaccine contained a "killed" virus). Some antivaccination zealots have told me that tens of thousands of people every year die from the toxins in the flu shot. Yet when I read the reports of the clinical trials of flu vaccines, I generally find that there were no deaths or serious adverse events among the people who got the flu shot. Nor have I ever met anyone who had a serious adverse reaction to a flu shot. Meanwhile, influenza kills thousands of people in the United States every year. Thus, the flu shot seems like a reasonable precaution. I would rather get a small dose of dead viruses than have to fight a huge infection with live viruses.

The word *influenza* came from the Italian word for influence. It originally meant that the disease was the result of the influence of something else, such as the stars or the weather. Cold and flu season occurs in the fall and winter, which correspond to the astrological signs of Libra through Pisces. By the mid 19th century, English-speaking people were using the word *influenza* to refer to any bad upper respiratory infection. Now we know that many unrelated viruses can cause upper respiratory infections. Doctors now reserve the words *influenza* and *flu* to mean influenza virus infections. In contrast, most cases of the common cold are due to a rhinovirus.

Influenza virus infects the lining of the respiratory tract. As a result, it produces the symptoms that are typical of a common cold, such as runny nose, sneezing, and coughing. These symptoms represent the body's attempt to rinse the infectious agent from the respiratory tract. Influenza virus infection can also produce fever and chills, muscle aches, headache, fatigue, and a general sick feeling. Those systemic symptoms result from the chemical messengers that the immune system produces in its attempt to fight the viral infection. That's why so many different diseases can produce the same set of cold-like or flu-like symptoms.

A common cold and the flu can produce similar symptoms. Both can cause sore throat, stuffy nose, coughing and sneezing. But in a case of the flu, the other symptoms—especially fever, chills, and headache and body aches—tend to be more common and more severe. The only way to tell for sure whether someone has a cold or the flu or some other viral respiratory infection is to test for the presence of the virus.

At first, microbiologists suspected that influenza was due to a bacterial infection. The great German microbiologist Richard Pfeiffer found a gram-negative rod-shaped bacterium (bacillus) in the phlegm of influenza patients. He named it *Haemophilus influenzae*. Most people called it Pfeiffer's bacillus. When the Great Pandemic of influenza broke out in 1918, many scientists still suspected that Pfeiffer's bacillus was the cause of the flu. However, an American pathologist named Martha Wollstein showed that many flu patients were not infected with Pfeiffer's bacillus. She concluded that Pfeiffer's bacillus did not cause the flu. It was merely an opportunistic infection. In other words, it thrived in patients who had been weakened by the flu. Thus, it could cause a deadly bacterial pneumonia in patients who would otherwise have survived the flu. (A particularly dangerous form of *Haemophilus influenzae* has been a major cause of bacterial meningitis in children. It is now preventable by vaccination, as I explain in chapter 32.)

In the 1930s, researchers at Britain's Medical Research Council proved that influenza is due to a virus. Through antibody tests, they showed that the influenza virus that caused the Great Pandemic of 1918-1919 must have been similar to a flu strain that was by then going around in pigs. When a new strain of "swine flu" emerged in 1976, public health authorities panicked. Fortunately, that strain of the flu did not lead to a pandemic.

Virologists eventually found that influenza viruses belong to a family called Orthomyxoviridae. Influenza viruses are enveloped viruses that have their genes encoded in a single strand of RNA. Like many single-stranded RNA viruses, influenza viruses can mutate fast. Not only is RNA less stable than DNA, but the cell's proofreading mechanisms that find and correct errors in double-stranded DNA cannot find and fix errors in RNA. A rapid mutation rate is actually an advantage for the influenza virus. Influenza viruses can mutate so quickly that their descendants can reinfect the same host in later years.

There are three species of influenza virus: A, B, and C. Influenza A is the one that causes the biggest problem for human health, especially because strains of influenza A virus can also infect other species of animals.

The influenza A viruses are sorted into strains according to two glycoproteins that are found in their envelope: hemagglutinin and neuraminidase. Hemagglutinin helps the influenza virus enter a new host cell. Neuraminidase helps the newly formed virions escape from the cell that produced them, so that they can infect a new cell.

The first form of influenza A virus to be identified was categorized as H1N1. At least 18 different forms of hemagglutinin have been discovered. Most of the influenza A strains that infect humans have H1, H2, or H3. Other forms of hemagglutinin are found in the influenza A viruses that infect birds, pigs, dogs, and horses. At least nine forms of neuraminidase have been discovered. Some of the drugs that have been developed for treating influenza work by blocking the activity of neuraminidase. Unfortunately, some dangerous strains of flu are developing resistance to the neuraminidase inhibitors.

Each strain of influenza is given a name that follows a set of rules set out by the WHO. First is the species (A, B, or C). Second is the host of origin, if the host is nonhuman. Third is the location where the strain was first isolated (e.g., Denver or Taiwan). Fourth is the strain number. Fifth is the year of isolation. Then, for influenza A viruses, the types of hemagglutinin and neuraminidase are given. An influenza virus isolated from a duck in Alberta, Canada, was called A/duck/Alberta/35/76 (H1N1). An influenza virus identified in a human being in Perth, Western Australia was named A/Perth/16/2009 (H3N2).

Traditionally, the annual influenza vaccine was trivalent, which means that it included the three flu strains (two strains of influenza A and one of influenza B) that were expected to cause the most serious public health problems in the upcoming flu season. However, the flu shot that I got for the 2015-2016 season was quadrivalent (four strains). Several new formulations of flu vaccine are now available. Healthy young patients can get a "live" vaccine in a nasal spray. There is also a high-dose injection for elderly patients. There is an egg-free version that is particularly useful for people who are allergic to eggs. There's also a formulation that is designed to be injected just under the skin, instead of into muscle.

Some flu strains differ only slightly from the strains that were going around last year. This kind of small mutation is called antigenic drift. The most serious strains of flu virus are the ones that have major changes from the viruses that had been circulating the year before. This major change is called antigenic shift. Antigenic shift can result when a single cell is infected by more than one kind of influenza virus, allowing the different strains to swap genes. The strains that result from an antigenic shift can be particularly dangerous.

Two basic kinds of influenza A virus strike terror into the heart of virologists. The first kind is any H1N1 that resembles the strain that caused the Great Pandemic of 1918-1919. Although that strain of flu virus was not isolated at the time, virologists eventually managed to identify its genes in a sample of tissue stored at the Armed Forces Institute of Pathology and in another sample recovered from the body of a flu victim who had been buried in permafrost in Alaska. The other terrifying kind of flu virus is any strain that has recently jumped from poultry or pigs to human beings. When poultry or pigs are grown on farms, especially on the same farm, they may exchange flu viruses with each other and with human beings. When two or more strains of flu virus infect the same cell, they can swap genes with each other. The result can be a hybrid flu virus that is very good at infecting and killing human beings.

Influenza epidemics cannot be contained through sanitation or hygiene. As people discovered during the Great Pandemic, quarantine is of limited value. Infected people become contagious for a day or so before they start to feel sick. Influenza is highly contagious because it causes coughing, which generates infectious airborne droplets. Because of its envelope, the influenza virus is fragile outside of the human body. It generally takes fairly close contact, usually within about 6 feet, to spread the flu. You can also catch the flu if you touch something that has been contaminated with flu virus and then touch your eyes, mouth, or nose. For that reason, frequent hand washing can help a little to prevent the spread of flu. Some drugs, such as amantadine and the neuraminidase inhibitors, have been used for reducing the severity of influenza virus infections. Unfortunately, influenza viruses have been developing resistance to amantadine, and the value of the neuraminidase inhibitors has been seriously questioned.

Vaccination is the only good way to prevent diseases that are spread by airborne droplets. Unfortunately, the influenza vaccines have limited effectiveness. Influenza vaccines are aimed at a moving target. To design an effective flu vaccine, virologists must accurately predict which strains of influenza virus will go around next year. If they make a good guess, the flu vaccine will be more effective. The flu vaccine may even provide some protection against flu viruses that have slight mutations from the vaccine strains. However, the flu vaccine will probably not cover an unexpected antigenic shift.

Fortunately, even if the vaccine strains provide only a partial match to the circulating flu viruses, the vaccine can provide some measure of protection because of cross-reaction and affinity maturation. Cross-reaction means that antibodies can bind to something other than the antigen for which they were originally made. If the match between the vaccine viruses and the circulating flu viruses is reasonably close, the vaccine may cause you to produce antibodies that cross-react with the circulating flu virus. This cross-reaction can give you some protection. It also allows for affinity maturation. As I explained in chapter 14, affinity maturation means that during an immune response, the B cells evolve to provide antibodies that provide a better and better fit to the infecting germ. The result may be a shorter and milder illness than you would have had if you had not been vaccinated.

Cross-reaction and affinity maturation can compensate for some degree of antigenic drift. However, they cannot compensate for antigenic shift, which is the major genetic change that results from reshuffling of the genes of unrelated flu strains. If a completely new, dangerous strain of flu emerges, virologists must rush to create a new vaccine. That's why virologists and public health officials get so worried about "bird flu" or "swine flu." Those dangerous viruses can cause a serious worldwide epidemic called a pandemic.

Tracing an influenza epidemic is like trying to nail Jell-O to the wall. Influenza is hard to diagnose because many different diseases produce "flu-like" symptoms. Even if you seek medical care, your doctor or nurse practitioner might not be able to tell whether you have a case of the flu or a bad cold, or perhaps a case of respiratory syncytial virus infection. There are tests for influenza virus infection, but they are expensive and they often give false-negative results, especially if they are run more than a week after the illness started. Because of this problem with diagnosis, and because many people with influenza do not seek medical care, it is hard to track influenza epidemics. There's a lot of guesswork involved in estimating the size of the influenza burden in any given year.

To monitor influenza epidemics, the WHO and the CDC have set up a surveillance system. Healthcare providers who participate in the system report the number of patients who have an influenza-like illness. Participating laboratories provide data on the kinds of influenza viruses they are finding. These reports help to tell us how widespread a flu epidemic is, and which strains of virus are involved. However, they don't give us reliable data on death rates.

It's easy to tell if someone is dead, but it's hard to tell whether a death was due (directly or indirectly) to influenza. Most doctors don't test for influenza. Nor do doctors have to include the influenza diagnosis on the death certificate if someone died of a complication of the flu. Nor would everyone who dies of a complication of the flu be included in the "influenza and pneumonia" category. Influenza could lead to a heart attack or a stroke. Nevertheless, epidemiologists with the CDC estimate that, since 1976, an average of about 30,000 Americans each year die of influenza and its complications. In a good year, the death toll may be as low as 3000. In bad years, it can be roughly 50,000. That's bad enough, but a serious flu pandemic could cause a breathtakingly high death rate.

The Great Pandemic of influenza that swept the world in 1918-1919 killed perhaps 40 million people worldwide—more people than any other disease outbreak in history. Some medical historians say that the Great Pandemic killed more people in 24 weeks than the AIDS epidemic killed in 24 years. Ordinary flu epidemics are most deadly among newborns and the elderly. The Great Pandemic also killed remarkably large numbers of healthy young adults. That's why epidemiologists get scared when they hear reports of young adults dying of influenza.

Public health authorities are taking two different approaches to dealing with the flu. One is to try to reduce the impact of the ordinary strains of flu that go around every year, especially in the fall and winter. The other is to stamp out dangerous new strains before they develop the ability to spread easily from person to person.

Most new strains of influenza arise in an area that extends from Malaysia and western Indonesia to Korea and Japan. Flu viruses can easily circulate all year long within this region because of overlapping flu seasons. In the temperate areas (Korea and Japan), the flu season tends to be during the winter. In the tropical areas, the flu season occurs during the rainy season. After circulating in eastern and southeastern Asia, a new strain of flu then makes its way to Europe and North America. Eventually, it reaches South America, which seems to be a dead end for influenza strains.

Virologists are continually watching for dangerous new flu strains to appear in eastern and southeastern Asia. Fortunately, many of the particularly deadly strains can be identified before they have developed the ability to spread easily from person to person. Thus, public health workers strive to identify and isolate patients infected with these deadly new strains. Virologists also try to predict which strains of flu are likely to be important in Europe and the United States in the following flu season.

Antivaccination activists have told me horror stories about how deadly the flu vaccine supposedly is, but their stories don't match the results of actual clinical trials of the vaccines. Most flu vaccines are a "killed" vaccine and are remarkably safe, especially in comparison to facing flu season unvaccinated. You cannot catch flu from a "killed" flu vaccine. There are some "live" flu vaccines, which are given as nose drops or a nasal spray instead of as an injection. The "live" vaccines are intended to create a real infection, but one that is usually too mild to cause symptoms. Nevertheless, pregnant women, people with a suppressed immune system, and people who are in contact with people with a suppressed immune system should not receive "live" vaccines. Some live flu vaccines should not be given to children under 5 years of age because of the risk of high fever leading to convulsions.

One concern that public health authorities have about influenza vaccines is a possible link to a neurologic disease called Guillain-Barré syndrome. As I explained in the Introduction, Franklin Delano Roosevelt's paralysis might have been due to Guillain-Barré syndrome, rather than due to polio. Guillain-Barré syndrome is serious but rare disease. About a third of the cases occur after a gastrointestinal infection with a bacterium called *Campylobacter jejuni*, and some occur after cases of influenza or influenza-like illness. The swine flu vaccine that was used in 1976 was associated with a small increase in the risk of Guillain-Barré syndrome, roughly one additional case per 100,000 vaccinated individuals. However, research suggests that the risk of getting Guillain-Barré syndrome from the flu vaccines used in recent years is less than one in 1 million.

Do people really want me to believe that a small dose of dead or weakened flu viruses is likely to be more harmful than a huge population of rapidly multiplying "live" viruses? As you might expect, the results of clinical trials of the vaccines show that being vaccinated is much safer than having the flu. Other kinds of studies have shown that a flu shot can reduce the risk of hospitalization or death in high-risk populations, such as people with diabetes or heart disease. Vaccinating pregnant women against influenza can dramatically reduce the risk that their babies will be hospitalized for influenza during their first 6 months, while they are still too young to be vaccinated.

Antivaccination activists spread a lot of misinformation about influenza vaccines. Among other things, they complain that each year's flu vaccine is a new product and has therefore never been tested. That claim is misleading. This year's vaccine may differ only slightly from last year's vaccine. Some components may be the same as last year's. The results of the clinical trials for each brand of flu vaccine can be found in the prescribing information for that product. Note that the clinical trials are big enough to show that the vaccine reduces the risk of influenza-related illness. However, these studies are generally not big enough to show whether vaccinated people are less likely to be hospitalized or to die because of flu. To see the effect of influenza vaccination on rates of hospitalization or death, you have to look at database studies. Such studies typically show that recent vaccination against the flu is associated with lower risks of hospitalization and death among sick people (such as diabetics) and the elderly.

Antivaccination activists don't seem to understand that much of the research on flu vaccination deals with questions of vaccination strategy, rather than the effectiveness of the vaccine per se. Public health authorities want to know who should be vaccinated first, especially if the supply of vaccine is limited. Should you focus on the people most likely to die, or the people most likely to spread the infection? You could focus on vaccinating the sick and the elderly. They are the most likely to die of the flu, but they are also the least likely to mount an effective immune response to the vaccination, which is why they can now be given a high-dose flu vaccine. On the other hand, if you vaccinate healthy schoolchildren and working adults, you are much more likely to reduce the spread of the disease. Epidemiologists want to know which approach would save the most lives, and which one would save lives most cost-effectively.

To answer these questions, you generally have to use mathematical modeling. You can't just count the number of vaccinated people and compare that to the number of deaths in any given year. You have to control for how contagious and how deadly that year's flu was, and how well that year's vaccine matched the flu that was circulating. You also have to account for the other serious respiratory viral infections, such as respiratory syncytial virus, which can easily be mistaken for influenza. It's hard to get clear answers from such messy data.

Influenza will never be eradicated. Human beings can catch influenza infections from farm animals (mainly pigs and poultry), as well as from wild animals. Also, the influenza virus mutates so rapidly that immunity to last year's flu strain might not protect you this year. Two approaches could theoretically help to avoid future flu pandemics. The first would be to persuade people to stop growing poultry and pigs in eastern and southeastern Asia. That would help to stop the flow of dangerous new genes into the flu strains that infect human beings. Of course, that scenario is never going to happen. However, public health authorities have started keeping track of influenza outbreaks in poultry and regulating the live poultry markets in Hong Kong. The other approach would be to develop an effective universal flu vaccine. A universal flu vaccine has been called the Holy Grail of virology.

The existing flu vaccines include some rapidly mutating proteins from the surface of the virus. To make a universal flu vaccine, you need to target a genetically stable protein. Some viral proteins can stay remarkably stable year after year. That's because they do something that is vital and has little or no room for error. Any mutation that interferes with their function would be weeded out by natural selection. In contrast, natural selection favors the mutations that are harmless to the virus but help to make the virus unrecognizable to a previously infected host.

A flu strain like the one that caused the Great Pandemic of 1918 is a terrifying prospect. Yet like the ordinary seasonal flu, that epidemic trailed off during the summer, only to flare up again in the fall. In tropical regions, the flu season is during the rainy season. These facts suggest that low levels of vitamin D, the sunshine vitamin, could increase the risk of influenza and other respiratory infections. However, sunbathing is not a substitute for vaccination.

30

Hepatitis B

Hepatitis means inflammation of the liver. In the 20th century, researchers discovered that several unrelated viruses could attack the liver. One of these viral illnesses was called *infectious* hepatitis because it can be easily spread by contaminated water or from person to person. It is now called hepatitis A. Another viral hepatitis seemed to be much harder to catch. Because it could be spread by blood transfusion, by sharing unclean needles, or through sexual contact, it was called *serum* hepatitis. It is now called hepatitis B. There are also several other forms of viral hepatitis, including hepatitis C, hepatitis D, and hepatitis E.

Hepatitis A can cause a serious illness, but its effects generally do not last long. Hepatitis B can also cause a serious acute illness that sometimes causes death from liver failure. Most people recover from the acute phase of hepatitis B. Unfortunately, some people go on to have a persistent infection. Not only do they serve as carriers of the infection, they can go on to suffer from scarring of the liver (cirrhosis) or even liver cancer. About 25% of the people with a persistent hepatitis B infection will eventually die of liver failure or liver cancer. Many people who have a chronic hepatitis B infection have no idea that they are infected.

Scientists have known since World War II that hepatitis B is caused by a virus that can be carried for a long time by seemingly healthy people. A terrible outbreak of hepatitis occurred among servicemen who had received a vaccine against yellow fever. This vaccine contained serum from blood that had been donated by seemingly healthy people. However, some of these people had a history of jaundice (yellowing of the skin and eyes), which is a sign of hepatitis. This finding provided evidence that hepatitis B virus could be carried by seemingly healthy people for a long time and that it could be transmitted by blood products. Much of our knowledge about the long-term effects of hepatitis B virus in adults came from studies of the men who were accidentally infected by this contaminated yellow fever vaccine in the 1940s.

When the military authorities realized that the yellow fever vaccine was contaminated with hepatitis B virus, they did two things: They switched to a yellow fever vaccine that did not contain human blood serum, and they gave that vaccine only to the men who were going to an area where yellow fever was a problem. Together, those two precautions solved the problem.

Today, both hepatitis A and hepatitis B can be prevented by vaccination. Thanks to widespread use of the hepatitis B vaccine, there have been sharp decreases in the number of hepatitis B infections and liver cancers in children. Besides being effective, the hepatitis vaccine is remarkably safe. Nevertheless, the hepatitis vaccine is controversial because it is given to newborns. People just don't like the idea of vaccinating babies against a disease that can be sexually transmitted. Yet the hepatitis B virus (HBV) can also be spread by sharing a washcloth or a toothbrush with an infected person. A toddler can catch hepatitis by being bitten by another toddler.

Before the hepatitis B vaccine became available, roughly 24,000 children per year became infected with HBV in the United States. As the use of the hepatitis B vaccine has expanded, the number of new cases of HBV infection has steadily dropped. It's extremely important to protect the very young against hepatitis B. The babies and young children who become infected with HBV are the people most likely to develop a persistent infection. Thus, they are the people most likely to serve as carriers of the virus and to go on to suffer and die from liver failure or liver cancer because of HBV infection.

Several treatments for chronic hepatitis B infections are available. Unfortunately, none of these drugs can cure the infection, and they all have serious side effects. However, they can reduce the risk of liver damage. In other words, it's far better to prevent hepatitis B than to try to treat it.

The hepatitis B virus is a member of the hepadnavirus family. Other hepadnaviruses cause liver infections in other species. The hepadnaviruses are enveloped viruses whose genes are in a double strand of DNA. Because of its fatty envelope, the hepatitis B virus cannot survive for long outside its host. That's why it takes such intimate contact to spread the virus. Like many other enveloped viruses, hepatitis B can cause a chronic infection.

The first vaccine against hepatitis B was developed by virologist Maurice Hilleman at Merck. Since hepatitis B can cause a chronic infection that leads to cancer, a "live" vaccine was unthinkable. Hilleman decided instead to try to isolate a protein from the surface of the hepatitis B virus. He wanted to create a vaccine that contained the viral protein but none of the infectious viral DNA. Hilleman collected blood from gay men and intravenous drug users—populations that were known to have a high risk of hepatitis B infection. Hilleman then developed a multistep purification process that isolated the hepatitis B surface antigen and killed every known virus. The first large-scale tests of the hepatitis B vaccine involved gay men. The vaccine was introduced in 1981.

In retrospect, it seems shocking that someone would have made a vaccine out of blood products from homosexual men and intravenous drug users, both of whom are at high risk for HIV infection, which had not yet been discovered. Some people have claimed that Hilleman's vaccine was responsible for spreading HIV within the gay community, but those accusations were false. Hilleman's purification and sterilization procedure really did kill all known viruses, including HIV. His vaccine did not spread AIDS. However, it did help to reduce the spread of hepatitis B, which is particularly dangerous for someone with HIV.

Nevertheless, Hilleman's vaccine was withdrawn from the market in 1986 because it was replaced by a safer and cheaper alternative. Pablo D.T. Valenzuela of Chiron Corporation put the gene for the hepatitis B surface antigen into brewer's yeast. He then got the yeast to produce large amounts of that protein. Valenzuela's vaccine contained the viral antigen. However, it had never been in contact with the actual virus. This recombinant vaccine is still in use today.

In the United States today, the recombinant hepatitis B vaccine is given to newborns. Babies who are born to mothers who have been infected with hepatitis B are also given a dose of antibodies to HBV (hepatitis B immune globulin), to prevent them from catching hepatitis B from their mothers. A series of boosters is then given when babies are 6 to 18 months of age.

The hepatitis B vaccine is one of the safest vaccines ever made. And since routine vaccination of newborns against hepatitis B began in the United States, the incidence of new cases of hepatitis B has gone down 82%, mainly among children. Of course, antivaccination activists oppose the use of the hepatitis B vaccine. They claim that it is inappropriate to give a vaccine against a sexually transmitted disease to infants. Yet hepatitis B can also be spread by nonsexual contact, such as one toddler biting another toddler. The younger a child is when he or she catches the hepatitis B virus, the more likely the child is to become persistently infected.

The use of the hepatitis B vaccine has led to sharp decreases in hepatitis B in countries where the disease had been highly endemic. In Taiwan, giving the vaccine to babies and young children has decreased the rate of childhood liver cancers. In fact, the success of the hepatitis B vaccine has led some people to hope that we can drive hepatitis B into extinction through vaccination.

31

Rotavirus

Rotavirus is a common cause of severe diarrhea in babies and young children. Worldwide, rotavirus diarrhea still causes nearly half a million deaths per year, mainly among babies and children under 5 years of age. Thus, the rotavirus vaccine has the potential to save hundreds of thousands of lives, mainly in poor countries. Thanks to advances in fluid therapy, the death toll from rotavirus diarrhea in the United States had dropped to only a few dozen per year, even before the first rotavirus vaccine became available. Nevertheless, roughly 70,000 babies and young children per year in the United States were still being hospitalized because of rotavirus diarrhea. Thanks to the widespread use of the rotavirus vaccine in the United States, hospitalizations for rotavirus diarrhea have gone down by about 90% since 2006.

Since the development of germ theory in the 1860s, doctors had suspected that most cases of vomiting and diarrhea were due to infections of the stomach and intestines. By the 1880s, it was obvious that some diarrheal diseases are caused by bacteria. In the 1940s, Jacob Light and Horace Hodes from Johns Hopkins University School of Medicine in Baltimore showed that some "filterable agent" (i.e., a virus) from children with diarrhea could also cause diarrhea in calves.

In 1973, an Australian virologist named Ruth Bishop used an electron microscope to look at tissue from the intestines of young patients with severe diarrhea. She saw that these tissue specimens were filled with viral particles that looked like tiny wheels. These viruses were called rotavirus because *rota* is the Latin word for wheel.

By the 1980s, it was clear that rotavirus is a major cause of severe diarrhea in babies and young children. It is endemic worldwide. In other words, it is present in all populations all the time. Nearly every human being gets at least one case of rotavirus infection by the time he or she is five years old. A person's first bout of rotavirus infection is usually the worst. People who survive it generally develop partial immunity. As a result, the later infections cause milder symptoms. In adults, a rotavirus infection may cause no symptoms at all. A person can have a contagious case of rotavirus infection without even feeling sick.

Unlike many gastrointestinal infections, rotavirus infections are just as common in societies with good sanitation as they are in societies with poor sanitation. That fact suggests that the virus can easily be transmitted from person to person. A single gram of feces from an infected person can contain 20 trillion rotavirus virions. However, it takes a dose of only 100 of those virions to give someone a case of rotavirus diarrhea.

Like other gut infections, rotavirus can be spread by the fecal-oral route. Thus, it could be spread by water that is contaminated with raw sewage. However, rotavirus can also be spread by people who do not wash their hands well after going to the bathroom, by contaminated objects, and possibly even by airborne droplets, especially if someone vomits. The rotavirus virions do not have an envelope, which explains why they can survive in the environment for up to 19 days after they leave their host. Vaccination is the only practical way to prevent diseases that are that easily spread.

It's ironic that rotaviruses were found to cause a serious disease. They belong to a family called the Reoviridae. The prefix *reo-* originally stood for "respiratory enteric orphan." These viruses were originally called orphan viruses because they did not seem to cause any disease. So it came as a surprise that rotavirus turned out to be responsible for so many cases of severe diarrhea in babies and young children.

Five species of rotavirus have been identified. They have been labeled A, B, C, D, and E. Rotavirus A is responsible for about 90% of the rotavirus infections in human beings. The rotavirus strains that are commonly found in human beings often swap genes with some of the rotaviruses that are found in livestock.

Rotavirus is a major cause of severe diarrhea in babies and young children worldwide. In countries with good healthcare systems, many babies and young children with rotavirus diarrhea end up in the hospital. These young patients are far more likely to survive a severe rotavirus infection if they get fluid replacement therapy, sometimes intravenously. In countries with poor health care systems, many babies and young children die of rotavirus diarrhea.

Vomiting and diarrhea cause dehydration. They also cause loss of electrolytes such as sodium and potassium. In the United States, pediatricians tell parents to give their children an electrolyte drink like Pedialyte when the children have diarrhea. The WHO and UNICEF have been teaching people all over the world how to make their own electrolyte drinks for sick people, especially for sick babies. This simple advice has saved the lives of countless babies. Nevertheless, some patients with severe vomiting and diarrhea need more fluid than they can keep down. They need intravenous fluids.

By the 1990s, it was clear that rotavirus infection was a major public health problem in the United States. Rotavirus was responsible for more than 400,000 doctor visits, more than 200,000 emergency room visits, and 55,000 to 70,000 hospitalizations every year. Thanks to advances in medical care, rotavirus causes only a few dozen deaths per year in the United States. However, the death toll from rotavirus diarrhea in poor countries remains shockingly high—nearly half a million deaths per year globally.

Humanity will probably never succeed in driving rotavirus into extinction. A rotavirus infection does not produce lifelong immunity.

You can be infected with rotavirus repeatedly. However, the later infections may be so mild that you don't even realize that you are infected. Yet you can still pass the virus on to other people. Although rotavirus will always be with us, vaccination against rotavirus can help prevent babies from getting so sick from rotavirus that they need hospital care.

The first vaccine against rotavirus (RotaShield) was introduced in 1998. However, it was taken off the market the following year because of a concern about a rare but serious side effect: intussusception. Intussusception is a telescoping of the intestine—one portion of the intestine slides inside the neighboring portion. This is a serious and potentially life-threatening problem. It causes severe abdominal cramping, along with vomiting. If the intestine becomes damaged, the patient might start passing bloody stool.

Fortunately, a radiologist can often correct an intussusception while doing the procedure that confirms the diagnosis: a contrast enema. By carefully adding air or fluid to expand the intestine, while watching the x-ray image of the intestine on a fluoroscope, the radiologist can make the intestine unfold. If this procedure does not work or if the wall of the intestine has been injured, the problem must be corrected surgically. Sometimes, the surgeon can simply unfold the intestine. However, a damaged portion of the intestine may need to be removed.

In the clinical trials, there were five cases of intussusception among the 10,054 babies who got the RotaShield vaccine and only one case of intussusception among the 4,633 babies who got the placebo vaccine. However, the difference between the groups (0.05% vs 0.02%) was so small that it could have been due to random chance. Nevertheless, intussusception is serious and can be deadly, so it was listed in the prescribing information as a possible adverse event. Thus, doctors were strongly encouraged to report any possibly vaccine-related case of intussusception to VAERS.

Nobody expected that intussusception would be a rare side effect of rotavirus vaccination, mainly because nobody realized that intussusception was a rare side effect of a natural rotavirus infection. After all, nearly everyone eventually gets at least one rotavirus infection by age 5, but intussusception is rare. Nevertheless, federal, state, and local health authorities worked together to see whether the RotaShield vaccine did increase a baby's risk of intussusception. A large health insurance company also studied its claims database to see whether babies who had been vaccinated with RotaShield were more likely to be hospitalized with intussusception.

Roughly 1.5 million babies in the United States were vaccinated with RotaShield while it was on the market. During that time, 15 cases of intussusception were reported to VAERS. The Minnesota Department of Health documented another five cases. All 20 of those babies were treated, primarily with minor procedures, and recovered.

After analyzing all of the available data, scientists concluded that the RotaShield vaccine did cause a few cases of intussusception: maybe one or two extra cases of intussusception for every 12,000 vaccinated babies. Yet even though roughly 1.5 million babies in the United States got the RotaShield vaccine, the overall number of cases of intussusception in the United States did not seem to go up. Yes, the RotaShield vaccine caused a few cases of intussusception. However, the wild rotavirus, which nearly everyone catches eventually, probably has a similar effect. Thus, even unvaccinated babies could end up with intussusception, after they caught a wild rotavirus infection.

After RotaShield was found to be causing a few cases of intussusception, the ACIP stopped recommending it and the manufacturer took it off the market. That decision was based on the balance of risk and benefits for babies in the United States. Rotavirus diarrhea was a major cause of hospitalization in the United States, but it was causing remarkably few deaths. Only about 60 babies per year were dying in the United States because of rotavirus infection. Thus, even a few cases of a potentially life-threatening side effect were enough to cause RotaShield to be taken off the market in the United States.

The decision to stop using RotaShield made sense for the United States. However, the balance of benefits versus risks would have been different in countries where rotavirus diarrhea was killing large numbers of young children. In those countries, the use of RotaShield would have saved many lives. Unfortunately, the public health authorities in many of those countries did not want to use a vaccine that had been rejected as unsafe in the United States. Tragically, that decision represented a missed opportunity to save about 2000 lives per day, every day, for the 7 years it took for the next rotavirus vaccine to become available.

There was no available vaccine against rotavirus from 1999, when RotaShield was taken off the market, until 2006, when RotaTeq was introduced. Another rotavirus vaccine, Rotarix, was approved in 2008. Each of these vaccines was developed through a different process, from different strains of rotavirus.

The risk of intussusception seems to be about 90% lower with RotaTeq than it had been with RotaShield. One study estimated only 1.5 extra cases of intussusception for every 100,000 babies vaccinated with RotaTeq. It's harder to get an accurate estimate of the risk of intussusception for Rotarix because fewer babies have received it. Meanwhile, the use of these rotavirus vaccinations has meant about 50,000 fewer hospitalizations for diarrhea among the roughly 4.3 million babies born in the United States in a given year.

As I read about the history of the rotavirus vaccine, I was struck by how concerned the FDA and CDC were about even the possibility of a rare but serious side effect of a childhood vaccine. The antivaccination activists claim that the FDA and CDC ignore tens of thousands of vaccine-related deaths. Antivaccination activists insist that the FDA and CDC allow dangerous, toxic products to stay on the market, just so that vaccine makers can make big profits. Yet when you read the actual scientific reports about the safety problems with actual vaccines and historical accounts of how decisions about vaccine policy were made, you can clearly see that the public health authorities in the United States take vaccine safety very seriously.

The rotavirus vaccines are "live" vaccines that are given by mouth. The goal is to produce a harmless gastrointestinal infection that will cause the body to produce a strong and long-lasting immune response. Like any "live" vaccine, the rotavirus vaccine should not be given to children with a suppressed immune system. The virus from the rotavirus vaccine can spread to other people. Thus, the vaccine might be withheld if someone in the household has an immune system disorder.

The most common adverse events after rotavirus vaccination are relatively mild and temporary: diarrhea and vomiting, upper respiratory infection, and bronchospasm (asthma-like wheezing). Serious side effects, such as intussusception, are extremely rare.

The rotavirus vaccines work. They reduce a child's need for hospitalization for a rotavirus infection by 89%. Vaccinated children also had 48% fewer emergency room visits and 12% fewer doctors' office visits. Besides helping to prevent illness and suffering, the rotavirus vaccine has helped to reduce healthcare costs. If you refuse to vaccinate your children against rotavirus, you will increase your own children's risk, and your friends' and neighbor's children's risk, of ending up in the hospital with a severe case of diarrhea.

32

Haemophilus influenzae Type B (Hib)

Until the late 1980s, *Haemophilus influenzae* type b (Hib) was responsible for about 80% of cases of bacterial meningitis in babies and young children. Nearly one in every 200 children in the United States got Hib meningitis by the time they were 5 years old. There were about 12,000 cases per year, mainly in children under the age of 5. Roughly 600 of those children died. About 4,000 of the survivors suffered from serious lifelong disability, such as severe mental retardation, blindness, or deafness. Fortunately, an effective vaccine introduced in 1987 has practically eliminated Hib from the United States and other industrialized countries. Since the introduction of the Hib vaccine, the incidence of Hib meningitis in the United States has gone down by more than 99%. Unfortunately, Hib is still a major public health problem in many poor countries.

As I explained in chapter 9, many different kinds of bacteria normally live on the inner and outer surfaces of the body without causing any trouble. When those bacteria start to cause inflammation or even tissue damage, the problem is described as an infection. The infection can invade areas of the body that are normally free from bacteria. When bacteria spread to the fluid that surrounds the brain and spinal cord, the result is a serious problem called bacterial meningitis. (The meninges are the membranes that cover the brain and spinal cord.) Hib was an important cause of bacterial meningitis in babies and young children. It could also cause epiglottitis, which is an inflammation of the flap of tissue that normally blocks the windpipe when you swallow. Epiglottitis can quickly strangle a baby to death.

If left untreated, Hib epiglottitis or Hib meningitis can kill the patient within a matter of hours after the first symptoms appear. Even with appropriate antibiotic treatment, about 3% of children with Hib meningitis die. The Hib infection can spread throughout the body, even to the bones and joints. As a result, a few survivors of invasive Hib infection lose toes, fingers, or limbs or need extensive skin grafting. About 20% of the survivors of Hib meningitis are left with permanent hearing loss or other problems with the nervous system. Even children who seem to have recovered may go on to have behavioral problems and poor performance in school.

Although the Hib infection can respond to antibiotics, the infection may already have caused serious problems by the time the diagnosis is made. Thus, it is far better to prevent the disease through vaccination than to try to cure it through antibiotics. However, people who have been exposed to someone with Hib meningitis may be given antibiotics. The purpose of the antibiotic treatment is to clear the Hib from their upper respiratory tract. Not only does this help to prevent them from getting sick from Hib, it helps to keep them from passing Hib on to other people.

Haemophilus influenzae was discovered in 1892 by the famous German microbiologist Richard Pfeiffer. When he did a Gram staining procedure on mucus from influenza patients, he found many short, pink rod-shaped bacteria (gram-negative coccobacilli). He called them *Bacillus influenzae* because he thought they were the cause of influenza. Eventually, Pfeiffer's bacillus was reclassified into the genus *Haemophilus*. Thus, it is now called *Haemophilus influenzae.*

By the 1920s, it was clear that *Haemophilus influenzae* was not the cause of the flu and was often found in the upper respiratory tract of healthy people. Like many potentially invasive bacteria, *Haemophilus influenzae* is a facultative aerobic bacterium. In other words, it prefers to use oxygen to burn fuel for energy. This preference for a high-oxygen environment explains why it thrives in the upper respiratory tract. However, *Haemophilus influenzae* can shift over to anaerobic metabolism, which doesn't consume oxygen. Thus, *Haemophilus influenzae* can survive in tissues with low oxygen levels, which explains why it can survive in deep tissue.

In the 1930s, an American microbiologist named Margaret Pittman figured out why so few of the people with *Haemophilus influenzae* in their respiratory tract got an invasive infection. Some strains of *Haemophilus influenzae* have a polysaccharide capsule, and some do not. There were six different types of capsule, which she labeled a through f. The nonencapsulated strains are sometimes called "nontypeable," even though genetic testing can now be used to tell them apart.

Any strain of *Haemophilus influenzae* can cause a local infection in the respiratory system, such as sinus infections, ear infections, bronchitis, or pneumonia. However, only the strains with a capsule can cause an invasive infection, such as blood infections (bacteremia), bone infections (osteomyelitis), and meningitis. Before the introduction of the Hib vaccine, most cases of invasive infection with *Haemophilus influenzae* were due to type b. Only a few were due to type a. Unfortunately, the Hib vaccine has no effect against type a. Thus, the few cases of *Haemophilus influenzae* meningitis that still occur in the industrialized countries are due mainly to type a.

It's not surprising that the encapsulated types of *Haemophilus influenzae* are responsible for causing invasive infections. As I explained in chapter 9, a capsule can help to protect a bacterium from the immune system, at least for a while. The capsule makes it easier for *Haemophilus influenzae* to make its way into the bloodstream and then into other tissues. The capsule also protects the *Haemophilus influenzae* from being attacked by white blood cells, at least until the body starts making antibodies that bind to that capsule. Eventually, however, the immune system figures out ways to defeat Hib. That's why invasive Hib infections occur mainly in young children.

The capsule of type B contains a polysaccharide called polyribosyl ribitol phosphate (PRP). By the 1930s, it was clear that human beings could develop natural immunity to type B and that antibodies to PRP played an important role in that protective immune response. Unfortunately, it is difficult to create a vaccine that would provoke an immune response to a polysaccharide.

During a natural infection, some of the cells involved in the immune system engulf the germ and break it apart. Then, they display bits of the germ on their surface, in a way that draws the attention of T cells. When the T cells get involved, the body can mount a stronger and longer-lasting immune response. Unfortunately, the T cells can get involved only when the antigen is a protein, not when it is a polysaccharide.

The B cells can learn to make antibodies against polysaccharides, but through a process that is believed to be independent of the T cells. However, the "T-independent" immune response has some important weaknesses. The most important, as far as Hib is concerned, is that it generally does not work in children who are less than 18 months old. Unfortunately, that is the age-group at highest risk for illness and death from Hib. Another problem is that the antibody responses from these T-independent immune responses generally don't last long, and they cannot be shifted into high gear by booster shots.

The first vaccine against Hib was introduced in the United States in 1985. Unfortunately, this vaccine was based on the polysaccharide from the capsule. As you might have guessed, it did not work in children under 18 months of age. In other words, the vaccine was least effective for the patients who needed it most. Since the polysaccharide vaccine was such a disappointment, scientists developed a conjugate vaccine.

You can make it easier for the immune system to develop antibodies to a polysaccharide if you bind that polysaccharide to a carrier protein, thus producing a conjugate. The carrier protein makes it possible for T cells to get involved in the immune response. Three different

Hib conjugate vaccines have been produced, each with a different carrier protein. The Hib conjugate vaccines produce strong and long-lasting protection, even in babies as young as 6 months of age. Until that point, babies are usually protected by the anti-Hib antibodies that they got from their mother.

The Hib vaccine is well tolerated. The side effects may include some redness, swelling, and warmth at the injection site. About 1 in 20 babies runs a fever after the vaccination. However, these side effects are generally mild and temporary.

Haemophilus influenzae is found only in human beings. There is no wild reservoir. The conjugate vaccine not only prevents disease from Hib, it keeps people from being carriers of Hib. Thus, it may be possible for us to drive Hib into extinction by vaccination, just as smallpox has been driven into extinction. Then, nobody would need to be vaccinated against Hib in the future.

33

Streptococcus pneumoniae (*Pneumococcus*)

S*treptococcus pneumoniae*, which is also called the pneumococcus, is a major cause of illness and death worldwide. Most of these illnesses and deaths are among the very young and the very old, as well as among people whose immune systems have been damaged in some way. Many strains of pneumococcus are becoming increasingly resistant to antibiotics. Thus, vaccination is becoming increasingly important for controlling pneumococcal disease.

The pneumococcus is often found in the mouth and throat of healthy people. It was first isolated in 1881 by two scientists who were working independently on two separate continents. In France, Louis Pasteur found it in the saliva of a patient with rabies. An army doctor in the United States named George Miller Sternberg found it in his own saliva. By the late 1880s, it became clear that the pneumococcus was also a major cause of pneumonia and other serious infections.

The pneumococcus is a coccus, which means that it is round. It is often found in pairs (diplococci). The pneumococcus is often described as lancet-shaped, which means that it is slightly pointed on one side.

The pneumococcus is gram-positive, which means that it shows up as dark purple when stained with the Gram staining procedure. A pale area surrounding each cell represents the polysaccharide capsule (for an explanation of bacterial capsules, see chapter 10).

Streptococcus pneumoniae is a facultative anaerobic bacterium. In other words, it does not need oxygen in the form of O_2 but it can tolerate the high-oxygen environment of the upper respiratory tract. Thus, it can survive in the upper respiratory tract but can also invade deeper tissues.

Besides causing infections of the respiratory tract, the pneumococcus can also cause blood infections (septicemia). From there, it can spread to the bones and joints and the heart. It can even enter the fluid that surrounds the brain. There, it produces inflammation of the meninges, which are the membranes that surround the brain and spinal cord. Thus, the pneumococcus is also a major cause of bacterial meningitis.

Attempts to develop a vaccine against the pneumococcus began as early as 1911. However, those early attempts were unsuccessful. It is hard to make an effective vaccine against the pneumococcus because the vaccine has to be aimed at the polysaccharide in the capsule. Also, there are at least 90 different serotypes of pneumococcus, each with its own polysaccharide. Immunity to one serotype does not necessarily protect you against another. For that reason, vaccine developers started trying to develop polyvalent vaccines, which provide protection against more than one strain.

At first, the pneumococcus was highly susceptible to antibiotics. Then, in the 1970s, antibiotic-resistant pneumococci started appearing. Some strains are resistant to more than one class of antibiotic. This emerging antibiotic resistance made the development of effective vaccines even more urgent.

The first pneumococcal vaccine was introduced in 1977. It included the polysaccharides from 14 different strains of pneumococcus. In 1983, it was replaced by a 23-valent vaccine that was designed to protect patients against the strains that were responsible for 88% of pneumococcal infections of the blood.

Unfortunately, polysaccharide vaccines do not work well in young children. As I explained in chapter 32, it's hard to develop an effective vaccine against a polysaccharide. The T cells cannot take part in the immune response unless the antigen includes a protein. To enlist the support of the T cells, you need to bind the polysaccharide in the vaccine to a protein. This combination of polysaccharide and protein is called a conjugate.

Conjugate vaccines are useful for preventing infection by the strains that are included in the vaccine, but only the strains that are included in the vaccine. The first conjugate pneumococcal vaccine was introduced in 2000. The first formulation covered only 7 strains (7-valent). A later version covered 10 strains. The current version covers 13 strains of pneumococcus. The 23-valent polysaccharide vaccine covers 12 of those strains, plus 11 others.

The CDC recommends the pneumococcal conjugate vaccine for all children younger than 5 years old and for adults with certain risk factors. The CDC currently recommends the 23-valent polysaccharide vaccine for adults age 65 and older, as well as for people 19 years and older with risk factors such as diabetes. The 23-valent vaccine is also recommended for people over 5 years of age who are at particular risk for pneumococcal infection.

Thanks to the pneumococcal conjugate vaccine, the number of pneumococcal infections among young children has gone down sharply. The number of invasive infections, such as pneumonia and meningitis, by the vaccine strains has gone down by more than 90%. Vaccinated children are also less likely to get earaches.

Vaccinating young children against pneumococcal infection has even helped to produce some herd immunity. Thus, it has decreased the risk of these infections in older children and adults. This decrease in infections, and especially the decrease in antibiotic-resistant infections, is important. It shows that vaccines can help to reduce the problem of antibiotic-resistant bacteria.

The pneumococcus is specifically adapted to living in human beings. There is no animal reservoir. Thus, vaccination could help to eliminate the worst strains of pneumococcus from the population.

The pneumococcal vaccines are generally well tolerated. Most of the side effects are mild and temporary, such as mild pain or redness at the injection site. Less than 1% of vaccinated patients experience fever, muscle aches, or more severe local reactions. Serious side effects, such as allergic reactions, are rare.

34

Chickenpox and Shingles

Chickenpox is a highly contagious disease that causes painful, itchy blisters. It is sometimes called varicella. Chickenpox results from infection with the varicella zoster virus (VZV). An effective vaccine against chickenpox was introduced in 1995.

Before the introduction of the chickenpox vaccine, nearly everyone caught chickenpox in childhood. There were roughly 3 to 4 million cases of chickenpox per year in the United States. Roughly 10,000 Americans per year were hospitalized for complications of chickenpox, including pneumonia and necrotizing fasciitis (flesh-eating bacteria). About 100 Americans died of chickenpox every year. Today, some antiviral drugs can help reduce the severity of a case of chickenpox, but it would be better to prevent the disease to begin with.

The older you were when you caught chickenpox, the worse the disease tended to be. Adults accounted for only 5% of chickenpox cases but 35% of the resulting deaths. Pregnant women are at particularly high risk for complications of chickenpox. Roughly 10% to 20% of pregnant women with chickenpox got pneumonia, and as many as

40% of them died of it. If a pregnant woman survived the chickenpox, there was up to a 2% chance that her baby would be born with congenital varicella syndrome: low birthweight, scarring of the skin, and problems with the limbs, brain, and eyes.

I caught a bad case of chickenpox when I was in sixth grade. It was horrible. I had an itchy, painful, blistering rash all over my body. I was told not to scratch the blisters, or they would leave scars. The soles of my feet hurt so badly that I could not walk. My throat was so sore that I could not swallow. The doctor told me to gargle with some warm water with aspirin in it. Of course, nowadays, people are warned not to give aspirin to chickenpox patients, for fear of causing a rare disorder called Reyes' syndrome.

For me, the one ray of hope was the idea that the horrible disease would go away on its own, never to return. Years later, I found out that that was not entirely true. Once you have been infected with the chickenpox virus, it stays with you for life. It hides in your nerve tissue, just waiting for some weakening of your immune system. Then it rises up again to create an agonizingly painful, itchy rash called shingles. Sometimes shingles is called zona because the rash is limited to only a particular zone.

Shingles usually appears as a red, blistering rash that forms a stripe on one side of the body. That's because the virus that has been living in the root of a spinal nerve travels down the length of that nerve to attack the skin. Thus, the rash appears only in the area supplied by that nerve. That area is a called a dermatome, which literally means a slice of skin (Figure 23).

People should go straight to the doctor at the first sign of a shingles attack, especially if it is on the face. If shingles attacks your eye, it can cause permanent blindness. Even shingles on a less critical region, such as the torso, can cause a serious problem. It can lead to a long-lasting agonizing pain called postherpetic neuralgia or neuropathic pain. Antiviral drugs can help to relieve the pain of shingles and reduce the chance that it will lead to postherpetic neuralgia.

VZV is a member of the herpesvirus family (Herpesviridae). It is sometimes called herpes zoster and sometimes herpesvirus-III. VZV is related to the viruses that cause cold sores and genital herpes. It is also related to the Epstein-Barr virus that causes mononucleosis. The herpesviruses are surrounded by a fatty envelope, which helps to explain why they are generally spread only by close contact and why they can cause a persistent infection.

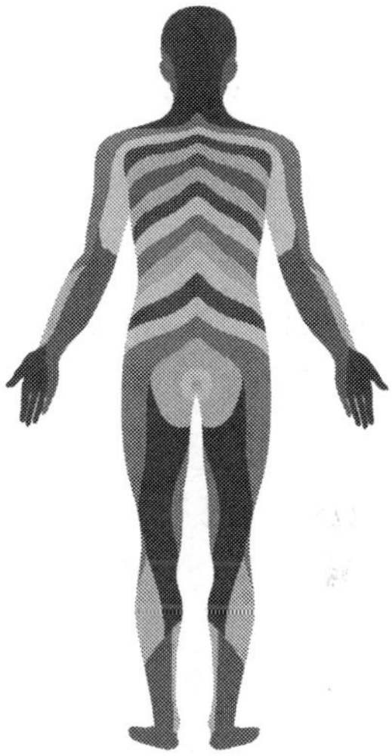

Figure 23. The area of skin served by a particular cranial or spinal nerve is called a dermatome. A shingles attack usually involves just one cranial or spinal nerve. As a result, the rash generally appears on only one side of the body, in the area of one dermatome.

People usually catch chickenpox by inhaling the airborne droplets that are produced when an infected person coughs. They can also become infected by touching something contaminated by the infected person's saliva or by the fluid from the blisters. People with shingles can spread the VZV, thus causing chickenpox. Shingles patients remain contagious until the blisters dry up.

Back when I had chickenpox, there was no treatment. Since then, some antiviral drugs including acyclovir and valacyclovir have been developed. These drugs can reduce the symptoms of chickenpox or shingles. They may also reduce the risk that a shingles outbreak will damage nerve fibers. To be effective, they must be started right away.

A shingles attack can cause lasting damage to the nerves. This damage is called neuropathy, which means nerve disease. Because of this nerve damage, the pain and other abnormal sensations of a shingles attack can linger for a long time after the rash disappears. Neuropathic pain can be severe. It does not respond to ordinary pain medications, even morphine. Some other kinds of drugs, including the drugs that are normally used for treating depression or epilepsy, are sometimes helpful in managing neuropathic pain.

There are two vaccines against VZV. They are both "live" vaccines. Therefore, they should not be given to pregnant women or to anyone with a weakened immune system. One of the VZV vaccines is intended to prevent chickenpox. The other is a stronger version of the same vaccine, for preventing shingles in someone who has probably already had chickenpox. (It would also prevent chickenpox in someone who never had it.) The ordinary chickenpox vaccine is not strong enough to serve as a booster for preventing shingles.

Antivaccination activists are against the use of the chickenpox vaccine. They claim that the chickenpox is no big deal. They insist that the vaccine contains dangerous poisons. They also claim that there is no need for a shingles vaccine. Some of them even claim that children should be allowed to have chickenpox, to boost their grandparents' resistance to shingles. What an appalling suggestion! I heard one antivaccination activist claim that smearing honey on a shingles rash works better than an antiviral drug. I hope that people don't take his advice!

Some people want to expose their children to natural chickenpox, instead of having them vaccinated against chickenpox. Some of these people recommend distributing lollipops that have been contaminated with an infected child's saliva. This strikes me as a cruel and reckless thing to do. Vaccination is far safer. Fortunately, the vaccine is so effective that chickenpox has become much less common. Thus, the antivaccination zealots will have much less of an opportunity to sicken their children.

Thanks to vaccination, we have 3.5 million fewer cases of chickenpox per year in the United States. The incidence of chickenpox among infants, who are too young to be vaccinated, has gone down by 90%. Hospitalizations due to chickenpox have decreased by 9000 cases per year. The vaccine prevents 100 deaths per year. We will not be able to eradicate VZV any time soon, because the virus is hiding out in the nerve roots of people who had been infected in the past. Nevertheless, chickenpox vaccination has saved lives and led to a dramatic decrease in the burden of the disease.

35

Meningococcal Disease

Neisseria meningitidis is called the meningococcus because it is a round bacterium (coccus) that is a major cause of bacterial meningitis. Bacterial meningitis is a serious, often deadly infection that inflames the meninges, which are the membranes that cover the brain and spinal cord. If you do a Gram staining procedure on spinal fluid from someone with meningococcal meningitis, you will see tiny pink (gram-negative) dots. However, doctors don't wait for these lab results to come back. When they suspect meningococcal meningitis, they start antibiotic treatment right away. An invasive meningococcal infection is a medical emergency. It can kill within hours of the first sign or symptom of illness.

If you look carefully at a specimen of stained meningococci, you may see that each cell is surrounded by a pale area, which represents its polysaccharide capsule. This capsule is like Harry Potter's cloak of invisibility. It helps the meningococcus hide from the body's white blood cells, at least for a while. Like its cousin *Neisseria gonorrheae*, which causes a sexually transmitted disease called gonorrhea, the meningococcus is specifically adapted to living on and in human beings. These two species of *Neisseria* are found nowhere else in nature. As you might expect, both species have found ways to avoid our immune defenses.

The meningococcus is aerobic, which means that it needs oxygen in the form of O_2. Thus, it should come as no surprise that the meningococcus normally lives in our upper respiratory tract. About 5% to 10% of adults have colonies of meningococcus in their upper respiratory tract. Fortunately, most people eventually become immune to the meningococcus on their own. If the person's immune system has been weakened by cigarette smoke or a respiratory infection, the *Neisseria meningitidis* can spread to other parts of the body.

The meningococcus can infect the lungs (pneumonia), and then the bloodstream (bacteremia or meningococcemia), and then the meninges (meningitis). Any bacterium that makes its way into the spinal fluid is probably all through the body. Thus, a meningococcal infection can involve the heart, the joints, and even the bones. The bloodstream infection can cause blood clots that can cut off circulation. The result can be the death of tissue.

Before the development of antibiotics, about 85% of invasive meningococcal infections resulted in death. Even with prompt antibiotic treatment, the case-fatality rate is still 10% to 14%. About 40% of people with meningococcemia die, even if they receive treatment. Survivors often have severe brain damage. They may end up deaf and prone to seizures. Some survivors need skin grafts. Some lose their hands, feet, and nose to gangrene.

Meningococcal disease spreads through direct person-to-person contact, through respiratory droplets or contact with saliva. In the United States, meningococcal disease is most common among young people living in crowded conditions, such as college students living in dormitories. People who have been exposed to someone with a known case of meningococcal disease are at higher risk for being colonized by the bacteria and possibly becoming sick from it. In the United States, the incidence of meningococcal disease seems to peak in the late winter and early spring. It also seems to follow a longer cycle that peaks every 7 to 10 years.

In the United States, meningococcus is an uncommon but serious disease. Tragically, meningitis has been far more common in the so-called meningitis belt of sub-Saharan Africa. In a normal year, meningococcal meningitis would strike about 5 to 10 out of 100,000 people per year in those countries. However, there were frequent epidemics, during which the incidence could be as high as 1000 cases per 100,000 people per year. In Africa, meningococcal disease is most common during the dry season (December through June). Because meningococcus can be easily spread by airborne droplets among crowds of people, meningococcal disease was often spread by people returning from a religious pilgrimage to Saudi Arabia. The Kingdom of Saudi Arabia does require visitors to have proof of vaccination against meningococcus. Unfortunately, the polysaccharide vaccine that has been available since the 1970s does not prevent people from being carriers of meningococcus.

It has been hard to develop safe and effective vaccines against meningococcus because the meningococcus hides inside its capsule. The vaccine makers must therefore target the large sugar molecules (polysaccharides) in that capsule. Yet as I explained in chapter 32, polysaccharide vaccines have important limitations. Polysaccharide vaccines tend to be ineffective in babies. Even in adults, the polysaccharide vaccines for meningococcus provide only 3 to 5 years of protection, and only against the strains that are represented in the vaccine. Also, the polysaccharide vaccines do not provoke a strong enough immune response to clear the meningococcus from the respiratory tract. As a result, even widespread use of the polysaccharide vaccine would not produce herd immunity.

Strains of *Neisseria meningitidis* can be sorted into 13 serogroups. Each has a different polysaccharide in its capsule. Serogroup B causes more than half of the cases of meningococcal disease in babies in the United States. Serogroups C, Y, and W135 cause about 75% of the cases in people age 11 years and older. Most cases in Africa are due to serogroup A. The polysaccharide vaccine that was introduced in the 1970s covers four serogroups of *Neisseria meningitidis* (A, C, Y, and W135).

Fortunately, some conjugate vaccines against meningococcus have been developed. In a conjugate vaccine, the bacterial polysaccharide is bound to a bit of protein. This bit of protein allows the immune system's T cells to get involved in the immune response. The result is a more powerful, longer-lasting immune response. Unlike the polysaccharide vaccine, the conjugate vaccine can enable the immune system to clear the *Neisseria meningitidis* from the upper respiratory tract. Thus, the conjugate vaccines can do more than keep the individual from getting sick from meningococcus. The conjugate vaccines may prevent the individual from carrying the meningococcus and passing it on to other people. Thus, the conjugate vaccines may make it possible to create herd immunity and possibly drive some strains of *Neisseria meningitidis* into extinction.

It has been difficult to develop a safe and effective vaccine against serogroup B, which has antigens that look a lot like human nerve tissue. The immune system generally does not make antibodies against the body's own tissue. Self-antibodies would cause the immune system to attack the body itself. The result would be an autoimmune disease. To develop a serogroup B vaccine that would be not only effective but safe, researchers used an approach called reverse vaccinology.

The entire genome of serogroup B had already been sequenced, which means that scientists have decoded all of its genes. As I explained in chapter 13, genes are just recipes for proteins. Once you know which amino acids are used in what order in making a protein, you can use a computer to predict the protein's shape. The vaccine developers then went through these proteins to figure out which ones would make good vaccine antigens. Then, the genes for those proteins can be put into a yeast or bacterium, so that large amounts of the protein can be produced cheaply.

Because of the seriousness of meningococcal disease, the FDA put the serogroup B meningococcal vaccines on a fast track for approval. The FDA even allowed emergency use of unlicensed meningococcal vaccine to stop outbreaks of meningococcal disease at Princeton University and the University of California, Santa Barbara. There are now two licensed vaccines against meningitis B in the United States.

Because of the introduction of the new vaccines against meningococcus B, national governments have been revising their recommendations for meningococcal vaccination. The CDC recommends vaccination against meningitis B for individuals 16 to 23 years of age. The CDC also has specific recommendations for people on college campuses that have recently had an outbreak of serogroup B meningococcal disease. The two available brands of vaccine against meningococcus B are not interchangeable. The patient should receive the same vaccine product for all doses.

In 1996 and 1997, the worst meningitis epidemic in African history swept across sub-Saharan Africa, killing 25,000 people. In response, an organization called PATH and the WHO launched the Meningitis Vaccine Project in 2010. This project was intended to eliminate meningitis as a public health threat from sub-Saharan Africa. The project has introduced MenAfriVac®, which is a conjugate vaccine that covers serogroup A. The vaccine was designed to tolerate temperatures of up to 40°C (104°F) for up to 4 days. Thus, it can be used in areas where vaccines cannot be reliably kept frozen. Not only does MenAfriVac® cost less than half as much as the polysaccharide vaccine, it is likely to produce herd immunity. In 2014, an infant version of MenAfriVac® that could be incorporated into routine childhood vaccination programs became available. By the end of 2014, more than 217 million Africans had been vaccinated against meningitis A. The Meningitis Vaccine Project has met its objectives and has been concluded. Meanwhile, PATH continues to work with African governments and global organizations to fight meningitis A in what had been the Meningitis Belt.

36

Other Vaccine-Preventable Diseases

The antivaccination zealots keep insisting that vaccines are ineffective and dangerous. Yet I have had two personal experiences that tell me otherwise. First, I worked for a veterinary journal that ran many articles about vaccination for farm animals. Big livestock producers would not bother to spend money to vaccinate their cattle and hogs and especially their poultry if the vaccines did not work. Second, I lived in a military town. The military would not bother to vaccinate the troops if those vaccinations undermined their troops' effectiveness. In fact, military people get more vaccinations than anyone else, partly because they are expected to travel to the ends of the earth at a moment's notice and partly because of the fear of biological weapons (e.g., anthrax).

The CDC maintains a Web page (www.cdc.gov/travel/destinations/list) that helps Americans figure out what vaccinations they need if they plan to travel overseas for various purposes. For example, if you were going to do disaster relief in Haiti, you should be up to date on your regular vaccinations, including your tetanus shot. You should also be vaccinated against hepatitis A, hepatitis B, and typhoid. If you are likely to be dealing with animals, you also need a rabies vaccination. You will also need a prescription for antimalarial drugs.

When you look at the vaccine recommendations for travelers, it's easy to see that the recommended vaccination schedule in the United States really is designed to promote public health, not to sell vaccines. Many vaccines that are needed overseas are not needed here. They are generally for diseases that are spread by unclean water (typhoid and cholera) or by mosquitoes (yellow fever and Japanese encephalitis).

37

Conclusion

In this book, I have described two serious interrelated problems. One is that human beings are suffering and dying from preventable disease. The other is that few people in our society know how to base their decisions on scientific evidence or even how to take part in reasonable conversations. In addition to outbreaks of whooping cough and measles, we are suffering from a grotesque epidemic of incivility. Back in the 1950s, Jonas Salk was hailed as a hero for inventing the first effective vaccine against polio. In 2009, Paul Offit, the co-inventor of the rotavirus vaccine, declined to do book signings for his new book because he had received so many death threats because of his advocacy of vaccination.

In 1796, a British doctor named Edward Jenner found an effective and surprisingly safe way to prevent people from catching smallpox, which was a leading cause of death back then. This discovery saved hundreds of millions of lives. It eventually allowed humanity to drive smallpox into extinction. Yet from the moment this discovery was made, a vocal opposition movement started trying to scare people away from taking advantage of it. If these antivaccination zealots had had their way, smallpox would still be killing and blinding people, and governments would still be struggling to contain outbreaks of that horrible, disfiguring, and often deadly disease.

From the very beginning, some religious zealots have insisted that vaccination is the work of the devil. Even today, many people feel that any kind of health care besides faith healing is an insult to God. Of course, they often frame their arguments in secular terms. Although they feel that vaccination is a spiritual pollution, they often talk about the chemicals in the vaccines, to appeal to a secular audience. Sadly, the people who are most at risk from the vaccine-preventable diseases are the children whose families belong to churches that preach against vaccination. Unvaccinated members of these churches often go overseas on mission trips. Thus, they can easily bring home diseases like measles, which can spread like wildfire among the unvaccinated children in their congregations.

Many advocates of alternative medicine—such as chiropractic, homeopathy, and "energy healing"—are also outspoken opponents of vaccination, typically because they believe that their healing systems are more effective and safer than vaccination. However, such approaches to medicine have been around for hundreds of years, and they never made a dent in the number of deaths due to infectious disease. Meanwhile, the medical and public health measures based on the germ theory of disease have saved hundreds of millions of lives, especially the lives of babies and young children. Thus, they doubled our life expectancy in the United States. Today, many people swear by homeopathy or some other alternative medicine approach for preventing infectious disease. In reality, they are taking advantage of the cocoon of safety provided by the vaccinated people all around them.

In the United States today, we are suffering from a breakdown of civility at all levels of society. By civility, I don't just mean politeness. I mean the use of evidence and logic to answer scientific questions and the use of mutual respect in resolving conflicts. As I argued in *Not Trivial: How Studying the Traditional Liberal Arts Can Set You Free*, this breakdown in civility is a predictable result of the defects of our educational system. Children do not learn much about history or biology, and they get no direct instruction in how to think logically. Nor do they learn much about civics, which is the study of the theoretical and practical aspects of citizenship. As a result, they don't know much about infectious disease or vaccination. Nor do they learn how the government could or should deal with threats to public health. After young people leave school, they are unlikely to catch up on the lessons they missed. Instead, they are bombarded with nonsensical conspiracy theories. For that reason, it will be hard to educate the public about the benefits of vaccination.

There have always been people who refuse to vaccinate their children. Fortunately, we can control the spread of communicable diseases, and even drive some of those diseases into extinction, even if a few children remain unvaccinated. We simply need to vaccinate enough people to stop the circulation of the diseases. To achieve that level of immunization, public health activists must help spread accurate information about the safety of the vaccines and the dangers posed by the vaccine-preventable diseases. Even if we cannot completely eradicate a disease, we must strengthen herd immunity so that the children who cannot be vaccinated, and the children of the parents who refuse to vaccinate, will still be protected.

Measles, mumps, and rubella are no longer endemic in the United States. However, we still have occasional outbreaks of measles and mumps. These outbreaks result when someone becomes infected overseas. We can limit the spread of those outbreaks within the United States by persuading more people in the United States to vaccinate their children. However, the best way to control those diseases is to drive the viruses that cause them into extinction, so that they can no longer be reimported.

I hope that by the time you read these words, polio and Guinea worm will be extinct. Measles, mumps, and rubella should be next on the list for extinction. What will you do to join in the fight to eradicate those diseases?

Index

A

D

E

I

J

K

L

M

N

O

P

Q

R

S

70967785R00215

Made in the USA
Columbia, SC
17 May 2017